Vancouver
Notes

for Internal Medicine

Vancouver Notes

for Internal Medicine

HIGH-YIELD CONSULT GUIDES

BRANDON TANG,
MD, MSc, EDITOR

MEIYING ZHUANG,
MD, EDITOR

JAMES TESSARO,
MD, MHPE, FRCPC, EDITOR

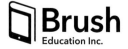

Brush
Education Inc.

Brush Education Inc.
www.brusheducation.ca
contact@brusheducation.ca

Cover and interior design: Carol Dragich, Dragich Design; Cover image: iStockPhoto, Natali_Mis

Library and Archives Canada Cataloguing in Publication

Title: Vancouver notes for internal medicine : high-yield consult guides / Brandon Tang, MD, MSc, editor, Meiying Zhuang, MD, editor, James Tessaro, MD, MHPE, FRCPC, editor.

Names: Tang, Brandon, editor. | Zhuang, Meiying (MD), editor. | Tessaro, James, editor.

Description: Includes bibliographical references and index.

Identifiers: Canadiana (print) 20220225753 | Canadiana (ebook) 20220225842 | ISBN 9781550598995 (softcover) | ISBN 9781550599008 (PDF) | ISBN 9781550599015 (EPUB)

Subjects: LCSH: Medical consultation—Handbooks, manuals, etc. | LCSH: Internal medicine—Handbooks, manuals, etc. | LCGFT: Handbooks and manuals.

Classification: LCC R727.8 .V36 2022 | DDC 610.69/6—dc23

We acknowledge the support of the Government of Canada
Nous reconnaissons l'appui du gouvernement du Canada |

Contents

Preface

On the educational journey to becoming a physician, each transition comes with growing confidence, expectations, and responsibility. One of the greatest challenges for newly minted clinical clerks and residents is acquiring the knowledge of processes needed to succeed in their new clinical roles.

Early in our training, we realized that there was a lack of guidance on how to perform consultations in internal medicine. Before seeing a patient, we would prepare ourselves by researching and annotating the key historical features, physical findings, and investigations to guide ourselves. It was hard to know where to begin.

Enter *Vancouver Notes.* The inspiration for this resource came from our own experiences as physician learners. This novel medical textbook consists of consultation guides (e.g., key history questions, physical examination manoeuvres, and investigations) that provide learners with an organized approach to common presentations in internal medicine (e.g., chest pain, pancreatitis). A resource like this would have saved us hours of preparation, enhanced our efficiency, and likely improved the organization and quality of our consultations.

The book is meant as a point-of-care reference, rather than a resource to read from end to end. For example, if you receive a referral for pancreatitis, our clinical guide outlines the key information you need to gather during your assessment. Typically, physician learners gather this knowledge throughout a rotation and acquire it tacitly, but our resource helps learners succeed by equipping them with this information from day one.

This first edition of *Vancouver Notes* was developed through the collective efforts of more than 90 resident physicians and faculty members at the University of British Columbia (UBC). We envision it as a legacy project that future generations of residents can add to, adapting the book to evolving needs in medical education. The book was developed in the midst of the global COVID-19 pandemic and is a true testament to our contributors' dedication and commitment. We would like to express our immense gratitude to everyone who worked on this book, and for the leadership of the Internal Medicine Residency Training Program at UBC, whose faculty supported us from the outset. Finally, we thank Brush

Education who have made it possible for this resource to reach the hands of trainees across Canada and worldwide.

To our readers, we hope this resource serves you well and we wish you the best of luck on your educational journey.

Disclaimer

The publisher, authors, contributors, and editors bring substantial expertise to this reference and have made their best efforts to ensure that it is useful, accurate, safe, and reliable.

Nonetheless, practitioners must always rely on their own experience, knowledge and judgement when consulting any of the information contained in this reference or employing it in patient care. When using any of this information, they should remain conscious of their responsibility for their own safety and the safety of others, and for the best interests of those in their care.

To the fullest extent of the law, neither the publishers, the authors, the contributors nor the editors assume any liability for injury or damage to persons or property from any use of information or ideas contained in this reference.

How to Use This Book

This resource is meant as a point-of-care reference for consultations in internal medicine.

It is a guide for collecting information during consultations, and for communicating crucial information to other health-care providers.

Don't read it from end to end. Read it strategically.

Here's how.

Start Here: General Guide for All Consultations

The general guide appears first in the resource because it applies to all consultations in internal medicine.

The general guide contains information that is not repeated from chapter to chapter.

So, read through this before you start working with the information in the other chapters.

Starting Points on Specialty Consultations

The "starting points" section at the beginning of each chapter applies to all consultations within a specialty. Guidelines for specific consultations (i.e., for presentations within a specialty) follow this opening section.

Like the general guide for all consultations, the starting points are worth scanning before you delve into specific presentations within a chapter.

The starting points describe information you need to capture, no matter the specific presentation.

The sections on specific presentations describe additional information you need to capture.

Presentations Within Specialties

The information in each section has a standard organization, with segments on reason for referral, past medical history, physical examination, and so on.

Each concludes with a segment on impression and plan, which focuses on communication: how to write up notes for consultations, and what to consider and include.

As you work through a section for a specific presentation, don't forget to scan the more general information in the general guide for all consultations and the starting points for the specialty.

At first, you may scan this general information frequently—and it is easy to scan. As you use the resource, though, it will become more and more familiar.

1

General Internal Medicine

Dr. Mitchell Vu
Dr. Elina Liu
Dr. Justin Lambert
Dr. Ben Schwartzentruber

REVIEWER
Dr. Yu Chiao Peter Chen

Start Here: General Guide for All Consultations

The consultation guides in this resource follow the general approach outlined in this section. They do not repeat all the information outlined here. We assume you will have this approach in mind for every consultation.

Identification

The identification of a patient is a way to communicate key information to other health-care providers.

It starts as the information you receive when a patient is referred to you for a consultation. As you learn about the patient during the consultation, you may change some of the information it contains.

To create an identification statement, summarize key features of the patient's current presentation, including highlights of relevant history. *For example:* "Robert is a 72-year-old man with a history of hypertension and diabetes presenting with progressive dyspnea and ankle swelling."

Reason for Referral

The reason for referral summarizes why a patient has been referred to you for a consultation. It describes the question that prompted the referral.

Keep an open mind about the patient's presentation during your consultation, however. Resist anchoring the consultation in the question that prompted the referral: the patient's number one problem may not be the reason they were referred.

History of Present Illness

Clarify the character, causes, and consequences of the patient's current presentation.

CHARACTER

Determine the mode of arrival: Determine how the patient arrived for care (e.g., whether they walked in or were brought by ambulance).

Clarify the sequence of events: Establish a time-ordered sequence of events leading up to the present, starting with when the patient was last at their baseline of health.

› The patient may present this information in a disorganized manner, but you must reorganize this information into a coherent story.

› This sequence may include elements usually found when discussing past and current diagnoses.

» For example, if the patient has acute decompensated heart failure (ADHF), determine their last hospital admission for ADHF, their last echocardiogram, and whether they are followed by a cardiologist or heart function clinic.

Clarify workup or management already in place: If your consultation takes place in the ED, determine any workup or management the patient has received.

Apply the mnemonic OPQRST AAA: This helps you better understand each presenting symptom. OPQRST AAA stands for: **O**nset, **P**rovocation, **Q**uality, **R**adiation, **S**everity, **T**emporal changes, **A**lleviating measures, **A**ssociated symptoms, **A**ggravating factors.

CAUSES

Identify pertinent positives and negatives: Highlight pertinent positives and negatives relevant to each presentation using the approach "Why does the patient have this disease?" and "Why are they presenting **now**?"

› For example, in ADHF, the underlying cause of heart failure may be ischemic cardiomyopathy; triggers for decompensation could include compliance with diet and medications, new ischemia, and so on.

Group symptoms by clinical syndrome: For example, symptoms related to COPD include increased dyspnea, cough, sputum production or purulence, and wheezing.

CONSEQUENCES

Clarify sequelae of the patient's current presentation.

• For example, for a fall: Was there a head injury? Are there focal neurological deficits?

REVIEW OF SYSTEMS
Screen for other symptoms with a systems-based approach.

Past Medical History
Determine all relevant chronic diseases: Clarify, if possible, severity, symptom control, and care providers (e.g., specialist, clinic), as in the following examples:
› **Angina:** severity on the Canadian Cardiovascular Society (CCS) scale; name of specialist providing care
› **Diabetes mellitus:** type 1 or 2; whether managed with insulin; most recent HbA_{1c}; name of hospital or endocrinology clinic providing care
› **COPD:** most recent pulmonary function tests; bronchodilator regimen; number of past exacerbations
› **AF:** $CHADS_2$ score[1]; rate and rhythm control agents; anticoagulation agents

Collect other key information:
› Explore in detail past medical issues relevant to the current presentation.
› Explore in less detail medical issues less relevant to internal medicine (e.g., cataracts, hernia repairs).
› Do not miss chronic issues that other health-care providers may have failed to document. This frequently happens with chronic kidney disease.
› Do not assume that a prescribed medication indicates a particular diagnosis: for example, not everyone on a PPI has GERD; not everyone on a loop diuretic has HF.

Past Surgical and Procedural History
Past surgeries and procedures require less detail than past diagnoses, unless they are immediately relevant to the current presentation.

Medications
• Group medications by indication (e.g., group HF medications, group diabetes medications).
• Note any recent changes to prescribed medications.
• Assess compliance.
• Ask about OTC medications, herbal medications, and supplements.

Allergies
Ask about allergies to medications, the type of reaction involved, how long ago the reaction occurred, and if the patient has ever rechallenged the medication or had a skin test for it.

Family History

- Determine what family members have had what disorders, and at what age.
- Family history may be less relevant in older adults who have chronic noncommunicable diseases.

Social History

- At minimum, ask about smoking, recreational drug use, and alcohol use.
- Consider asking about sexual and travel history.
- Consider asking about occupation, housing situation, and financial supports.

Functional History

In frail patients, or patients with comorbidities, determine the patient's ability to carry out ADLs and IADLs, including their ability to manage their own medications.

Code Status

- Determine the patient's goals of care (e.g., code status discussion, advance directives).
- If the patient has no previously expressed wishes and cannot communicate their goals of care, identify a person who can act as a substitute decision maker for the patient.

Physical Examination

The starting points of a physical exam always include ABCs (airway, breathing, circulation), vital signs, and general impression. The exam then proceeds system by system. It finally inventories lines and tubes.

For systems, consider leading with the organ system of interest. For example, if the patient has abdominal pain, lead with an abdominal exam; if dyspnea, lead with a cardiovascular or respiratory exam. The level of detail needed for each exam depends on the patient's active issues.

Airway, breathing, circulation (ABCs): Always start with this.

Vital signs: Obtain and note their trend since the patient presented for care.

General impression: Does the patient look well or unwell?
  › For example, are they alert, sitting up in bed, and conversing? Are they diaphoretic, sprawled on the bed, and only responding when you shout in their ear? Are they pale and unresponsive?

Head, ears, eyes, nose, throat: Assess for pupil size, pupillary response to light and accommodation, sinusitis, oral lesions, dental caries, and lymphadenopathy.

Cardiovascular: Assess for heart sounds, presence of murmurs and thrills, perfusion, height and character of JVP, and edema.
› If a murmur is present, determine its character, the location where it is loudest, its grade, and any radiation.
› In some cases, examine peripheral and central pulses and assess their regularity; and assess the warmth of skin, capillary refill, and changes of chronic venous or arterial disease.

Respiratory: Always assess the work of breathing and breath sounds, and look for adventitious sounds.
› Are there findings of COPD?
› Is PE possible? Are there findings of DVT in the peripheral vascular system?

Abdominal: Always assess shape (e.g., flat or distended) and bowel sounds; look for tenderness and masses; and screen for hepatosplenomegaly.
› If tenderness is present, assess for peritoneal findings (e.g., rebound, guarding).
› Perform a DRE if indicated.

GU: Assess for tenderness at the costovertebral angle, presence of a Foley catheter, appearance of urine, and bladder fullness and tenderness.

Neurological: Conduct a basic screening exam, which assesses orientation (person, place, time), cranial nerves, sensation in the extremities (using a light touch screen), and strength in all 4 limbs.
› If the presenting issue is neurological, a more detailed exam is required.

Musculoskeletal and dermatological:
› If rashes are present, note the character of the lesions and the location of the rash.
› Look for swollen or tender joints, if relevant (i.e., in the context of infection or inflammation).
› Assess for tenderness along the spine.

Lines and tubes: Check for peripheral IV access, central lines, Foley catheters, telemetry devices, and so on.

Investigations

RELEVANT PAST INVESTIGATIONS
- Check if past investigations establish a baseline of health or illness, especially in the context of the current presentation.
- Examples of past investigations include laboratory work, infectious disease status (e.g., HIV, viral hepatitis), imaging, and age-appropriate malignancy screening.

FOR EVERYONE

- Always consider a CBC with differential, a standard electrolyte panel, and tests for urea and creatinine.
- Also consider tests for liver enzymes and function, an extended electrolyte panel (Mg, Ca, PO_4), and a coagulation profile (INR, PTT).

FOR ALMOST EVERYONE

ECG: Note rate, rhythm, axis, evidence of old or new ischemia, conduction abnormalities, and QTc (relevant for medications).

Chest x-ray: This is relevant to all cardiac, respiratory, and infectious presentations, and a host of others.

IF CLINICALLY INDICATED

Knowing which additional investigations to order comes with experience.

- In general, order tests for anything that will change management within the next 24 hours. Most other things can wait.
- Order additional tests with purpose: be mindful of how each test ordered affects the patient and how it changes your management.

Impression and Plan

GENERAL BREAKDOWN

Start with a summary: You could look at this as your revised patient identification statement, based on key insights about the patient from your consultation. It should include pertinent positives and negatives that lead to your provisional diagnosis and management. *For example:* "Robert is a 72-year-old man with shortness of breath, orthopnea, and leg edema, found to be hypoxemic (requiring 2 L of supplemental oxygen), and with a chest x-ray showing new bilateral pleural effusions consistent with ADHF."

Organize issues by priority:
> Put the most important issue first.
> Use the same basic structure for each issue: 1) differential diagnosis, 2) causes and consequences, 3) workup and management.

Be precise: Try to use the most precise diagnostic terminology that is warranted. For example, if a patient has dyspnea and is also hypoxemic, the issue is hypoxemia, which is an objective correlate of the patient's dyspnea; if they are also found to have PE, then the issue is PE, which explains both dyspnea and hypoxemia.

List needed subspecialty consultations: Include these if subspecialty input is required.

ISSUES BREAKDOWN

Issue #1

- This is always the most serious or life-threatening issue, which may or may not be the reason for referral. *For example:* "Issue #1: ADHF. Left ventricular ejection fraction is 35% due to ischemic cardiomyopathy. Decompensation likely due to medication noncompliance. Start furosemide 40 mg IV twice daily. Hold ACEIs given acute kidney injury; restart ACEIs on discharge. Continue home beta-blocker. Restrict fluid and sodium. Repeat echocardiogram: most recent was 4 years ago."
- Follow a similar framework for all your active issues, including most likely etiology, differential diagnosis, investigations, and management.
- Rank the remaining issues after issue #1 in order of severity.

Multifactorial Issues

Many issues will be multifactorial in etiology, in which case include the likely contributors. *For example:* "Issue #2: AKI. Multifactorial: prerenal from use of ACEIs and NSAIDs with possible renal acute tubular necrosis. Send specimens for UA and microscopy. Obtain a bladder scan to screen for postrenal causes. Hold ACEIs and stop NSAIDs. Treat HF as above. Consider renal US if not improving."

Chronic Issues

- Consider including these, because not all chronic issues are managed appropriately (e.g., drug choice, dosing).
- Always include these if your plan affects aspects of their management.

Stable Issues

Consider including these to reinforce that current management is appropriate and does not need to be changed. *For example:* "Issue #3: AF. Persistent. Nonvalvular. $CHADS_2$ = 3. Anticoagulated on apixaban 5 mg twice daily. Rates 70–90 on home bisoprolol 5 mg daily. Continue home medications."

Uncertain Diagnosis

If the diagnosis is uncertain—which is often the case initially—include pertinent positives and negatives from the clinical exam and investigations to support or refute each possibility in the differential diagnosis. *For example:* "Issue #4: Leg redness and swelling. Suspect peripheral edema from HF and chronic venous stasis dermatitis. Patient was referred for possible bilateral cellulitis, but is afebrile with normal WBC and no tenderness. Hold antibiotics for now, treat HF, and monitor for improvement."

BEST PRACTICES

The following best practices are relevant to every patient, particularly in the inpatient setting.

Goals of care or code status: Make sure this information is in place.

DVT prophylaxis: Is it needed? Consider contraindications, existing therapeutic anticoagulation, and the risk status of the patient (IMPROVE score[2]). If a patient needs anticoagulation, what will you give them? Consider renal function.

Allied health-care providers: These could include social work, physical therapy, occupational therapy, and wound care.

Patient disposition: Does the patient need admission to hospital? If so, does internal medicine fit their needs best? Can they be safely discharged with follow-up?

Altered Level of Consciousness

These notes are in addition to the **general guide for all consultations** on page 1.

In patients presenting with altered level of consciousness (aLOC), an accurate history can be difficult to gather. You can often piece together a thorough consultation with collateral history from friends, family, bystanders, and emergency medical services. Collateral information can drastically change your management decisions, so it is definitely worth the effort.

Identification

Follow the **general guide for all consultations**.

Reason for Referral

Possible reasons for referral include:

- workup and management of a patient presenting with aLOC of undetermined cause
- monitoring for complications after an ingestion causing aLOC (e.g., after ingestion of TCAs)

History of Present Illness

TIMELINE OF EVENTS

Clarify:

- when the patient was last at their cognitive baseline
- what was happening prior to the change in level of consciousness (LOC)

- other symptoms experienced around the time LOC changed (e.g., fluctuations in LOC or associated symptoms)
- if found down, how long the patient was down
- whether they have had similar episodes of aLOC in the past

DIMS-RE MNEMONIC

DIMS-RE (**D**rugs, **I**nfections, **M**etabolic abnormalities, **S**tructural disease, **R**etention, **E**ncephalopathy) is commonly used to recall the differential diagnosis in aLOC. When the cause of aLOC is unknown, it helps structure history questions.

Drugs:
> › What prescribed medications does the patient take? Have they missed or taken extra doses?
> › Have there been any recent changes to prescription medications?
> › Has the patient received any new medications in hospital, or stopped any home medications?
> › Does the patient use alcohol, marijuana, or other substances?
> » Determine: how much and for how long; routes of administration; last use; previous complications from substance use.

Infections: Check for the following symptoms:
> › fever, chills, or rigors (these suggest general infection)
> › headache, neck pain, nausea, photophobia, or behaviour changes (meningitis or encephalitis)
> › cough, rhinorrhea, pharyngitis, or dyspnea (respiratory infection)
> › abdominal pain, nausea, vomiting, or diarrhea (abdominal infection)
> › dysuria, hematuria, urinary urgency, frequent urination, abnormal vaginal discharge, or suprapubic pain (GU infection)
> › tooth pain or recent dental work
> › new skin rashes, wounds, or sore joints

Metabolic abnormalities: Questions depend on the metabolic abnormality identified through investigations.

Structural disease:
> › Are there features of seizure associated with the episode of aLOC (e.g., tongue biting, urinary incontinence, gaze deviation, repetitive jerking movements)?
> › Does the patient have neurological symptoms or deficits?
> › Is there a history of risk factors for seizure: past head trauma, childhood seizures, or past stroke?
> › Are there constitutional symptoms or red flag features of headache that suggest underlying malignancy or inflammatory conditions?

Retention:
> › Is the patient constipated?

> Does the patient have lower urinary tract symptoms: increased frequency of voiding, nocturia, weak stream, intermittency, incomplete emptying, or straining?

Encephalopathy:
> Does the patient have symptoms of cancer associated with known paraneoplastic encephalitis?
> Does the patient have new severe hypertension?
> Does the patient have symptoms of progressive hepatic encephalopathy (day-night reversal, increasing abdominal distention)?

Past Medical History

DIMS-RE can help structure questions about past medical history, including a past history of:

- substance use or mental health conditions
- infections
- conditions associated with immunocompromise (e.g., diabetes, chronic use of steroids or other immunosuppressants, past chemotherapy, HIV)
- chronic disease (e.g., cirrhosis, chronic kidney disease, obstructive airway disease)
- malignancy
  > If yes, determine: when the patient was diagnosed, the stage of disease, and treatment received.
- seizures or head trauma
- stroke or neurocognitive impairment
- poorly controlled hypertension

Past Surgical History

Check for:
- recent procedures (these can be a source of infection)
- past neurosurgery

Medications

Review the patient's use of:
- prescribed medications, including when prescriptions were last filled and amounts of medication provided to the patient
  > Obtain collateral history, as necessary, to clarify if the patient was taking medications as prescribed: Is overdose a possibility?
- OTC medications (e.g., antiemetics, antihistamines, muscle relaxants)
- supplements and vitamins

Allergies

Follow the **general guide for all consultations.**

Family History

Check for aLOC.

Social History

Ask about the patient's living arrangements, employment history, and functional status.

Physical Examination

Airway: Note that assessing and maintaining the patient's airway is particularly important.

GCS: Use this to assess LOC.

Vital signs

Neurological:
> Perform a cranial nerve exam.
> Look for rigidity and clonus.
> Perform a motor and sensory exam.
> Check central and peripheral reflexes.
> Look specifically for asterixis if there is concern for metabolic encephalopathy.
> Look for evidence of meningitis (e.g., neck stiffness, photophobia, and signs such as jolt accentuation, Kernig sign, and Brudzinski sign).

Respiratory: Look for signs of infection and obstructive airway disease.

Cardiovascular: Assess perfusion and check for stigmata of endocarditis.

Abdominal: Check for signs of peritonitis or chronic liver disease.

GU: Check for costovertebral angle tenderness and suprapubic tenderness.

Dermatological (skin and soft tissue): Conduct a total body skin exam, looking for rashes and signs of infection.

Investigations

LABORATORY INVESTIGATIONS

CBC: WBC count and differential are especially important.

Glucose: This rules out symptomatic hypoglycemia.

Electrolytes (Na, K, Cl, HCO_3) and extended electrolytes (Ca, Mg, PO_4): Assess for abnormalities and calculate the anion gap.

Creatinine and urea: Compare the results to baseline.

Liver enzymes (AST, ALT, ALP, GGT) and liver function (albumin, bilirubin, INR, PTT): Check for chronic disease or reasons for hepatic encephalopathy.

Coagulation panel

Venous blood gas: Check for carbon dioxide retention.

CK, lactate, and prolactin: These may be elevated immediately after a seizure.

Serum toxicology screen (alcohol, acetylsalicylic acid, acetaminophen) and urine drug screen

Serum osmolality: This allows you to calculate the osmolar gap.

Carboxyhemoglobin: Pursue this on suspicion of carbon monoxide poisoning.

Thyrotropin (TSH): Consider whether to also investigate T_3 and T_4.

Cortisol: Ideally, this would be morning (AM) cortisol.

MICROBIOLOGY

Septic workup: Pursue this on concern for infection, or in the undifferentiated patient, including:
> › blood cultures
> › urinalysis (with or without urine cultures, as indicated)
> › sputum culture (if the patient has respiratory symptoms)
> › CSF culture and viral PCR (if LP is performed)

IMAGING

Compare new imaging to previous imaging, if available.

CT of the head: This is commonly done to look for structural causes of aLOC (e.g., intracerebral hemorrhage, stroke, mass, increased intracranial pressure, infection).

MRI of the head: Consider this to better assess for some specific conditions including posterior reversible encephalopathy syndrome, herpes simplex encephalitis, and autoimmune vasculitis.

Abdominal x-ray: Some clinicians order this to look for fecal loading.

Bladder scan: Order this to look for urinary retention.

OTHER INVESTIGATIONS

LP: Order a standard workup (e.g., opening pressure, cell count, differential, protein, glucose, Gram stain, and culture) and consider ordering HSV PCR, *Cryptococcus* PCR, acid-fast bacillus test, mycobacterial culture, cytology, and others as indicated.

ECG: Consider telemetry on concern for ingestion.

EEG: Consider this on suspicion of seizure or nonconvulsive status epilepticus.

Impression and Plan

GENERAL APPROACH
- Include the suspected cause of aLOC.
- Be mindful of the patient's disposition:
  › Concerns about the patient's ability to protect their own airway may mean the patient should stay in the ED or be admitted to critical care.
  › Concerns about ingestion with potential for arrhythmia may mean the patient should stay on telemetry.

TREATMENT
The treatment specifics you outline will depend on the cause of aLOC. The DIMS-RE mnemonic helps clarify a list of issues to always consider.

Drugs:
  › On concern about toxic ingestion, call poison control.
  › Always consider possible coingestions (e.g., with alcohol, check the osmolar gap to look for the presence of toxic alcohols).
  › Consider antidotes for certain drugs (e.g., naloxone for opioids; fomepizole for ethylene glycol and methanol; flumazenil for benzodiazepines; cyproheptadine for serotonin syndrome).
  › Consider what drugs dialysis could remove.
  › Consider withdrawal from drugs as a cause for aLOC: in particular, watch for alcohol and benzodiazepine withdrawal.
  › Limit the use of additional sedating medications.
  › Order drug levels when available, but do not rely too heavily on them as they can be misleading.

Infection:
  › Have a low threshold of suspicion when considering whether to order a septic workup (e.g., blood cultures, urine cultures, chest x-ray).
  › Ensure an antimicrobial regimen sufficient to cover possible sources of infection.
  › Meningitis treatment requires high doses of antimicrobials to penetrate the blood-brain barrier.
    » Consider coverage for listeria in patients older than 50, pregnant women, and immunocompromised individuals.
    » Consider treatment with dexamethasone on suspicion of pneumococcal meningitis: treatment should start before or with the first dose of antibiotics.
    » Consider empiric antiviral coverage for HSV and antifungal agents in at-risk groups.

Metabolic abnormalities:
  › Always check the patient's glucose level.
  › With sodium derangement, be cautious of rapid correction.

› Consult a respiratory therapist about possible noninvasive positive pressure ventilation if you are concerned about narcosis related to hypercapnia.

› Consult a nephrologist if you have concerns that uremia in the setting of renal failure, or certain toxic ingestions, are contributing to the patient's aLOC as these conditions may require dialysis.

› When no cause is identified, consider testing for endocrine and autoimmune conditions.

Structural disease:

› Rule out structural causes early.

» Perform a neurological exam and order imaging promptly: structural causes may require urgent intervention (e.g., intracerebral hemorrhage, abscess, stroke).

› If you suspect seizure, be mindful of medications that may lower the patient's seizure threshold further.

Retention:

› Is there evidence of fecal retention that requires laxatives, or urinary retention that requires a Foley catheter?

Encephalopathy:

› Is there evidence of posterior reversible encephalopathy syndrome (PRES) that would require emergent treatment of hypertension?

› Are there signs of hepatic encephalopathy that would warrant treatment with lactulose?

Hypertensive Crisis

These notes are in addition to the **general guide for all consultations** on page 1.

Identification

Follow the **general guide for all consultations**.

Reason for Referral

Crucial information in the referral includes hypertensive urgency versus emergency, and presenting BP. *For example:* "Patient referred for assessment of hypertensive emergency with BP 220/120, found to have significant acute kidney injury with hematuria."

• **Hypertensive urgency:** This is hypertension without end organ damage.

• **Hypertensive emergency:** This is hypertension with end organ damage or dysfunction, including stroke, intracerebral hemorrhage, encephalopathy, HF, MI, acute kidney injury, retinal hemorrhage, and aortic dissection.

- **Presenting BP:** In urgency, this should be > 180/120 mmHg without signs of end organ damage or dysfunction.

History of Present Illness

Determine how the hypertension was discovered: For example, was it identified at home, at a doctor's office, or incidentally on physical exam?

Identify red flags for secondary causes of hypertension: See sidebar.

Conduct a review of systems assessing for causes: Ask about:
› endocrine disorders: Cushing syndrome; hypo- or hyperthyroidism; pheochromocytoma (symptoms include pallor, palpitations, headache, diaphoresis)
› sleep apnea
› pregnancy
› pain crisis

Conduct a review of systems assessing for consequences: Ask about:
› **Neurological symptoms:** stroke, PRES (symptoms may include headaches; unilateral weakness; changes in vision; confusion; dysarthria or aphasia; paresthesias; vertigo; nausea and vomiting)
› **Cardiac symptoms:** chest pain, difficulty breathing
› **Vascular symptoms:** back pain, abdominal pain
› **Renal symptoms:** hematuria, flank pain, oliguria or anuria
› **Response to management in the ED:** peak BP and MAP; antihypertensive management; changes in symptoms and BP after treatment

|||||||||||||||||||||||||||||||||||||||||||||||||||||||||||||||||||||||||||||||||||||||||||||||||||||||||||||||||

RED FLAGS FOR SECONDARY CAUSES OF HYPERTENSION

Acute rise in BP, with previously well-controlled hypertension

Younger than 30

Poorly controlled hypertension with more than 3 antihypertensives, including a diuretic

Past Medical History

Determine the past history of hypertension:
› At what age was the patient's hypertension diagnosed?
› How was it diagnosed?
› How high was the initial BP?
› How difficult has control of BP been?
› How many medications has the patient been on, and how quickly were the medications escalated?
› Which medications have been effective and ineffective?

› What previous episodes of hypertensive urgency or emergency has the patient had?

› What is the patient's typical BP at home?

Assess for other entities: Be sure not to miss entities that may give you a hint about the etiology, such as:

› fibromuscular dysplasia

› endocrinopathies (hyper- or hypothyroidism, Cushing disease, pheochromocytoma, hyperparathyroidism)

› renal disease

› aortic disease

› atherosclerosis

› conditions associated with MEN-2a/2b, including medullary thyroid cancers, hyperparathyroidism, neuromas

› chronic hypokalemia

› sleep apnea

› metabolic syndrome

Past Surgical History
Follow the **general guide for all consultations.**

Medications
- Determine the start date, and time of last dose, for each current antihypertensive.
- Determine the patient's compliance with current medications.
- Ask about medications that can cause hypertension, such as OCs and antidepressants (especially monoamine oxidase inhibitors).
- Ask about herbal medications and OTC medications.

Allergies
Follow the **general guide for all consultations.**

Family History
Check for:
- hypertension, including age of onset
- MEN-1, MEN-2a/2b

Social History
Ask about:
- occupation
- factors affecting the patient's ability to adhere to medications (e.g., financial constraints, cognitive impairment)
- diet and exercise

- alcohol use, tobacco use
- recreational drug use, particularly sympathomimetic drugs such as amphetamines and cocaine; and withdrawal from alcohol, opioids, and benzodiazepines

Physical Examination

BP:
> Ensure BP is taken correctly, with the patient at rest and the arm at heart level.
> Determine current BP, peak BP, and bilateral arm BPs.

Other vital signs

Orientation:
> If indicated, apply GCS criteria and/or assess the patient's cognition.
> Often screening for orientation to person, place, and day (month and year) suffices.

Body habitus: Assess for obesity or evidence of Cushing syndrome.

Head, ears, nose, throat:
> Look for flare hemorrhages and/or papilledema on funduscopy.
> Perform a cranial nerve exam.
> Check for moon facies and a dorsocervical fat pad.

Thyroid-related systems:
> Assess the patient's reflexes.
> Look for:
  » skin, hair, nail changes
  » thyroid bruits
  » thyroid nodules or goiter
  » eye changes (ophthalmoplegia, lid lag, restricted extraocular movement, proptosis)
  » pretibial myxedema

Cardiovascular: Perform a full cardiovascular evaluation, including manoeuvres to assess for:
> pulses
> size and location of point of maximal pulse
> pulse deficit (this may indicate aortic dissection)

Respiratory: Assess for pulmonary edema.

Abdominal: Look for:
> costovertebral angle tenderness
> abdominal bruits

Neurological: Assess gait, and strength and sensation in bilateral upper and lower extremities.

Musculoskeletal: Check for ecchymoses, proximal muscle wasting, and violaceous abdominal striae.

Investigations

LABORATORY INVESTIGATIONS

CBC with differential, creatinine, urea, electrolytes (Na, K, Cl, HCO_3), liver enzymes (AST, ALT, ALP, GGT):
› Check for significantly increased creatinine (more than 50%) after starting ACEIs or ARBs, which would suggest renovascular disease.
› Order hemolysis tests if evidence of anemia or thrombocytopenia.

Ca: If elevated, order parathyroid hormone.

Mg, PO_4

Troponin

Plasma renin-to-aldosterone ratio: This is particularly useful in patients with chronic hypokalemia.

Thyrotropin (TSH)

Cortisol: Perform 2 tests for hypercortisolemia on suspicion of Cushing syndrome.
› Test options include midnight salivary cortisol, 24-hour urine cortisol, and low-dose dexamethasone suppression.
› Note that stress can falsely elevate results for these tests (which is a particular issue for inpatients).

Urine: Order:
› urinalysis and microscopy, urine albumin-to-creatinine ratio
› 24-hour urine studies (metanephrines, normetanephrines, catecholamines, cortisol)

IMAGING

Chest x-ray: This screens for widened mediastinum or pulmonary edema.

CT of the chest (aortogram) or transesophageal echocardiography: Pursue this on concern for features of dissection (e.g., stabbing chest pain radiating to the back, pulse deficit, BP asymmetry).

CT of the head: This assesses for bleeding in patients with neurological symptoms.

MRI of the head: Pursue this in patients with symptoms suspicious for PRES (confusion, visual changes).

Renal Doppler ultrasound: Pursue this on suspicion of fibromuscular dysplasia or renovascular disease.

CTA or MRA of the abdomen: These assess for renovascular disease.

OTHER INVESTIGATIONS

ECG: Use this to assess for signs of LV hypertrophy (evidence of chronicity) and acute or chronic ischemia.

Impression and Plan

GENERAL APPROACH

Describe the patient's history with hypertension: Specify:
› age of diagnosis
› red flags
› home antihypertensives

Document their presenting BP and MAP.

Clarify urgency versus emergency for this case: Does the patient have signs of end organ damage (i.e., neurological, cardiovascular, or renal signs)?

Clarify precipitants for the hypertensive crisis:
› Why does the patient have a hypertensive crisis now?
› Examples of precipitants include medication noncompliance and change in diet.

Document pending investigations: List investigations ordered to assess for causes and consequences of the patient's hypertension.

TREATMENT

Describe target BP:
› Aim for a 10% to 15% drop in MAP in the first hour, and a total 25% drop in the first 24 hours.
› **Caution:** Reducing BP too quickly may cause harm to the organs that regulate perfusion: the brain and kidneys.
› Note target BPs for these special cases:
  » **Intracranial hemorrhage:** systolic BP < 160 mmHg or as determined by neurosurgery
  » **Aortic dissection:** BP < 120/80 mmHg and heart rate 60 beats per minute within 20 minutes
  » **Ischemic stroke:** "permissive hypertension" < 220/120 mmHg, or < 180/105 mmHg with thrombolysis

List agents of choice to achieve target BP depending on context:
› **Urgency:** Oral agents to consider include captopril, labetalol, and hydralazine.
› **In cases of HF:** Consider a nitro patch and furosemide, and avoid beta-blockers until compensated.
› **Emergency:** IV agents to consider include hydralazine, labetalol, and nitroprusside.
› **In cases of aortic dissection:** IV labetalol or esmolol are first-line therapies to meet both BP and heart-rate targets; on reaching the maximum beta-blocker dose, nitroglycerin or nitroprusside may be added.
› *Note:*
  » Treatment may depend on the cause or consequence of hypertension.

» Beta-blockers alone are contraindicated in the setting of pheochromocytoma or cocaine-induced hypertension.

Outline a strategy for monitoring the patient:
> Clarify the frequency and type of monitoring required, and consider the best location for monitoring: a critical-care setting may be required for invasive monitoring (e.g., arterial line and/or infusions through a central line).
> If urine output decreases with a dramatic drop in MAP, this may be secondary to poor renal perfusion.

Obstetric Medicine

These notes are in addition to the **general guide for all consultations** on page 1.

Identification

Crucial obstetrical information is captured in the acronym GTPAL (number of **gestations**, **term** pregnancies, **preterm** pregnancies, **abortions**, **live** births), and the gestational age of the fetus (expressed as number of weeks plus additional days). *For example:* "Anne is a 32-year-old woman, G1T0P0A0L0 at 28+3 weeks gestational age with chronic hypertension presenting with shortness of breath."

Reason for Referral

• Anything medical can happen to pregnant and postpartum women.
• Be on the watch for: hypertension, gestational diabetes, eclampsia, liver disorders of pregnancy, VTE, thyroid disorders, hyperemesis, and bleeding disorders.

History of Present Illness

Identify:
• when and how pregnancy was achieved (ask about fertility medications, IVF)
• whether this is a single or multiple pregnancy
• the course of the pregnancy and medical care during the pregnancy (including who is providing care: midwife, general practitioner, obstetrician)
• the character of presenting symptoms (onset, severity, stable versus progressive, aggravating and alleviating factors)
• symptoms suggesting preeclampsia (headaches, visual changes, chest pain, shortness of breath, right upper quadrant pain, nausea, vomiting, changes to urine output)

- symptoms that would prompt urgent referral for obstetrical care (bleeding, decreased fetal movements, contractions, and ruptured membranes)

Past Medical History

PAST OBSTETRIC HISTORY
Determine:
- dates and relevant medical issues of previous pregnancies
- use of fertility aids or IVF for previous pregnancies
- how and where the patient's children were born (spontaneous vaginal delivery or caesarian section at home or in hospital)

OTHER PAST HISTORY
Review the following systems and issues:
- **Cardiovascular:** chronic hypertension, gestational hypertension, cardiomyopathies, valvular disease
- **Endocrine:** diabetes mellitus (clarify type 1 or type 2), gestational diabetes mellitus, thyroid disease, obesity
- **Hematological:** VTE, anemia, bleeding disorders
- **Autoimmunity:** SLE, findings of anti-SSA autoantibodies, antiphospholipid antibody syndrome, other
- **Infections:** HIV, HBV, HCV, STIs (current or previous)
- **GI:** liver disease
- **Respiratory:** asthma, smoking
- **Gynecological:** endometriosis, cervical cancer screening, other

Past Surgical History
Ask about:
- gynecological surgeries
- other surgeries

Medications
Relevant medications include:
- prepregnancy medications
- medications during pregnancy
- prenatal vitamins
- prophylaxis already prescribed for preeclampsia or VTE

Allergies
Follow the **general guide for all consultations.**

Family History
Determine the obstetric history of all first-degree relatives, if known.

Social History
- Be aware of the increased risk of intimate partner violence during pregnancy and screen for this, if appropriate.
- Ask about:
    › the patient's regular physical activity and activity tolerance before and after pregnancy
    › social, emotional, and financial supports
    › smoking, and use of alcohol and recreational drugs, before and after pregnancy

Physical Examination
Vital signs: Remember that normal BP decreases approaching the second trimester and rises slightly (i.e., returns to normal) in the third trimester.

Cardiovascular: Check for signs or symptoms of HF or chronic hypertension; jugular venous distension; lower extremity edema or sacral edema; third or fourth heart sounds; displaced apical beat (note that some changes may be physiologic).

Respiratory: Assess the work of breathing, and for crackles and wheezes.

Abdominal: Check for right upper quadrant tenderness and jaundice.

GU: Check for urine output and costovertebral tenderness.

Neurological: Check for focal deficits and seizures.

Dermatological: Check for rashes, excoriations, petechiae, and bleeding from IV sites.

Investigations

RELEVANT INVESTIGATIONS FROM EARLIER IN PREGNANCY
Review the results of previous investigations and compare them with results from current investigations, including: obstetrical US; infectious disease screening; CBC; renal function (creatinine, eGFR); liver enzymes (AST, ALT, ALP, GGT) and liver function (albumin, bilirubin, INR, PTT); thyrotropin (TSH); oral glucose tolerance; urinalysis; and urine protein-to-creatinine ratio.

FOR EVERYONE
Blood chemistry: Follow the general guide for all consultations, *but note:*
    › Expected hemoglobin and creatinine levels are **lower** in pregnancy.
    › Mild neutrophilia is common throughout pregnancy and peripartum.
Urinalysis and urine protein-to-creatinine ratio (or 24-hour protein)

IF CLINICALLY INDICATED
Peripheral blood smear: This is relevant to anemia and HELLP syndrome.

Uric acid, LDH, INR, PTT: These are relevant to preeclampsia.

Thyroid function: Order thyrotropin (TSH) with or without T_3 and T_4; anti-thyroid peroxidase antibodies (anti-TPO antibodies); and thyrotropin receptor antibody (relevant to Graves disease).

β-HCG: This is relevant to hyperemesis and molar pregnancy.

Oral glucose tolerance test: This is relevant to gestational diabetes mellitus (HbA_{1c} is less accurate in pregnancy).

Echocardiogram: Pursue this on concern for peripartum cardiomyopathy.

BNP: Note that normal ranges in pregnancy are not well validated.

Abdominal US: Pursue this on concern for liver disorders of pregnancy.

Pelvic US: Pursue this on concern for molar pregnancy.

Doppler US of the legs: Pursue this on concern for VTE.
> › If US findings are negative despite clinical suspicion of VTE, order a V/Q scan (perfusion portion only).
>> » A CT pulmonary embolism study is acceptable if a V/Q scan is unavailable.
> › Note that D-dimer testing is not recommended.
> › Consider a chest x-ray if the differential diagnosis includes other causes of dyspnea.

Impression and Plan

Before prescribing any new medications, review their safety in pregnancy and breastfeeding.

GESTATIONAL OR CHRONIC HYPERTENSION

- Treat severe, acute hypertension with labetalol (IV), immediate-release nifedipine (oral), or hydralazine (IV).
- Treat chronic hypertension with labetalol (oral), methyldopa, or long-acting nifedipine.

PREECLAMPSIA

- Characterize the severity of the preeclampsia and describe organ involvement.
- Manage acute hypertension as above.
- Prescribe magnesium sulphate, if indicated, to prevent and treat eclampsia.
- Consult with specialists in obstetrics and maternal-fetal medicine: delivery is definitive management of preeclampsia.
- If the presentation has no severe features, consider inpatient expectant management.

HEART FAILURE

- Prescribe furosemide for diuresis: pregnant women respond well to low doses.

- ACEIs and ARBs are contraindicated in pregnancy.

VENOUS THROMBOEMBOLISM

Prescribe a low molecular weight heparin (or unfractionated heparin) for the current episode and prophylactic doses for future pregnancies.

ASTHMA

Follow standard management (do not withhold steroids for severe asthma).

HYPOTHYROIDISM

- This includes subclinical hypothyroidism.
- Targets are unique to pregnancy, often < 2.5 mU/L for thyrotropin (TSH), but consult local guidelines.
- Monitor thyrotropin every 4 to 6 weeks.

HYPERTHYROIDISM

- Gestational transient thyrotoxicosis should resolve by 14 to 18 weeks; consider treatment with beta-blockers (propranolol) for a short time to control symptoms, if needed.
- Consider pelvic US to rule out molar pregnancy.
- For Graves disease, stop antithyroid medications, if possible; if not, prescribe propylthiouracil in the first trimester, and methimazole after that.

DIABETES MELLITUS

- Consider a trial of lifestyle measures.
- Tight glycemic control improves outcomes for mother and baby.
- Insulin is often the first-line therapy, though there is increasing evidence for metformin.

POSTPARTUM HEMORRHAGE

- Defer to obstetric specialists.
- For patients with an underlying bleeding disorder, prescribe oxytocin, tranexamic acid, or packed RBCs or other blood products (e.g., von Willebrand factor concentrate, recombinant factor VIIa).

HEPATIC DISORDERS

For intrahepatic cholestasis of pregnancy, prescribe ursodiol or emollients.

HELLP SYNDROME

- Treat with magnesium sulphate to prevent eclampsia.
- Treat hypertension.
- If the gestational age is more than 34 weeks, discuss delivery; if less than 34 weeks, and the mother and fetus are stable, consider treating with betamethasone and delaying delivery up to 48 hours.

ACUTE FATTY LIVER OF PREGNANCY
- Provide supportive care.
- Discuss timing of delivery with obstetric specialists.
- Consider consulting GI specialists about liver transplantation.

Perioperative Medicine

These notes are in addition to the **general guide for all consultations** on page 1.

Identification

Key features of the patient's current presentation include:
- age
- relevant comorbidities
- type of surgery the patient is undergoing
- indication for the surgery
- urgency of the surgery (i.e., elective, urgent, or emergent)

Reason for Referral

- Note that the reason for referral may be nonspecific in a medically comorbid patient: the request may be "please optimize."
- Crucial information includes:
  › the setting for the consultation (preoperative or postoperative)
  › the specific question posed by the surgical team (e.g., whether it regards cardiovascular risk, perioperative medication management, elevated troponin)

History of Present Illness

BOTH PREOPERATIVE AND POSTOPERATIVE ASSESSMENT

- Identify the indication for the surgery, the surgeon, and the date of surgery. *For example:* "Dr. Smith is to perform an elective left total hip arthroplasty for osteoarthritis under general anesthesia 2 weeks from now."
- If the surgery relates to a medical condition, provide an appropriate history (e.g., an appropriate cancer history in the context of surgical oncology; a cardiac history in the context of CABG surgery).
- Conduct a review of systems with a focus on cardiovascular and pulmonary disease. Assess for:
  › pulmonary hypertension
  › right-sided heart failure
  › obstructive sleep apnea (use the screening mnemonic STOP BANG)
  › exercise capacity (quantify this as METs: e.g., 2 flights of stairs = 4 METs)

- Conduct a frailty screen: review ADLs and IADLs.

PREOPERATIVE ASSESSMENT ONLY

Screen for contraindications to urgent surgery: Most are unstable
cardiac conditions, including:
  › flow-limiting cardiac condition, including severe aortic stenosis,
    mitral stenosis, and hypertrophic cardiomyopathy with obstruction
    (look for angina, syncope)
  › active HF
  › current ACS
  › unstable arrhythmia

Screen for indications to delay elective surgery: Examples include:
  › poorly controlled type 2 diabetes
  › poorly optimized cardiac or respiratory condition
  › recent PCI requiring dual antiplatelet therapy

POSTOPERATIVE ASSESSMENT ONLY

- Assess the course of the patient's postoperative health.
- Review the patient's anesthesia record, if available (i.e., vital signs during
  surgery; medications, fluids, transfusions given during surgery).

Past Medical History

GENERAL APPROACH

Ask about diagnoses related to the perioperative concern and the specialists involved, and about other comorbidities (e.g., diabetes).

PARTICULAR CONCERNS FOR THIS CONSULTATION

Hemostasis: Ask about:
  › anticoagulation therapy, the indication for therapy (e.g., AF, VTE,
    coagulopathy), date of diagnosis for the indication, relevant risk
    scores (e.g., $CHADS_2$), and current treatment
  › bleeding diathesis (e.g., von Willebrand factor deficiency, hemophilia,
    immune thrombocytopenia)

Cardiovascular disease: Identify the patient's most recent
  investigations (including those with normal results) and note
  features of concern, including:
  › **ECG:** signs of ischemia (current or past), chamber enlargement,
    arrhythmias
  › **Echocardiogram:** EF, significant valvular pathology, signs of
    pulmonary hypertension (e.g., elevated pulmonary arterial systolic
    pressure, RV systolic pressure)
  › **Coronary angiogram:** stents (identify type and date placed), residual
    occlusive disease

> **Other cardiac tests:** stress test for evidence of coronary ischemia, Holter monitor for evidence of arrhythmia, other tests

Respiratory conditions: Determine:
> results of the patient's most-recent pulmonary function tests (e.g., FEV_1)
> level of disease control (e.g., number of COPD exacerbations in the last year)

Renal function: Determine the patient's baseline.

Rheumatic conditions: Determine:
> disease severity, and active or recent treatments
> **in particular,** previous steroid use, and current use of biologic agents, including when the patient took their last dose

Cognitive impairment: This is important for delirium risk.

Past Surgical History
Identify previous surgeries and complications.

Medications
- **All medications:** Establish the indication, when therapy started, and patient compliance.
- **Anticoagulants:** Establish when the patient took their last dose.

Allergies
Follow the **general guide for all consultations**.

Family History
Check for:
- conditions related to the patient's past medical history and indication for surgery
- conditions related to the patient's ability to use anesthetics (e.g., malignant hyperthermia)

Social History
Follow the **general guide for all consultations**.

Physical Examination
Cardiovascular, respiratory, and abdominal:
> Perform a focused exam to identify poorly controlled disease and screen for conditions that could alter perioperative care.
> Depending on the indication for surgery, perform a more detailed exam of the relevant system (but avoid interfering with dressings in postoperative patients, except in cases of infection).

› Features to watch for include:
  » **Severe aortic stenosis:** late-peaking systolic murmur; soft or absent S2; brachioradial delay; apical-carotid delay
  » **Severe mitral stenosis:** diastolic rumble (best auscultated at the apex)
  » **Pulmonary hypertension:** loud pulmonic valve closure (P2), RV heave
  » **Obstructive sleep apnea:** large tongue; elevated BMI or neck circumference
  » **HF:** edema, crackles, jugular venous distension

Investigations

LABORATORY INVESTIGATIONS

CBC, creatinine, INR, PTT

Other investigations: Pursue investigations relevant to the clinical context, including those relevant to comorbidities (e.g., HbA_{1c} for diabetes).

IMAGING

- Review previous cardiac investigations (e.g., echocardiogram, angiogram, stress test).
- Review previous pulmonary investigations (e.g., pulmonary function test, chest imaging, sleep study).

CARDIOVASCULAR RISK ASSESSMENT

Baseline ECG: Consider this for preoperative patients.

Postoperative ECG: Have this performed in the recovery room for patients older than 65, or with a revised cardiac risk index (RCRI) score greater than 1.[3]

Preoperative BNP: Pursue this in patients aged 45 to 64 with cardiovascular disease.[3]

Investigations to avoid: Avoid ordering preoperative cardiac imaging or stress tests for risk stratification.
  › **Exception:** Consider an echocardiogram on suspicion of flow-limiting valvular lesions (severe aortic or mitral stenosis).

Impression and Plan

PREOPERATIVE PATIENTS

- Summarize the planned procedure and your overall evaluation. *For example:* "Mr. Smith is a 68-year-old man with a history of CAD who is being evaluated for an elective hip arthroplasty in 2 weeks. We recommend proceeding with the surgery as scheduled."
- Organize the plan by preoperative and postoperative care, or by organ system.

|||||||||||||||||||||||||||||||||||||||||||||||||||||||||||||||||||||||||||||||||||||||||||||||||||||||||||||||||||||

GUIDELINES ON SURGERY SCHEDULING[3]

Emergency surgery: Do not delay.

Urgent surgery: Recommend delay only for unstable cardiac conditions.

Elective surgery: Consider recommending delay for poorly controlled medical conditions (e.g., diabetes, HF), or in the context of high risk for uncontrolled bleeding due to transient anticoagulation or antiplatelet requirements.

Medication Management

Choice of medication may vary depending on the type of surgery planned, the patient's risk for uncontrolled bleeding, and other factors.

Anticoagulants and antiplatelet agents in general: Guidelines for perioperative management depend on the type of anesthesia used.
> Guidelines for neuraxial anesthetic tend to be more conservative.
> For questions or concerns about anticoagulation or antiplatelet agents, always speak with the surgeon and the anesthesiologist.

Anticoagulants:
> Timing of discontinuation will depend on the agent's half-life and the patient's renal function.
> Bridging of anticoagulation is typically only done in the setting of active VTE, a mechanical valve, recent cerebrovascular accident, and AF with a $CHADS_2$ score greater than 4. Refer to relevant guidelines (e.g., Thrombosis Canada).

Antiplatelet agents[4,5]:
> Stop clopidogrel and ticagrelor 5 to 7 days, and prasugrel 7 to 10 days, before surgery. In some cases, acetylsalicylic acid (ASA) can be continued perioperatively depending on the surgery and surgeon.
> If the patient has had a recent PCI, delay elective procedures at least 3 months after insertion of drug-eluting stents, and 1 month after insertion of bare-metal stents.
> In the context of urgent surgery, delay for antiplatelet washout if possible.

Beta-blockers: Continue these if they are a preexisting medication, but patients should not start them immediately before surgery.[6]

CCBs: The decision to hold or discontinue these may depend on BP control.

ACEIs and ARBs: Hold 24 hours before surgery.[3]

Noninsulin diabetes medications: Hold doses on the morning of the surgery. Hold sodium-glucose contransporter-2 (SGLT2) inhibitors at least 3 days in advance.

Insulin:
> › Continue long-acting insulin at one-half to two-thirds of home dosing.
> › For lengthy surgery (e.g., more than 2 meals missed), consider IV insulin. Discuss this option with the anesthetist.

Statins: Continue these.

Steroids: In patients with adrenal insufficiency or those chronically on steroids, consider stress dosing.

Cardiac Risk Stratification

- Document the patient's RCRI score (calculate this with the Canadian Cardiovascular Society algorithm). Communicate the patient's cardiac risk to the patient and surgical team.
- List further investigations required, if any, and provide recommendations based on the results.
  > › For example, if the patient's preoperative BNP is elevated, order tests for troponin every day for 3 days after surgery.

Respiratory Risk Stratification

- Document the patient's postoperative risk for respiratory complications (e.g., pneumonia, respiratory failure). The ARISCAT score and Arozullah score are common estimators.[7]
- Evidence shows that most efforts to prevent postoperative respiratory complications are ineffective, but you should communicate the patient's risk to the patient and surgical team.

Delirium Risk

- Limit the use of medications that commonly cause delirium, especially in patients with preexisting cognitive impairment.
- Outline nonpharmacological interventions to reduce delirium: ensure the patient has their usual sensory aids with them in hospital (e.g., hearing aids, glasses); promote family visitation.

Venous Thromboembolism Prophylaxis

The surgical team usually determines this based on the type of surgery.

POSTOPERATIVE PATIENTS

- Clarify with the surgical team whether they want you to manage postoperative issues, or to provide advice for them to manage the issues. Document this in your plan.
- Closed-loop communication about who will follow up any issues or investigations is key. Document the strategy in your plan.

Cardiac Issues

Myocardial Injury After Noncardiac Surgery (MINS)

- Monitor for MINS in patients with an RCRI score greater than 1; or who are older than 65; or who are aged 45 to 64 with cardiovascular disease.

- Monitoring entails an ECG in the postanesthesia care room and daily ECGs for 48 to 72 hours.[3]
- If the patient's preoperative BNP level is > 92 pg/mL, or their NT-proBNP is > 300 pg/mL, order postoperative tests for troponin every day for 48 to 72 hours.[3]
- If MINS is detected, ASA and statins are recommended.[3]

Acute Coronary Syndrome
- Management of ACS often depends on the patient's recent surgeries, stability, and toleration of antiplatelet therapy.
- The management plan is often a joint decision among those providing cardiac, internal medicine, and surgical care.

Atrial Fibrillation
- Provide a workup for triggers such as postoperative infection, hypovolemia, ACS, HF, and PE.
- Consider rate control.
- Consider anticoagulation, but note that there are no clear guidelines for postoperative AF: patients seem to have the same stroke risk as for paroxysmal AF.

Respiratory Issues
Outline standard treatment for any issues that emerge (e.g., pneumonia, COPD exacerbation).

Delirium
See also Altered Level of Consciousness in this chapter.
- Outline an approach to look for causes.
- Minimize medications that commonly cause delirium, but treat pain appropriately.
- Limit the use of lines and tubes, ensure the patient has their usual sensory aids, and promote early mobilization.

Infection
- Order appropriate cultures and initiate empiric antibiotics.
- If infection develops at the surgical site, obtain appropriate imaging and discuss source control with the surgical team.

Venous Thromboembolism
See also Venous Thromboembolism (chapter 9).
- Note that D-dimer testing has no diagnostic value for VTE in the postoperative setting.
- Always discuss anticoagulation therapy with the surgical team before initiating treatment.

Acute Kidney Injury

Outline a standard workup:

- Monitor urine output, and order urinalysis, urine microscopy, and renal US, if indicated;
- Treat volume status with IV fluids or diuresis, as required.

Medications

Most home medications can resume postoperatively, with some caveats:

- **Anticoagulation and antiplatelet agents:** Restart these when the surgical team deems them without risk for uncontrolled bleeding.
- **Insulin and oral hypoglycemic agents:** Restarting home medications depends on when the patient begins to eat again.

References

1. Gage BF, Waterman AD, Shannon W, et al. Validation of clinical classification schemes for predicting stroke. JAMA. 2001;285(22):2864-70. doi:10.1001/jama.285.22.2864
2. Rosenberg D, Eichorn A, Alarcon M, et al. External validation of the risk assessment model of the International Medical Prevention Registry on Venous Thromboembolism (IMPROVE) for medical patients in a tertiary health system. J Am Heart Assoc. 2014;3(6):e001152. doi: 10.1161/JAHA.114.001152
3. Duceppe E, Parlow J, MacDonald P, et al. Canadian Cardiovascular Society guidelines on perioperative cardiac risk assessment and management for patients who undergo noncardiac surgery. Can J Cardiol. 2017;33(1):17-32. doi: 10.1016/j.cjca.2016.09.008
4. Tanguay J, Bell A, Ackman M, et al. Focused 2012 update of the Canadian Cardiovascular Society guidelines for the use of antiplatelet therapy. Can J Cardiol. 2013;29(11):1334-45. doi:10.1016/j.cjca.2013.07.001
5. Thrombosis Canada. Perioperative management of antiplatelet therapy [Internet]. Whitby, ON: Thrombosis Canada; 2019 Feb 11 [cited 2020 May 10]. 5 p. Available from: https://thrombosiscanada.ca/wp-content/uploads/2019/02/Perioperative-Management-of-Antiplatelet-Therapy-2019-February-11.pdf
6. POISE study group; Devereaux P, Yang H, Yusef S, et al. Effects of extended-release metoprolol succinate in patients undergoing non-cardiac surgery (POISE trial): a randomised controlled trial. Lancet. 2008;371(9627):1839-47. doi:10.1016/S0140-6736(08)60601-7
7. Canet J, Gallart L, Gomar C, et al; ARISCAT Group. Prediction of postoperative pulmonary complications in a population-based surgical cohort. Anesthesiology. 2010;113(6):1338-50. doi:10.1097/ALN.0b013e3181fc6e0a

2

Allergy and Immunology

Dr. Arun Dhir
Dr. Pauline Luczynski
Dr. Jian Weng
Dr. Juan Camilo Ruiz

REVIEWER
Dr. Raymond Mak

ALLERGY

Starting Points: Allergy Consultations

These notes are in addition to the **general guide for all consultations** on page 1.

Identification

Key information in the identification statement for allergy consultations includes:

- ethnicity
- age
- sex
- occupation
- comorbidities

Reason for Referral

- Examples of reason for referral include possible food, drug, or environmental allergy, or reaction to physical agents (e.g., cold).
- Pay attention to notes about possible triggers: specific drugs, specific foods.

Table 2.1. Key Features of Hypersensitivity Reactions

TYPE	PATHOPHYSIOLOGY	ONSET AFTER EXPOSURE	KEY FEATURES
1	IgE	Rapid: within 1 hour	Pruritic rash, hives, lip and tongue swelling, change in voice quality, abdominal pain, nausea/vomiting, diarrhea Anaphylaxis (most severe presentation): dizziness, shortness of breath, wheezing/stridor, sensation of throat closure, syncope Previous exposure to a suspected drug (usual: however, sensitization may occur as a result of exposure to a cross-reacting compound)
2	Cytotoxic, antibody mediated	At least 5–8 hours	**Drug-induced hemolytic anemia:** dyspnea, fatigue, pallor, jaundice, dark urine, splenomegaly, bounding pulses, palpitations **Drug-induced thrombocytopenia:** petechial bleeding in skin and buccal mucosa, splenomegaly, hepatomegaly **Drug-induced neutropenia or agranulocytosis:** symptoms of infection, fever, stomatitis, pharyngitis, pneumonia, sepsis
3	Immune complex deposition	At least 1 week	Associated with prolonged drug administration Onset: at least 1 week after exposure Serum sickness: fever, urticarial or purpuric rash, arthralgias, glomerulonephritis Cutaneous small-vessel vasculitis: purpura/petechiae, fever, urticaria, arthralgias, lymphadenopathy Arthus reaction: localized skin necrosis, swelling, erythema (peaking by 24 hours after exposure)

Continued on p. 35

Table 2.1. *Continued from p. 34*

TYPE	PATHOPHYSIOLOGY	ONSET AFTER EXPOSURE	KEY FEATURES
4	Cell mediated	Delayed: at least 48–72 hours; sometimes weeks (can be less than 24 hours on reexposure)	**SJS/TEN** Prodromal symptoms: fever (> 39 C) and general malaise Skin tenderness, erythema, blistering, epidermal necrosis, desquamation, mucositis Skin lesions that start on the face and thorax before spreading to other areas, and that typically spare scalp, palms, and soles **DRESS** Fever (38-40 C), lymphadenopathy, facial edema, hepatitis and end organ damage Morbilliform eruption that progresses rapidly to an infiltrated erythema with follicular accentuation (> 50% body surface area) **AGEP** Rapid development (within 24 hours of exposure) of small pustules Lesions that generally begin on the face or intertriginous areas and extend to the trunk and limbs

Abbreviations: AGEP: acute generalized exanthematous pustulosis; DRESS: drug reaction with eosinophilia and systemic symptoms; SJS: Stevens-Johnson syndrome; TEN: toxic epidermal necrolysis

History of Present Illness

Determine:

- what triggered the patient to seek care
- what the suspected allergen is and how the patient was exposed to it
- features of any skin lesions (associated tenderness, appearance, distribution, time of onset, and progression)
- other key features of the reaction (see Table 2.1)
- the temporal relationships between symptoms and the administration of specific drugs (examine the patient's medical record)

Past Medical History

Review risk factors for drug hypersensitivity, which include age (adulthood), sex (female), atopy, underlying disease (e.g., SLE, HIV), and specific genetic polymorphisms.[1]

Medications

- Pay particular attention to newly initiated medications.
- For medications suspected as allergens, determine:
  › the indication for the medication
  › the dose and route of administration
  › previous exposures to the medication

Allergies

Ask about previous positive skin tests, patch test reactions, and results from any in vitro lymphocyte proliferation assays.

Family History

Follow the **general guide for all consultations.**

Social History

Check for:

- Asian or South Asian ancestry (relevant to Stevens-Johnson syndrome [SJS] and toxic epidermal necrolysis [TEN])
- possible environmental exposure to an allergen or chemical
- alcohol and drug use, smoking, occupational exposures

Physical Examination

See Table 2.2 for key findings.

Investigations

CBC with differential: Order this for all patients.
Autoimmune panel: Consider this for type 3 and type 4 reactions.
Other investigations: See Table 2.3.

Impression and Plan

GENERAL APPROACH

- Clarify whether the presentation is consistent with an immunologic response. If so, what type?
- Clarify possible offending agents.
- Document the severity of the reaction and what organ systems are involved.
- Stop or substitute all suspect medications; monitor the patient for symptom improvement after stopping these medications.
- Recommend a graded drug challenge when the benefit of a medication may outweigh the risk of a renewed reaction (this is mostly done in type 1 hypersensitivity).

TYPE 1 IgE-MEDIATED REACTION

Consider referral for skin testing.

Table 2.2. Key Findings in Hypersensitivity Reactions

TYPE	KEY FINDINGS
1	**Absence** of fever Flushing, angioedema, urticarial rash Anaphylaxis: dyspnea, wheeze/bronchospasm, stridor, reduced peak expiratory flow, hypoxemia, hypotension, tachycardia, angioedema, abdominal pain, vomiting, diarrhea
2	Clinical presentation: wide variations in severity **Drug-induced hemolytic anemia:** hyperdynamic state (tachycardia), tachypnea, pallor, jaundice, splenomegaly **Drug-induced thrombocytopenia:** petechial bleeding in skin and buccal mucosa; splenomegaly; hepatomegaly **Drug-induced neutropenia or agranulocytosis:** symptoms of infection; fever; stomatitis; pharyngitis; pneumonia; sepsis
3	**Serum sickness:** severe arthralgias and myalgias disproportionate to degree of swelling; urticarial lesions **CSVV:** palpable purpura and/or petechiae that are nonblanching, particularly in the lower extremities
4	**SJS/TEN** Body surface area affected: SJS, less than 10%; TEN, more than 30% Diffuse erythema; ill-defined, coalescing erythematous macules with central dusky purpura; bullae and blister formation; epidermal necrosis and/or desquamation with Nikolsky sign and possibly Asboe-Hansen sign Temperature > 39 C; hypotension; mucositis **DRESS** Body surface area affected: > 50% Morbilliform eruption, lymphadenopathy, symmetric facial edema and erythema Hepatomegaly, jaundice, tachypnea, hypoxemia **AGEP** Nonfollicular, pinhead-sized pustules on a background of edematous erythema with flexural predilection; possible facial edema Temperature > 38 °C Severe cases: possible atypical target lesions, coalescent pustules, and superficial erosions similar to SJS/TEN; possible involvement of mucous membranes (unusual)

Abbreviations: AGEP: acute generalized exanthematous pustulosis; CSVV: cutaneous small-vessel vasculitis; DRESS: drug reaction with eosinophilia and systemic symptoms; SJS: Stevens-Johnson syndrome; TEN: toxic epidermal necrolysis.

Urticarial Reactions

- These can be treated with a nonsedating H1 antihistamine, at levels up to 4 times the standard dose.
- H2 blockers are generally unhelpful.
- *See also* Urticaria in this chapter.

Table 2.3. Key Investigations for Hypersensitivity Reactions

TYPE	INVESTIGATIONS
1	Specific antigen skin-prick testing Anaphylaxis: • Serum tryptase in blood samples collected within 4-6 hours of the event confirms the event. • A baseline tryptase level in the future for particularly severe reactions may be helpful to rule out systemic mastocytosis.
2	Drug-induced hemolytic anemia, thrombocytopenia: LDH, bilirubin, DAT, peripheral blood smear
3	Creatinine; urea; urinalysis and microscopy; liver function tests; HBV/HCV serologies Biopsy of skin lesions (if present)
4	**SJS/TEN** Creatinine, urea, glucose, ESR, CRP Bacterial and fungal cultures if wounds are present Chest x-ray to assess for pneumonia and interstitial pneumonitis Biopsy of skin lesions with large (> 4 mm) punch biopsy or saucerization (deep shave biopsy) **DRESS** Creatinine, urea, UA, liver function tests, HBV/HCV serology Peripheral smear EBV, CMV, HHV-6, HHV-7, mycoplasma PCR (if indicated) Chest x-ray to assess for interstitial pneumonitis and/or pleural effusion Skin biopsy (if present) **AGEP** Pustular smear for bacterial culture (if indicated)

Abbreviations: AGEP: acute generalized exanthematous pustulosis; CMV: cytomegalovirus; CRP: C-reactive protein; DAT: direct antiglobulin test; DRESS: drug reaction with eosinophilia and systemic symptoms; EBV: Epstein-Barr virus; ESR: erythrocyte sedimentation rate; HBV: hepatitis B virus; HCV: hepatitis C virus; HHV: human herpesvirus; LDH: lactate dehydrogenase; PCR: polymerase chain reaction; SJS: Stevens-Johnson syndrome; TEN: toxic epidermal necrolysis; UA: urinalysis

Angioedema or Persistent Symptoms, Despite H1 Antihistamines
Administer a brief course of oral glucocorticoids.

Anaphylaxis
- Provide treatment immediately:
  › Administer IM epinephrine 0.3–0.5 mg.
  › Consider intubation if evidence suggests impending airway obstruction.
  › Initiate supplemental oxygen.
  › Obtain IV access and give IV fluids if needed.
  › If refractory, consider epinephrine infusion.

- Adjuvant therapies include H1 antihistamine, glucocorticoids, and inhaled bronchodilators.
- Patients on beta-blockers may require glucagon infusion.
- Monitor patients for hemodynamic stability and biphasic reaction.
- On discharge, provide patients with an anaphylaxis emergency plan, a prescription for an epinephrine autoinjector, and referral to an allergist.

TYPE 2 ANTIBODY-DEPENDENT CYTOTOXICITY

Drug-Induced Hemolytic Anemia
- Expect hemoglobin to improve in a few days to weeks after drug discontinuation.
- Consider a transfusion of packed RBCs for severe anemia (hemoglobin < 70 g/L).

Drug-Induced Thrombocytopenia
- Consider tests for drug-dependent antiplatelet antibodies.[2]
- For life-threatening bleeding, consider IVIG.
- For bleeding other than petechiae or purpura, but not severe, consider glucocorticoids.

Drug-Induced Neutropenia
- Neutropenia usually resolves within 1 to 3 weeks after cessation of the offending drug.[3]
- Consider treatment with G-CSF if the patient is ill from infection and you suspect bone marrow suppression.

TYPE 3 IMMUNE-COMPLEX REACTION

Serum Sickness
- Fever and arthralgias resolve, and new skin lesions stop forming, within 48 hours of stopping the offending medication.
- Antihistamines can treat pruritus.[1]
- Administer NSAIDs as analgesics and antipyretics.
- For severe symptoms, consider a short course of glucocorticoids.

Small-Vessel Vasculitis
- Expect resolution within days to a few weeks after drug discontinuation.
- Treat the associated underlying infection.

TYPE 4 CELL-MEDIATED REACTION
- Order genetic screening for HLA genotypes.
- Consider patch testing with drug preparations.
- Monitor patients for progression of skin lesions (mark the borders of lesions).

||||||||||||||||||||||||||||||||||||||||||||||||||||||||||||||||||||||||||||||||||||||||||||||||||||||||||||||||||||||||||||||||||||||

HLA SCREENING FOR DELAYED-ONSET HYPERSENSITIVITY

HLA-B*15:02 (increased risk of SJS/TEN with carbamazepine and other aromatic anticonvulsants)

HLA-B*15:11 (increased risk of DRESS with carbamazepine)

HLA-A*31:01 (increased risk of DRESS with carbamazepine)

CYP2C9*3 (increased risk of SJS/TEN with phenytoin, carbamazepine)

SJS/TEN

- Assess the severity of illness and the prognosis with the SCORTEN score.
- Consider for admission to the burn unit or ICU.
- Consider cyclosporine 3–5 mg/kg/day if you are treating the patient within 24 to 48 hours of symptom onset.[4]
- Provide supportive care for wounds and ophthalmic symptoms, fluid and electrolyte management, temperature management, and pain control.
- Monitor patients for pulmonary edema and super infections.

DRESS

- The extent of involved BSA is an important marker of disease severity: use Lund-Browder charts or the rule of nines for estimation.[5]
- Administer topical corticosteroids for pruritus and skin inflammation.
- For liver involvement:
  › Order serial liver enzymes and liver function tests.
  › Consider a hepatology consultation.
  › Severe hepatitis, particularly jaundice, may require liver transplant evaluation.
- For lung or kidney involvement:
  › Administer systemic corticosteroids (e.g., prednisone 0.5–2 mg/kg/day).
- Monitor the patient for other organ involvement, including myocarditis and pericarditis; GI bleed; pancreatitis; autoimmune thyroiditis; and encephalitis and meningitis.

AGEP

- Symptoms usually resolve without treatment within 1 to 2 weeks after drug discontinuation.
- Administer topical corticosteroids for pruritus and skin inflammation.
- Other organ involvement is not common.

Angioedema

These notes are in addition to the **general guide for all consultations** on page 1, and the **starting points for allergy consultations** at the beginning of this chapter.

Identification

Follow the **general guide for all consultations** and the **starting points for allergy consultations**.

Reason for Referral

The referral may seek to confirm angioedema and/or clarify appropriate management.

History of Present Illness

Determine key characteristics: Distinguish angioedema from other forms of edema.
> The swelling in angioedema is asymmetric and nonpitting.
> It is not gravitationally dependent.
> It has diffuse margins with normal colour or slight erythema of skin.
> It typically involves the upper respiratory and GI tracts.
> The onset is minutes to hours, with resolution in hours to days.

Clarify the disease course:
> Check whether the patient has had previous, similar episodes. If so, for how long and how often?
> Check whether any episodes have been life-threatening.

Assess the severity: Inquire about features of anaphylaxis, such as urticaria, pruritus, dyspnea, wheezing, nausea, vomiting, diarrhea, presyncope, and syncope.

Distinguish between histamine-mediated and bradykinin-mediated angioedema:
> **Histamine-mediated angioedema:** The onset is within minutes; it lasts less than 24 hours, has associated urticaria and flushing, and responds to antihistamines and corticosteroids.
> **Bradykinin-mediated angioedema:** It does not present with urticaria or pruritus, lasts more than 48 hours, and may present with pain or burning; it may also present with severe abdominal pain due to bowel wall angioedema.

Clarify triggers: Ask about:
> medications
> exposures (e.g., cold, dental work)
> allergens (e.g., insect stings, foods)
> menstruation
> stress or anxiety

Clarify impacts: Ask the patient how the reaction affects their quality of life.

llllllllllllllllllllllllllllllllllllllllllllllllllllllllllllllllllllllllllllllllllllllllllllllllllll
RED FLAGS IN ANGIOEDEMA

- Angioedema affecting the larynx, upper airway, and tongue can result in airway obstruction and asphyxiation.
- Acquired angioedema can be associated with B-cell lymphoproliferative disorders; check for symptoms such as fever, night sweats, and weight loss.

Past Medical History
- Check for allergies and a history of anaphylaxis.
- A history of autoimmune conditions or lymphoproliferative disorders raises suspicion for acquired angioedema.
- Check for infections (e.g., *Helicobacter pylori*, dental granulomata).

Medications
Perform a careful review of the patient's medications—including new or recently discontinued medications, and dose changes—with particular attention to:
- ACEIs
- neprilysin inhibitors
- NSAIDs
- estrogens

Allergies
Follow the **general guide for all consultations** and the **starting points for allergy consultations**.

Family History
Check for episodic swelling or recurrent abdominal pain: this raises suspicion for an underlying hereditary angioedema disorder (however, about 25% of cases occur de novo).

Physical Examination
- If present, note the distribution of the angioedema.
- Check for signs of histamine angioedema, such as urticaria, flushing, and hypotension.
- Assess for erythema marginatum (seen with nonhistaminergic angioedema).

Investigations

Choose investigations based on the differential diagnosis.

BRADYKININ-MEDIATED ANGIOEDEMA (NO URTICARIA)

This includes idiopathic, hereditary, acquired, and ACEI-mediated angioedema.

CBC, basic chemistry with liver function, CRP, ESR

C4 level: Use this as a screen.[6]

› If low, order C1 inhibitor antigen, function of C1 inhibitor, and C1q.

› Further genetic testing may be indicated if levels are normal (e.g., gain of function mutation to factor XII).

Serum protein electrophoresis: Gammopathy may indicate acquired angioedema.

US or CT scan: This can visualize suspected intestinal angioedema.

Workup for infection, malignancy, or autoimmune disease: Pursue these based on clinical history and physical examination.

Genetic screening: Offer this in cases of hereditary angioedema.

HISTAMINE-MEDIATED ANGIOEDEMA

Angioedema With Prominent Urticaria

See Urticaria in this chapter.

Angioedema With Anaphylaxis

Serum total tryptase: This may help confirm the episode as mast cell mediated.

Angioedema Due to Allergen

Skin-prick testing: Consider this for the presumed trigger and specific IgE levels.

Impression and Plan

GENERAL APPROACH

• Classify the angioedema (histaminergic versus bradykinin) based on history, physical examination, and investigations.

• All attacks of the upper airways are emergencies and should be treated immediately.

• If a trigger can be identified, avoiding or treating the causative condition is effective.

HEREDITARY AND ACQUIRED ANGIOEDEMA[7,8]

Acute Treatment

• Therapies include:
  › plasma-derived or recombinant C1 inhibitor (Berinert)
  › bradykinin B2 receptor antagonist (icatibant)

› kallikrein inhibitor (ecallantide: not available in Canada)
- Note that frozen plasma can be used if other therapies are not available.

Short-Term Prophylaxis
This can be considered prior to triggering exposures, and before medical or dental procedures, and includes:
- plasma-derived C1 inhibitor
- attenuated androgens (e.g., danazol) and antifibrinolytics (e.g., tranexamic acid) (less evidence supports these treatments)

Long-Term Prophylaxis
- First-line agents include scheduled plasma-derived C1 inhibitor and anti-plasma kallikrein antibody (lanadelumab).
- Other agents include attenuated androgens and antifibrinolytics (less evidence supports these treatments).

In All Cases
Advise the patient to wear a medical alert bracelet.

ACEI-INDUCED ANGIOEDEMA
- Discontinue the ACEI and monitor the patient.
- Acute treatment is the same as for hereditary and acquired angioedema.

ANGIOEDEMA WITH ANAPHYLAXIS
- Treat with IM epinephrine, IV fluids, oxygen, and protect the airway.
- Prescribe an epinephrine autoinjector and provide patients with an emergency plan.

ANGIOEDEMA WITH URTICARIA
- *See also* Urticaria in this chapter.
- Treat with antihistamines and corticosteroids.

IDIOPATHIC HISTAMINERGIC ANGIOEDEMA[9]
- Consider a trial of nonsedating antihistamines.
- Consider off-label use of other agents in acute or refractory cases.

IgE-Mediated Penicillin Allergy
These notes are in addition to the **general guide for all consultations** on page 1, and the **starting points for allergy consultations** at the beginning of this chapter.

Identification
Follow the **general guide for all consultations** and the **starting points for allergy consultations**.

Reason for Referral

The referral may seek to confirm penicillin allergy and/or clarify appropriate management.

History of Present Illness

Review reaction specifics:
> › What was the reaction?
> › How long ago was the reaction?

Review medication specifics:
> › What was the route and dose of the triggering medication?
> › How many doses did the patient receive prior to the reaction?
> › What was the indication for the medication?

Assess for IgE-mediated symptoms:
> › **Dermatological:** urticaria, angioedema, flushing
>> » *Pearl:* Hives move throughout the skin, and a single hive should not be present for more than 24 hours.
> › **GI:** crampy abdominal pain, diarrhea, emesis
> › **Cardiovascular:** presyncope, syncope, BP < 90 mmHg
> › **Respiratory:** shortness of breath, throat tightness, wheeze
> › **Ear, nose, throat:** rhinorrhea, congestion, sneezing, hoarseness, drooling

Identify red flags for severe cutaneous adverse reaction (SCAR) and severe non-IgE-mediated reaction: See sidebar.

Clarify the timeline:
> › Over what period of time did the reaction develop? (IgE-mediated reactions occur less than 1 hour after exposure.)
> › How long did the reaction last?
> › Were any other medications taken around the time of exposure? Were they newly started?
> › Was there a delayed rash?
>> » "Delayed benign drug rash" is a common, nonallergic rash. It is typically a diffuse maculopapular rash.

Clarify management taken: When the reaction occurred, how was it managed?

Review lab results: If lab results are available, assess for evidence of the following:
> › hemolytic anemia (found in type 2 hypersensitivity)
> › eosinophilia (associated with type 4 hypersensitivity)
> › hepatic or renal dysfunction (associated with type 4 hypersensitivity)

Ask about reexposure:
> › Was the patient exposed to the medication again following the reaction? If so, what happened?
> › Has the patient taken any other penicillins since the reaction?

Determine tolerance for other drugs: Has the patient tolerated cephalosporins? Carbapenems?

||||||||||||||||||||||||||||||||||||||||||||||||||||||||||||||||||||||||||||||||||||||||||||||||||||||||||||||||||||||||||||||||

RED FLAGS: SEVERE CUTANEOUS ADVERSE REACTION (SCAR) AND SEVERE NON-IgE-MEDIATED REACTION

Blistering, skin peeling (desquamation)

Fevers

Mucosal involvement

Conjunctival injection

Pustules

New onset arthralgias

Erythema multiforme (target-shaped lesions)

End organ damage, such as transaminitis, acute kidney injury, or lung involvement

---

Past Medical History

- Underlying atopic conditions (e.g., allergic rhinitis, asthma) are not risk factors for developing penicillin allergy; however, they may aggravate IgE-mediated drug allergies and they increase the risk of fatal anaphylactic reaction.
- Previous allergic reactions to medications increase the likelihood of developing other reactions, and raise the possibility of multiple drug allergy syndrome (a condition characterized by allergies to multiple, chemically distinct medications, often antibiotics).
- EBV infection, HIV, and hematologic malignancies may alter immune function and predispose patients to allergic reactions.[1]

Medications

Ask about:
- **Medications that interfere with testing:** Antihistamines, antidepressants, antipsychotics, and glucocorticoids can cause false negatives.
- **Beta-blockers:**
  › These reduce the effectiveness of epinephrine in treating anaphylaxis, which is particularly important if a drug challenge will be pursued.
  › Note the indication for beta-blockers (e.g., hypertension versus arrhythmia).

Allergies

- Determine reactions to medications: what medications, the type of reactions, how long ago, and if the patient has ever rechallenged the medications or had skin tests for them.
- Clarify how many medications and antibiotics have caused reactions (relevant to multiple drug hypersensitivity syndrome).

Family History
Family history of penicillin allergy does not confer a higher individual risk of penicillin allergy.[10]

Physical Examination
- This is generally of limited value if the reaction took place in the past.
- Examine cutaneous lesions, if present:
  › What is their distribution? (Do they affect the folds?)
  › Are they diffuse or localized?
  › Are there hives (raised, pruritic lesions)?
  › If a blistering reaction, is Nikolsky sign present? (This is the separation of blisters from underlying skin, which is a red flag for a non-IgE reaction.)
- Check for lymphadenopathy and splenomegaly (seen in non-IgE reactions).

Investigations
Previous lab results: Review these from around the time of the reaction for evidence of cytopenias, renal dysfunction, and liver enzyme derangements (associated with type IV hypersensitivity).

Skin test:
  › Pursue this if the history suggests an IgE-mediated reaction.
  › Skin tests are generally intradermal, given the higher sensitivity of this method compared to skin prick.

Serum tryptase:
  › In suspected anaphylaxis, an elevated serum tryptase level helps confirm the diagnosis.
  › Obtaining a tryptase level after anaphylaxis has resolved is also important to exclude mastocytosis, which is a risk factor for severe anaphylaxis.

Impression and Plan
GENERAL APPROACH
- Note that this segment presents a general guide for management: it should not replace clinical judgement.
- In severe cutaneous reactions, or severe IgE-mediated reactions, obtain guidance from an allergist.
- Begin by considering the findings from the history and investigations: classify the reaction as 1) an IgE-mediated reaction, 2) a nonallergic reaction, 3) a mild reaction without features of an IgE-mediated reaction, or 4) a serious delayed reaction (type 2, 3, or 4).

IgE-MEDIATED REACTION

This plan covers patients whose history suggests an IgE-mediated reaction; **or** patients with no obvious mucous membrane involvement, skin desquamation, or organ involvement (i.e., patients not experiencing type 2, 3 or 4 reactions), but whose reactions otherwise lack detail.

- It is safe to give these patients cefazolin, aztreonam, and third-, fourth-, and fifth-generation cephalosporins.
- If a penicillin, or a first- or second-generation cephalosporin, is strongly indicated or superior to alternatives, pursue skin-prick testing.
- If the patient reports isolated mild hives, without other symptoms of an IgE-mediated reaction (particularly if the reaction took place 10 years ago or in childhood), the patient has minimal risk of a recurrent serious reaction. Consider pursuing a direct oral challenge in consultation with an allergist.
  › Direct oral challenge of medications in low-risk patients is an active area of research. Only health-care providers with a strong understanding of drug allergy and the ability to deal with possible reactions should conduct them.
- If no other options are available, consider temporary drug desensitization, again in consultation with an allergist. This is a temporary procedure that can induce short-term tolerance.
- If an allergy has been confirmed, educate the patient about avoiding the offending medication: provide them with a list of generic names and brand names of the medication and of possible cross-reactive medications.
- Patients with severe reactions (e.g., anaphylaxis) should wear a medical alert bracelet.

NONALLERGIC REACTION

This plan covers patients who may experience an adverse effect, such as nonspecific GI symptoms or yeast vaginitis. Some patients may simply have a positive family history but no exposure to penicillins.

- Do not avoid penicillins and related antibiotics.
- Remove the allergy label from the patient's record.

MILD REACTION WITHOUT FEATURES OF AN IgE-MEDIATED REACTION

This plan covers patients who may have had a maculopapular eruption, or who have no recollection of the reaction, and who test negative for an IgE-mediated reaction.

These patients can take:
- third-, fourth-, or fifth-generation cephalosporins, carbapenem, aztreonam, or unrelated non-beta-lactams
—or—
- penicillin, or first- or second-generation cephalosporins, after an initial test dose given with a standardized procedure

SERIOUS DELAYED REACTION (TYPE 2, 3, OR 4)
This plan covers patients with SJS, TEN, DRESS, acute interstitial nephritis, hemolytic anemia, drug-induced cytopenias, and serum sickness.
- Avoid penicillins, cephalosporins, and carbapenems.
- Consider a cautious trial of aztreonam (monobactam).

Urticaria

These notes are in addition to the **general guide for all consultations** on page 1, and the **starting points for allergy consultations** at the beginning of this chapter.

Identification

Follow the **general guide for all consultations** and the **starting points for allergy consultations**.

Reason for Referral

The referral may seek to confirm urticaria and/or clarify appropriate management.

History of Present Illness

Confirm that the lesions are urticaria:
- › It can be helpful to show images of urticaria compared with other rashes to your patient.
- › Key characteristics of urticaria include:
  - » raised erythematous wheals with associated flare
  - » pruritus (often)
  - » associated angioedema

Distinguish acute versus chronic urticaria:
- › **Symptoms last less than 6 weeks:** acute urticaria
- › **Symptoms last more than 6 weeks:** chronic urticaria

Identify red flags: See sidebar.

Identify triggers: In about 50% of patients with acute urticaria, a
cause cannot be identified (idiopathic urticaria). Possible triggers
include:
> physical stimuli, including scratching (dermatographism), cold, heat,
  sunlight, pressure, delayed pressure (relevant to physical urticaria)[6]
> viral illness (very common trigger)
> parasitic infections (more common in developing countries)
> medications
> foods, including milk, eggs, peanuts, tree nuts, fish, shellfish
  (typical allergens; onset of symptoms is usually within 1 hour of
  consumption)

Clarify management taken: Determine therapies the patient has tried
and their effectiveness.

Clarify sources of exposure:
> Has the patient started any new medications?
> Do they have any infectious symptoms?
> Have they been exposed to latex, contact allergens, or insect bites?
  (Ask about these exposures specifically.)
> Screen for parasitic infection: ask about abdominal pain, GI
  symptoms, and travel history (travel history may not signify).[11]

Clarify impacts: How does the urticaria affect the patient's quality of
life?

||||||||||||||||||||||||||||||||||||||||||||||||||||||||||||||||||||||||||||||||||||||||||||||||||||||||||||||||||||||||||||||||||
RED FLAGS IN URTICARIA

Painful lesions, bruising, lesions
that last more than 48 hours
(these suggest urticarial
vasculitis)

Fevers, night sweats, weight loss
(lymphoproliferative disorders, malignancy)

Sicca symptoms, uveitis, lymphadenopathy, arthralgias,
other skin lesions, fevers
(autoimmune disorders)

Past Medical History
Assess for autoimmune conditions such as hypothyroidism, RA, vitiligo,
and SLE.

Medications
- NSAIDs are a common cause of chronic urticaria.
- Opiates and narcotics can cause urticaria due to direct mast cell
  activation.

Allergies

Follow the **general guide for all consultations** and the **starting points for allergy consultations.**

Family History

Check for a history of hives, recurrent fevers, and neurosensory loss. This raises suspicion for autoinflammatory syndromes (e.g., familial cold autoinflammatory syndrome).

Physical Examination

- If lesions are present, note their distribution, shape, and size.
- Check for bruises and/or discolouration.
- Check for lymphadenopathy and hepatosplenomegaly.

Investigations

Choose investigations based on the differential diagnosis.

CHRONIC SPONTANEOUS URTICARIA

This is generally diagnosed by history and physical examination. Pursue investigations if there is concern for a secondary cause.

General screening for secondary causes includes:
› CBC, CRP
› antithyroid antibodies (found in 45% of patients), optional

Based on history and exam, screen for the following:
› autoimmune disease (e.g., systemic lupus erythematosus, rheumatoid arthritis)
› chronic infections (parasitic infections are generally believed to be significant; consider also screening for viral hepatitis, HSV, *Helicobacter pylori*)
› stool ova and parasites if the patient has GI symptoms or exposures

If atypical features are present on history, consider the following:
› for urticarial vasculitis (painful lesions, residual hyperpigmentation): skin biopsy, complement levels (these are low in urticarial vasculitis)
› for Schnitzler syndrome, chronic urticaria with gammopathy (fevers, arthralgia, organomegaly, night sweats, weight loss): serum protein electrophoresis

ALLERGIC URTICARIA

Pursue skin-prick testing to presumed trigger and specific IgE levels.

PHYSICAL URTICARIA

Pursue challenge testing (e.g., ice cube test for cold urticaria; scratching the skin for dermatographism; hot bath testing for cholinergic urticaria; weight pressure for delayed-pressure urticaria).

Impression and Plan

THE IMPORTANCE OF RULING OUT OTHER SYSTEMIC DISEASE

Remember that urticaria can be a sign of many different diseases: before diagnosing chronic urticaria, make sure you have ruled out other systemic disease such as autoimmune disease and malignancy.

MANAGEMENT OF CONFIRMED URTICARIA

- Classify the urticaria based on history, physical examination, and investigations.
- If a trigger can be identified, avoidance is effective.
- In chronic spontaneous urticaria, patients should avoid NSAIDs, alcohol, and opiates. Dietary changes are not helpful.
- Initial therapy generally includes regular new generation H1-receptor antihistamines. Depending on response to therapy, patients may take up to 4 times the standard dose.
- Advise patients to avoid Benadryl (diphenhydramine) because of its anticholinergic effects and association with impaired cognitive performance.[12]
- For refractory cases, consider oral corticosteroids, and immunosuppressive or immunomodulatory agents (e.g., omalizumab, cyclosporine).
- More than two-thirds of new-onset urticaria is self-limiting.[13]

IMMUNOLOGY

Suspected Immunodeficiency

These notes are in addition to the **general guide for all consultations** on page 1.

Identification

Follow the **general guide for all consultations** and the **starting points for allergy consultations**.

Reason for Referral

- The referral may seek to confirm suspected immunodeficiency and clarify management.

- Other common concerns include:
  › recurrent infections (e.g., sinus, ear, and lung infections; abscesses)
  › opportunistic infections
  › abnormal lab results (e.g., hypogammaglobulinemia, possible lymphopenia)
  › suspicious family history
  › genetic testing results

History of Present Illness

GENERAL HEALTH AND DEVELOPMENT
Did the patient have any concerns during their neonatal period or early childhood?

INFECTIONS
- How old was the patient when they first developed infections?
- What sort of infections has the patient had?
- How frequent?
- How severe? Did they need IV antibiotics, hospitalization, or ICU?
- How did they respond to treatment? Is there a history of multiple or prolonged courses of antimicrobials?

IMMUNIZATIONS
- Could the infections have been prevented with vaccines? Has the patient had infections after live vaccines?
- What is the patient's immunization history? (Note that you can check this online in some jurisdictions.)

CAUSES
The range of presentations is broad and variable. This section presents some typical clinical presentations.

T-Cell and Combined Immunodeficiencies
Combined refers to abnormalities in both T cells and antibody production.
- These are less common in adults.
- They are associated with chronic diarrhea and failure to thrive.
- Patients have lymphopenia and neutropenia.
- Patients have recurrent opportunistic infections (e.g., thrush, *Pneumocystis jiroveci* pneumonia, CMV).

B-Cell or Humoral Immunodeficiencies
- These are the most common forms of immunodeficiency, and are often diagnosed in adulthood.
- Patients have reduced or absent immunoglobulin levels, or normal-to-increased immunoglobulin levels with abnormal function.

- They have recurrent bacterial infections (*Streptococcus pneumoniae, Haemophilus influenzae*), usually present as sinopulmonary infections.
- They may have chronic giardia.
- The immunodeficiency may be comorbid with autoimmune or granulomatous disease, GI disease, and/or bronchiectasis.

Innate Immunodeficiencies
- These are typically present early in life, but may occur later in life.
- Patients have pneumonias, abscesses, and skin infections.
- Chronic granulomatous disease (a defect in the neutrophil and macrophage oxidative burst), in particular, is associated with catalase-positive bacterial infections and fungal infections (e.g., *Aspergillus* infection); it is X-linked and autosomal recessive.

Complement Disorders
- This is the most rare form of immunodeficiency.
- It may have a similar presentation to B-cell or humoral immunodeficiencies.
- It involves defects in the early complement cascade, which lead to bacterial infections and autoimmunity.
- Terminal complement deficiency leads to *Neisseria* infections.

Disorders of Immune Dysregulation
- Patients present with fever and organ-specific inflammation as opposed to infections (e.g., hemophagocytic lymphohistiocytosis, autoimmune lymphoproliferative syndrome).
- Cytopenias, elevated platelets, and inflammatory markers may correlate with episodes.
- These disorders have early onset, and are associated with very early onset inflammatory bowel disease.

REVIEW OF SYSTEMS
Conduct a thorough head-to-toe review of systems.

Past Medical History
Check for:
- evidence of immune dysregulation, such as atopy and autoimmunity
- hematologic malignancies and other malignancies
- secondary immunodeficiency risk factors (e.g., type 2 diabetes, HIV infection, liver disease, kidney disease, poor nutrition, history of chemotherapy)

Medications
- Obtain a detailed history of antibiotic courses the patient has had. Focus on how often these have happened and whether the patient needed IV antibiotics.

- Ask about chemotherapy, and immunosuppressive or immunomodulatory medications (e.g., rituximab).
- Ask about anticonvulsants: these can cause hypogammaglobulinemia.

Allergies
Ask about allergies to penicillin, azithromycin, and trimethoprim: these medications may be required for infection prophylaxis.

Family History
- Draw a genetic family tree, showing at least 2 generations. Ask about consanguinity.
- Focus on genetic patterns (e.g., X-linked diseases, affecting only males).
- Check for a history of immunodeficiency, autoimmunity, recurrent infections, deaths from infection, and lymphoproliferative disease.
- Check for early neonatal or childhood deaths.

Social History
Ask about smoking status, alcohol use, occupation, and relevant exposures.

Physical Examination
General impression:
- Note any dysmorphic features.
- Check growth parameters in children.

Head, ears, nose, throat:
  › Check the ears and nose for signs of infection.
  › Check for the presence of tonsils, lymphadenopathy.
  › Examine the mouth for thrush.

Dermatological:
  › Check for ectodermal dysplasia and eczema.
  › Note any cutaneous lesions suggestive of infection (e.g., tinea pedis, warts).

GI: Check for splenomegaly.

Cardiorespiratory: Check for crackles and wheezes.

Investigations
STARTING POINTS
Rule out secondary immunodeficiency, if suspected: Screen for type 2 diabetes, HIV, cystic fibrosis, nephrotic syndrome, protein-losing enteropathy, and cirrhosis.

Start with CBC, differential, peripheral blood smear:
  › Neutropenia may indicate congenital neutropenia, cyclic neutropenia, or aplastic anemia.
  › Lymphopenia may indicate T-cell disease.

› Leukocytosis between infections may indicate leukocyte adhesion deficiency.
› Thrombocytopenia in male infants may indicate Wiskott-Aldrich syndrome.
› Anemia may indicate anemia of chronic disease or autoimmune hemolytic anemia.
› Howell-Jolly bodies (residual nuclear fragments in RBC) may indicate splenic impairment.
› Giant granules may indicate Chediak-Higashi syndrome.

FURTHER INVESTIGATIONS

• Make decisions about further investigations based on history and clinical suspicion.
• Genetic testing, and tests for specific protein presence or function, may be required.

T-Cell and Combined Immunodeficiencies

Lymphopenia is generally the first indicator.

Lymphocyte proliferation assays and flow cytometry: Consider these for further evaluation of cell count and function.

B-Cell or Humoral Immunodeficiencies

Serum immunoglobulin levels (IgG, IgA, IgM, IgE):
› IgG < 2 g/L suggests significant antibody deficiency, but may occur in protein-losing enteropathies or nephrotic syndrome.

Specific antibody titres:
› Absent response to vaccines suggests humoral deficiency.
› IgG titres to specific antigens can be assessed in immunized patients by measuring antibody titres before and after administration of vaccine antigens (commonly tetanus and diphtheria).
› A 2-fold or more increase at 2 to 3 weeks suggests antibody deficiency regardless of immunoglobulin levels.
› Consider measuring natural antibodies (e.g., antistreptolysin O, heterophile antibodies).

Flow cytometry: Pursue this for B-cell enumeration.

Innate Immunodeficiencies

Neutrophil function assays: Examples include dihydrorhodamine 123 response and stimulation assays for cytokine response.

Complement Disorders

C2, C3, C4 levels

Functional complement activity assays (CH50, AH50)

Impression and Plan

GENERAL APPROACH

- Formulate a differential diagnosis based on the history and available investigations, considering both primary and secondary causes.
- An important part of your assessment is determining whether the patient truly has an immunodeficiency, and, if so, identifying potential causes of secondary immunodeficiency.
- Management depends on the type of immunodeficiency.[14]
- For vaccine strategies, in all cases, refer to the Canadian Immunization Guide from the Public Health Agency of Canada.[15]

COMBINED IMMUNODEFICIENCY

- Treat infections, and provide antimicrobial prophylaxis and immunoglobulin replacement (IV or subcutaneous).
- Patients should avoid live attenuated vaccines.
- Pursue hematopoietic stem cell transplant in severe combined immunodeficiency (SCID).
  › Pursue gene therapy in X-linked SCID.

B-CELL IMMUNODEFICIENCIES

- Provide immunoglobulin replacement (IV or subcutaneous).
- Provide prophylactic antibiotics (covering *Streptococcus pneumoniae* and *Haemophilus influenzae*).
- Monitor for complications based on disease (e.g., hearing, pulmonary function, malignancy, autoimmune disease).

INNATE IMMUNODEFICIENCIES

- For phagocyte disorders, provide antibiotic and antifungal prophylaxis.
- Chronic granulomatous disease, consider BMT.
- Provide antimicrobial prophylaxis.

References

1. Joint Task Force on Practice Parameters; American Academy of Allergy, Asthma and Immunology; American College of Allergy, Asthma and Immunology; Joint Council of Allergy, Asthma and Immunology. Drug allergy: an updated practice parameter. Ann Allergy Asthma Immunol. 2010;105(4):259-73. doi: 10.1016/j.anai.2010.08.002
2. Arnold D, Curtis B, Bakchoul T. Recommendations for standardization of laboratory testing for drug-induced immune thrombocytopenia: Communication from the SSC of the ISTH. J Thromb Haemost. 2015;13(4):676-8. doi: 10.1111/jth.12852
3. Heit W, Heimpel H, Fischer A, et al. Drug-induced agranulocytosis: evidence for the commitment of bone marrow haematopoeisis. Scand J Haematol. 1985;35(5):459-68. doi: 10.1111/j.1600-0609.1985.tb02813.x

4. Arévalo J, Lorente J, González-Herrada C, et al. Treatment of toxic epidermal necrolysis with cyclosporin A. J Trauma. 2000;48(3):473. doi: 10.1097/00005373.200003000-00017

5. Lee H. Drug reaction with eosinophilia and systemic symptoms (DRESS). Mockenhaupt M, ed. UpToDate [Internet]. 2020 [cited 2020 May 17]. Available from: https://www.uptodate.com/contents/drug-reaction-with-eosinophilia-and-systemic-symptoms-dress?search=dress&source=search_result&selectedTitle=1~150&usage_type=default&display_rank=1#H27761127

6. Kanani A, Betschel S, Warrington R. Urticaria and angioedema. Allergy Asthma Clin Immunol. 2018;14(59):115-27. doi: 10.1186/s13223-018-0288-z

7. Betschel S, Badiou J, Binkley K, et al. The international/Canadian hereditary angioedema guideline. Allergy Asthma Clin Immunol. 2019 Nov 25;15:72. doi: 10.1186/s13223-019-0376-8

8. Busse P, Christiansen S. Hereditary angioedema. N Engl J Med. 2020;382(12):1136-48. doi: 10.1056/NEJMra1808012

9. van den Elzen M, Go M, Knulst A, et al. Efficacy of treatment of non-hereditary angioedema. Clin Rev Allergy Immunol. 2018;54(3):412-31. doi: 10.1007/s12016-016-8585-0

10. Kern R, Wimberley N Jr. Penicillin reactions: their nature, growing importance, recognition, management and prevention. Am J Med Sci. 1953;226(4);357-75. doi: 10.1097/00000441-195310000-00001

11. Arik Yilmaz E, Karaatmaca B, Sackesen C, et al. Parasitic infections in children with chronic spontaneous urticaria. Int Arch Allergy Immunol. 2016;171(2):130-5. doi: 10.1159/000450953

12. Gray S, Anderson M, Dublin S, et al. Cumulative use of strong anticholinergics and incident dementia: a prospective cohort study. JAMA Inter Med. 2015:175(3);401-7. doi: 10.1001/jamainternmed.2014.7663

13. Sackesen C, Sekerel B, Orhan F, et al. The etiology of different forms of urticaria in childhood. Pediatric Dermatology. 2004;21(2):102-8. doi: 10.1111/j.0736-8046.2004.21202.x

14. McCusker C, Upton J, Warrington R. Primary immunodeficiency. Allergy Asthma Clin Immunol. 2018;14(Suppl 2):61. doi: 10.1186/s13223-018-0290-5

15. Public Health Agency of Canada. Immunization of immunocompromised persons: Canadian Immunization Guide [Internet]. Ottawa: Public Health Agency of Canada [updated 2020-12-24; cited 2021 July 28]. Available from: https://www.canada.ca/en/public-health/services/publications/healthy-living/canadian-immunization-guide-part-3-vaccination-specific-populations/page-8-immunization-immunocompromised-persons.html

3

Cardiology

Dr. Eric Wong
Dr. Jaihoon Amon
Dr. Shekoofeh Saboktakin Rizi
Dr. Ren Jie Robert Yao
Dr. Abdulaziz Alshaibi
Dr. Soohyun Alice Chang

REVIEWER
Dr. Christopher B. Fordyce

Starting Points: Cardiology Consultations

These notes are in addition to the **general guide for all consultations** on page 1.

Identification

Key information in the identification statement includes age, sex, and pertinent cardiac risk factors.

Reason for Referral

The referral may seek to confirm a cardiac disorder (e.g., AF, MI) or to clarify appropriate management.

History of Present Illness

SYMPTOMS

Focus on the presenting symptom. In addition, always ask about:

- **Pain:**
  › Characterize the pain (e.g., duration, severity, radiation, ameliorating factors).
  › If angina, characterize the angina (e.g., whether it occurs at rest, whether exertion triggers it).

› Ask about atypical features (e.g., neck pain; left facial pain; "heartburn"; features relevant to peripheral vascular disease such as claudication symptoms).

- **Arrhythmia:** Ask about palpitations or fluttering sensations; the time course and frequency of these symptoms; and associated neurological symptoms.
- **Syncopal symptoms:** Has the patient had blackouts, fainting, dizziness, or falls?
- **HF symptoms:** Ask about dyspnea at rest and with exertion; weight gain; peripheral edema; orthopnea; paroxysmal nocturnal dyspnea; and oliguria.

RISK FACTORS

Risk factors are either **modifiable** (e.g., smoking, hypertension, diabetes, dyslipidemia, CKD, sedentary lifestyle) or **nonmodifiable** (e.g., family history, pregnancy, menopause).

- **For diabetes:** Check the patient's most recent HbA_{1c}.
- **For dyslipidemia:** Check LDL and cholesterol levels.
- **For chronic kidney disease:** Check the baseline creatinine level.

Past Medical History

Start with the patient's cardiac history: Ask about:
› CAD, including the most recent cardiac catheterization results
› ACS, including onset and type (e.g., STEMI, NSTEMI, unstable angina)
› PCI (stents and type)
› CABG, including the reason for CABG, number of grafts, and follow-up medical management
› presence of devices (permanent pacemaker, ICD, cardiac resynchronization therapy) and specifics of type
› percutaneous or surgical valve repair or replacement (mechanical or bioprosthetic)
› previous ablation procedures
› vascular surgery
› transplant surgery (heart, other organs)

Ask about hematological disorders: These include bleeding disorders and thrombotic disease.

Ask about inflammatory conditions: These include gout, recent malignancy, SLE, RA, rheumatic fever, and radiation to the chest.

Past Surgical History

Ask about other surgeries.

Medications

Ask about:
- **Cardiac medications:**
  - › These include antiplatelets, ACEIs, beta-blockers, CCBs, ARBs, antiarrhythmic medications, anticoagulants, antihypertensives, and statins.
  - › For each, clarify the dose, route, and when last taken.
- **Diabetes medications:** These include sodium-glucose cotransporter-2 (SGLT2) inhibitors, glucagon-like peptide 1 receptor (GLP-1) agonists, and other agents.
- **Other medications:** Ask about biotin (high levels of biotin interact with troponin assays).

Allergies

In addition to standard questions, ask specifically about allergies to, or intolerances for, cardiac medications, including:
- antiplatelets or anticoagulants (bleeding)
- statins (myalgias, myositis)
- ACEIs (angioedema)

Family History

Check for:
- CAD in first-degree relatives (in males younger than 55; in females younger than 65)
- sudden cardiac death (ask about drownings and single-operator vehicle accidents)
- infiltrative diseases (amyloidosis)
- lipid disorders, such as familial hypercholesterolemia

Social History

Ask about:
- smoking, alcohol use, drug use (e.g., cocaine)
- occupation (i.e., the level of physical activity it involves)
- ethnicity
- diet (i.e., healthy, nonhealthy)
- physical activity

Physical Examination

General appearance: Does the patient look unwell or acutely ill?
Vital signs:
  › Check temperature, HR, BP in both arms, and respiratory rate.

› Note tachycardia, bradycardia, wide/narrow pulse pressure, difference in bilateral BP, and orthostatic hypotension.

Inspection: Check for:
› signs of hypoperfusion (cold extremities, abnormal level of consciousness)
› respiratory distress
› peripheral edema
› elevated JVP, chest excursions, scars, devices

Palpation:
› Check peripheral pulses and apical impulse.
› Check for heaves and thrills.

Auscultation:
› Assess for heart sounds, murmurs (characterize these).
› Check the lungs for crackles.

Investigations

LABORATORY INVESTIGATIONS

CBC

Creatinine, electrolytes, Mg

Endocrine tests: HbA_{1c}, thyrotropin (TSH)

Lipid panel

Other laboratory investigations: Pursue these as relevant to the clinical context (e.g., troponin in ACS, BNP in heart failure).

OTHER INVESTIGATIONS

ECG:
› Look for baseline ECG findings (e.g., rhythms, LVH, LBBB, RBBB, Q waves).
› Interpret the most recent ECG in a systematic way, for example:
» rate, rhythm, axis, intervals (PR, QT, QRS)
» hypertrophy (LV, LA, RV)
» ischemia (ST changes, new LBBB, T-wave inversions)

Echocardiography: Check the most recent echocardiogram findings (e.g., EF, diastolic dysfunction, significant valvulopathy, ratio of pulmonary hypertension to pulmonary artery systolic pressure [PHT:PASP]).

Coronary angiography: Check the most recent result for percentage of obstruction in coronary arteries and presence of stents.

Impression and Plan

Summarize the patient's risk profile:
› Characterize symptoms: use the Canadian Cardiovascular Society (CCS) class for angina,[1] and the New York Heart Association (NYHA) functional classes for HF.[2]

› Describe your impression.

Describe the patient's disposition and how to respond:
› How sick is the patient?
› Is the patient hemodynamically stable?
› Do they need vasopressors or inotropic support?
› Do they need cardiac monitoring? (This would be appropriate in the context of VT, long pauses of more than 3 seconds, or high-degree heart block.)

Include risk stratification for ACS patients:
› Characterize the urgency for management using relevant validated tools or calculators (e.g., thrombosis in myocardial infarction [TIMI] risk score[3]; the Global Registry of Acute Coronary Events [GRACE] score[4]).
› Recommend an appropriate risk stratification strategy.

Assess atherosclerotic cardiovascular risk among stable patients: Use a validated clinical tool (e.g., the Framingham risk score[5]) and treat accordingly.
› **Low risk:** primary prevention
  » Examples include smoking cessation; weight loss; increased physical activity; risk-factor modification (hypertension, diabetes, dyslipidemia); statin therapy for statin-indicated conditions such as diabetes.
  » Acetylsalicylic acid (ASA) is not recommended.
› **Moderate risk:** statin therapy according to CCS guidelines
› **High risk:** secondary prevention
  » Examples include treating dyslipidemia (high-dose statins); controlling hypertension (target BP < 120/80 mmHg) and diabetes (target HbA_{1c} less than 7%); and recommending lifestyle changes (increased physical activity, weight loss, smoking cessation, healthy diet).
  » Pharmacologic therapy may include ASA; ACEI (all patients); beta-blockers for patients with an EF less than 40% or who are 3 years post-ACS; and SGLT2 inhibitors. (*Note:* avoid NSAIDs due to increased risk of adverse cardiovascular events.)

Atrial Fibrillation

These notes are in addition to the **general guide for all consultations** on page 1, and the **starting points for cardiology consultations** at the beginning of this chapter.

Identification

Key information in the identification statement includes the patient's age, and whether the patient has valvular AF (rheumatic mitral stenosis, prosthetic heart valve, or mitral valve repair) or nonvalvular AF.

Reason for Referral

Examples of reason for referral include unstable AF (hypotensive, cardiogenic shock), AF with rapid ventricular response (RVR), and newly diagnosed AF.

History of Present Illness

Clarify why the patient has sought care: For an inpatient, clarify why the patient was admitted to hospital.

Clarify the onset of symptoms: Some patients can tell when their AF began because of symptoms that include palpitations, lightheadedness, exercise intolerance, chest discomfort, and dyspnea.

Look for precipitating factors:
 › HF exacerbation (symptoms include dyspnea, orthopnea, paroxysmal nocturnal dyspnea, peripheral edema, and weight gain)
 › medication noncompliance
 › anemia
 › hypovolemia
 › electrolyte disturbances
 › risk factors for DVT and PE
 › thyroid disease
 › obstructive sleep apnea
 › postoperative acute stress
 › sepsis
 › alcohol intake ("holiday heart syndrome")

Past Medical History

Clarify AF history:
 › Is this a new diagnosis of AF?
 › If not, determine what management strategies have been tried in the past (e.g., rate control versus rhythm control; cardioversion; ablation procedures).
 › Distinguish valvular AF (rheumatic mitral stenosis, prosthetic heart valve, or mitral valve repair) and nonvalvular AF.
 › Check for the date of the patient's last echocardiogram.
 › Determine the patient's CHADS65 score.
 › If anticoagulation therapy is indicated, is the patient taking it? If not, why not?

Clarify other cardiac history:
 › **HF:** Check the date of the patient's last echocardiogram.
 › **CAD:** Check the last angiogram results (e.g., for CCTA results, stents, CABG).

Past Surgical History

Follow the **general guide for all consultations** and the **starting points for cardiology consultations.**

Medications

Check for:

- anticoagulants, in particular warfarin versus direct oral anticoagulants (DOACs)
- rate-control medications (beta-blockers or nondihydropyridine CCBs)
- antiarrhythmics
- other cardiac medications (e.g., antiplatelets, ACEIs and/or ARBs, spironolactone, furosemide, angiotensin receptor-neprilysin inhibitors, SGLT2 inhibitors)
- noncardiac medications

Allergies

Follow the **general guide for all consultations** and the **starting points for cardiology consultations.**

Family History

Check for CAD and arrhythmia.

Social History

Ask about:

- alcohol use, especially recent binge drinking that could lead to AF
- drug use, especially amphetamines and cocaine
- smoking
- occupation
- factors limiting the patient's ability to adhere to, or pay for, medications

Physical Examination

Vital signs: Make sure to document vitals at the time of seeing the patient and, if seeing the patient in the ED, vitals at the time of triage.

Volume status: Check this to assess if the patient is in acute HF (you may find bedside US helpful).

Cardiovascular: Conduct a focused cardiac exam; note that auscultating murmurs may be difficult if the patient is experiencing tachycardia.

Other systems: Conduct a brief physical exam of other systems.

Investigations

LABORATORY INVESTIGATIONS

CBC

Electrolytes, extended electrolytes
Renal function
Liver enzymes and liver function
BNP, troponins (with timeline)
Thyrotropin (TSH)
D-dimer

OTHER INVESTIGATIONS
Cultures
ECG: Use this to:
> distinguish AF from other conditions (e.g., frequent premature atrial contractions, premature ventricular contractions, multifocal atrial tachycardia)
> rule out an ischemic event that precipitated AF

IMAGING
Chest x-ray: This can identify signs of HF or consolidation.
CT pulmonary angiogram: This is to rule out PE.
Echocardiogram: Compare the results with previous echocardiograms, if available.

Impression and Plan

DIFFERENTIAL DIAGNOSIS
AF can present in a number of clinical scenarios. A key element of your plan is to clarify the relevant scenario. This supports your primary diagnosis, which you should present along with 1 or 2 top differentials, and treatment recommendations.

Unstable Atrial Fibrillation
- This presents with hypotension, severe HF, and active ischemia.
- Treatments include synchronized cardioversion; provide anticoagulation therapy for 4 weeks after cardioversion due to myocardial stunning and increased risk of clot formation.

Atrial Fibrillation With Rapid Ventricular Response
- **Without HF:**
  > Treat with beta-blockers or nondihydropyridine CCBs.
  > Provide IV administration (which is quick acting, but has a short half-life) and concomitant oral medication (which is long acting and will act as rate control after the IV medication wears off).
- **With HF:**
  > Treat with furosemide first; if the AF persists, then beta-blockers (in mild HF).

> Avoid beta-blockers in patients with severe HF (pulmonary edema requiring oxygen).
> In severe HF, consider a trial of digoxin (but not in patients with poor renal function).

POORLY CONTROLLED ATRIAL FIBRILLATION

If AF remains poorly controlled despite optimum doses of beta-blockers or CCBs, consider:

- chemical or electric cardioversion
- transesophageal echocardiography to rule out left atrial appendage thrombus prior to cardioversion in cases of: 1) valvular AF, 2) nonvalvular AF presenting within 12 hours, but after a recent stroke or TIA, 3) nonvalvular AF presenting within 12 to 48 hours with a CHADS65 score of 2 or higher, or 4) nonvalvular AF lasting more than 48 hours since onset.

NEW DIAGNOSIS OF ATRIAL FIBRILLATION

In AF that has been diagnosed within the past 12 months, recent evidence suggests that rhythm control is superior to rate control.[6] Consider referring these patients to specialists in cardiology or electrophysiology.

CHRONIC MANAGEMENT OF ATRIAL FIBRILLATION

Rate Control Versus Rhythm Control

- In most patients, rate control has a lower incidence of adverse effects and makes no difference in mortality compared to rhythm control.[6,7] Aim for a target heart rate lower than 100 beats per minute.[8]
- An exception to this rule is when patients experience significant symptoms while in AF. Try a rhythm control strategy to alleviate the patients' symptoms, which can be achieved by a pill-in-pocket approach, maintenance antiarrhythmic medications, or ablation.

Anticoagulation

Recommended treatment includes:

- warfarin in valvular AF
- no oral anticoagulants in nonvalvular AF where the CHADS score equals 0
- direct oral anticoagulants in nonvalvular AF when the CHADS score is greater than 0
- placement of a left atrial appendage closure device in patients who cannot tolerate oral anticoagulants due to bleeding risk

Elevated Troponin

These notes are in addition to the **general guide for all consultations** on page 1, and the **starting points for cardiology consultations** at the beginning of this chapter.

Identification

- Key information in the identification statement includes pertinent cardiac history (CAD, HF, AF).
- If the patient has no known CAD, it should describe risk factors for CAD (e.g., hypertension, dyslipidemia, diabetes, smoking, family history) and the presenting complaint.
- Note that the presenting complaint may not be cardiac related (e.g., in the context of sepsis, infection, or a postoperative patient).

Reason for Referral

Examples of reason for referral include ACS, elevated troponin, chest pain, unstable angina, and suspected MI.

History of Present Illness

Identify the main reason the patient is seeking care: clarify the quality and severity of the patient's presentation.

Assess cardiac symptoms:
> For stable CAD, characterize the chest pain based on the 3 usual indicators: retrosternal pain, pain induced by stress or exercise, and pain relieved with rest or nitroglycerin.
>> Typical angina presents with 3 indicators; atypical chest pain presents with 2 indicators; and noncardiac chest pain presents with 1 indicator.
> Assess for:
>> palpitations
>> symptoms of presyncope or syncope
>> peripheral edema
>> shortness of breath

Determine the patient's baseline functional status and exercise capacity: Base this on CCS class and NYHA class.

Identify CAD risk factors, if no known CAD: These include hypertension, smoking, dyslipidemia, diabetes, and family history of cardiac disease.

Work through noncardiac causes of elevated troponin: These include:
> risk factors for PE
> history of renal or liver failure
> stroke symptoms

› use of cocaine, methamphetamines, other drugs
› infectious symptoms

Identify interventions the patient has already received: Examples include IVF, nitroglycerin, and diuretics.

Past Medical History

Determine:

- cardiac-related history (CAD, HF, valvulopathy)
- pertinent investigations (echocardiograms, ECGs, Holter monitors, stress tests, myocardial perfusion imaging [MIBI], cardiac MRIs, CCTAs, coronary angiograms)
- primary cardiologist

Medications

Check for:

- ACEIs, ARBs, beta-blockers, mineralocorticoid receptor antagonists, Entresto, ivabradine, diuretics (indicated for HF)
- dual antiplatelet therapy (DAPT), statins (indicated for CAD)
- DOACs, warfarin (indicated for anticoagulation; specify INR target based on particular indication)
- other medications

Allergies

Follow the **general guide for all consultations** and the **starting points for cardiology consultations.**

Physical Examination

Vital signs:

› Determine vitals on presentation and when you assess the patient.
› Take BP on both arms.

Cardiovascular:

› Conduct a general inspection for devices, scars.
› Assess JVP: height, waveform, accelerated junctional rhythm response.
› Assess for normal heart sounds: S1/S2.
› Assess for extra heart sounds: S3/S4.
› Check for murmurs: assess location, grade, timing, radiation, and change with manoeuvres.
› Conduct a peripheral exam: look for edema, and cold versus warm extremities.

Respiratory: Look for evidence of pulmonary edema (crackles).

Abdominal: Look for evidence of ascites and hepatomegaly.

Investigations

LABORATORY INVESTIGATIONS

CBC

Electrolytes, extended electrolytes

Renal function

Liver enzymes and liver function

BNP, troponins: Include timeline.

OTHER INVESTIGATIONS

Cultures

ECG: Compare with previous ECGs, if available, with particular attention to any clear ischemic changes.

IMAGING

Check for any previous cardiac imaging (in case of omissions during the past medical history).

Chest x-ray

CT pulmonary angiogram

Impression and Plan

DIFFERENTIAL DIAGNOSIS

A key aspect of your plan is your primary diagnosis, along with 1 or 2 top differentials.

Chest Pain

1. Cardiac
   a. Ischemic: unstable angina, NSTEMI, STEMI
   b. Nonischemic: pericarditis, myocarditis, valvular
2. Noncardiac (life-threatening causes to rule out): tamponade, aortic dissection, pneumothorax, pulmonary emboli, esophageal rupture

Troponin Elevation

1. Cardiac
   a. Ischemic: type 1 (unstable angina, NSTEMI, STEMI), type 2 (MI secondary to either increased oxygen demand or decreased supply [e.g., sepsis, hypotension or hypertension, anemia, arrhythmias, heart failure, others])
   b. Nonischemic: peri- or myocarditis, valvular, aortic dissection, others
2. Noncardiac
   a. GI: hepatic failure
   b. Respiratory: PE
   c. Renal: renal failure
   d. Neurological: stroke or intracranial process

MANAGEMENT

Type 1 Myocardial Infarction[9,10,11,12]

Management principles for ACS include:

- oral ASA (325 mg once, followed by 81 mg daily)
- oral ticagrelor (180 mg once, followed by 90 mg twice per day; clopidogrel is an alternative)
- low-target unfractionated heparin (60 units/kg IV bolus [maximum 4000 units], followed by 12 units/kg/hour [maximum 1000 units] for 48 hours, or until PCI if there is ongoing chest pain)
- ACEI or ARB (e.g., oral perindopril 2–4 mg daily, or oral ramipril 2.5 mg daily)
  - › Note: Contraindications include hypotension and poor renal function.
- beta-blocker (e.g., metoprolol 25 mg daily)
  - › Note: Contraindications include bradycardia, atrioventricular block, severe bronchospasm, and acute HF.
- statin (e.g., oral atorvastatin 80 mg daily)
- cardiac catheterization based on risk stratification (TIMI risk score[3] and GRACE score[4])
- pain management (sublingual nitroglycerin spray every 5 minutes [maximum 3 doses] and morphine 2–4 mg IV every 5 to 15 minutes as needed)
- investigations (ECG and troponin levels; trend every 2–4 hours in acute setting)

Type 2 Myocardial Infarction

Treat underlying causes.

- This often requires risk stratification with MIBI, CCTA, stress test, or cardiac catheterization, either while in hospital or as an outpatient.

Noncardiac Etiology of Elevated Troponin

Treat underlying causes.

Heart Failure

These notes are in addition to the **general guide for all consultations** on page 1, and the **starting points for cardiology consultations** at the beginning of this chapter.

Identification

Key information in the identification statement includes the patient's age; EF, in the context of known HF; cardiovascular risk factors; past cardiac episodes; and cardiac surgical history.

Reason for Referral

Examples of reason for referral include shortness of breath, pulmonary edema, peripheral edema, worsening exercise capacity, and assessment for CHF.

History of Present Illness

Assess baseline functional status and exercise capacity: Characterize with the NYHA classification.

Clarify timing of onset: Check whether new symptoms began within days to weeks versus months to years.

Ask about HF symptoms: These include shortness of breath on exertion (SOBOE), orthopnea, paroxysmal nocturnal dyspnea, and peripheral edema.
> A practical question to ask is: How many pillows do you sleep on at night? Is this new for you?
> Ask about weight gain and leg swelling.

Ask about ischemic symptoms: These include chest pain or SOBOE (this can be anginal equivalent), chest pain in the past, and chest pain that is relieved by rest or nitroglycerin.

Ask about rhythm-type symptoms: These include palpitations and presyncope.

For patients with known HF, look for exacerbating factors such as:
> acute ischemia
> recent URTI or other infection
> compliance with diet (low salt, fluid restriction) and medications
> recent excessive alcohol use
> changes in medications or in weight
> worsening valvular disease

Be aware of mimics: These include PE; tamponade or pericardial constriction; severe liver disease (cirrhosis); and renal dysfunction (nephrotic syndrome).

Past Medical History

CARDIAC HISTORY

Assess cardiac risk factors: Ask about diabetes; hypertension; dyslipidemia; obesity; and inflammatory conditions such as gout and RA.

Clarify previous cardiac events: Ask about previous MIs; and previous cardiac investigations, especially echocardiograms, ECGs, Holter monitors, stress tests, MIBI, cardiac MRI, CCTA, and coronary angiograms.

Clarify previous cardiac consultations: Ask about follow-ups with cardiology, visits to heart function clinics, and cardiac workups.

OTHER PAST MEDICAL HISTORY

Focus on previous history of cancer and chemotherapy: Check for anthracycline, trastuzumab, and newer immunotherapy.

Review infectious history: Check for HIV, TB, Chagas disease, and rheumatic heart disease exposure and risk factors.

Review metabolic diseases: Check for thyroid dysfunction and others.

Review pulmonary disorders: Check for lung diseases, and risk factors for pulmonary hypertension and RV failure.

Review renal history and baseline renal function: This affects appropriate medications and dosing.

Past Surgical and Procedural History

Determine cardiac surgical history: This is an important step and involves checking for:

› congenital heart disease
  » Discern the anatomy as well as possible, and determine the surgeon who performed the procedure and the cardiologist who provided care.
› coronary interventions (PCIs, previous angiograms, CABG)
› valvular interventions
› previous ablations and electrophysiological interventions

Determine what cardiac devices the patient currently has: These may include:

› permanent pacemaker (PPM)
› ICD or cardiac resynchronization therapy defibrillator
› LVAD

Medications

Group medications by indication:

- **ACEI/ARB, beta-blocker, mineralocorticoid receptor antagonists:**
  › Check for recent changes in these medications.
  › Ask about:
    » sacubitril-valsartan, ivabradine
    » SGLT2 inhibitor
    » hydralazine and nitroglycerin for poor renal function
    » other afterload reducing agents and antihypertensives
    » home diuretic
- **CAD:** ASA, DAPT, statins
- **Anticoagulation:** DOAC, warfarin (determine INR target)
  › Determine the indication for anticoagulation.
- **Rhythm control:**
  › propafenone or flecainide
  › sotalol
  › amiodarone (determine duration and indication)
- **Other medications**

Allergies
Follow the **general guide for all consultations** and the **starting points for cardiology consultations.**

Family History
Check for:
- premature coronary artery disease
- cardiomyopathies, HF, or sudden death (particularly in the young)

Social History
Ask about:
- alcohol use, drug use (e.g., stimulants), smoking
- occupation
- factors limiting the patient's ability to adhere to, or pay for, medications
- home situation, ADLs, and IADLs, especially for elderly patients
- travel history, country of origin, and immigrant or refugee status (relevant when considering rheumatic heart disease and Chagas disease)

Physical Examination
Vital signs: Obtain the patient's BP (systolic and diastolic), heart rate (regular versus irregular), oxygen saturation, temperature, and weight.

Cardiovascular:
- › Check for devices and sternotomy scars.
- › Assess the patient's volume status: check JVP elevation and perform an abdominojugular reflux test.
- › Check for peripheral edema: lower extremities, sacrum, scrotum.
- › Auscultate for mitral regurgitation (common), and presence of S3 or S4.
- › Assess the temperature of the patient's extremities as an indicator of perfusion (warm versus cold).

Respiratory: Check for evidence of pulmonary edema: crackles to bilateral bases, decreased air entry to bases, and dullness to percussion suggest effusions.

Abdominal: Check for ascites and hepatomegaly.

Findings that suggest alternative diagnoses for shortness of breath: These include:
- › evidence of pulmonary hypertension
- › evidence of PE (calf tenderness, isolated RV failure)
- › evidence of COPD or asthma

Investigations

LABORATORY INVESTIGATIONS

CBC

Electrolytes and extended electrolytes: Pay special attention to K, especially in the context of acute kidney injury or use of diuretics.

Renal function: Renal function affects diuretic dosing and medication management.

Thyrotropin (TSH)

BNP, troponin: Order this for patients with chest pain.

Liver enzymes: These assess for congestive hepatopathy.

Lactate with or without mixed venous saturation: This helps assess for cardiogenic shock.

Extended Workup for Heart Failure in Cases of Unclear Diagnosis
Consider further laboratory investigations depending on history and clinical suspicion.

HIV

Serum protein electrophoresis

Serum free light chain assay

Iron studies (transferrin saturation, ferritin)

Ceruloplasmin

Infectious workup and cultures

OTHER INVESTIGATIONS

ECG: This assesses for ischemic changes and chamber enlargement, and rate and rhythm irregularities.

IMAGING

Chest x-ray: This assesses for cardiomegaly, pulmonary edema, pleural effusions, and other pathologies.

Echocardiogram: Pursue this in patients who have no recent echocardiogram and on suspicion of HF.

Further workup for ischemia: Further workup is based on symptoms and suspicion for CAD.

MRI: This can help resolve uncertainty about the etiology of HF (e.g., infiltrative cardiomyopathy, myocarditis).

Pyrophosphate scan: Pursue this in the context of high suspicion for amyloidosis.

Impression and Plan

DISTINGUISHING HEART FAILURE FROM OTHER DISORDERS

- Consider the differential diagnosis for shortness of breath.

- List supportive evidence for HF from BNP level, history, and physical examination.

EMERGENT MANAGEMENT OF HEART FAILURE

- In patients with severe respiratory distress, and in the context of a confident diagnosis of HF, consider noninvasive ventilation (if there are no contraindications) with bilevel positive airway pressure or CPAP.
- If the patient has concurrent hypertension and overload, consider giving IV furosemide and afterload reduction with nitroglycerin patch or infusion.

SEVERITY OF HEART FAILURE

Use the Forrester classification:

- **Warm and wet:** These patients are overloaded and decompensated, but stable, and should be treated on the ward with diuresis.
- **Cold and wet, or tending to cardiogenic shock:** These patients may need inotropic support and higher-level monitoring.

ETIOLOGY OF HEART FAILURE

- HF has many possible etiologies and the diagnosis is important; consider further investigations if the etiology is uncertain.
- A brief list of etiologies includes:
  › ischemic HF
  › hypertension, diabetes
  › tachyarrhythmia-induced HF
  › valvular heart disease
  › pericardial disease
  › substance-induced HF (alcohol, stimulants)

GUIDELINE-DIRECTED TREATMENT OF HEART FAILURE

There is a difference in management between HF with reduced EF (HFrEF), where EF is less than 40%, and HF with preserved EF (HFpEF), where EF varies within the normal range.[13]

- In the acute setting, provide patients who are overloaded and decompensated with diuresis.
- Address the cause of CHF (e.g., revascularize for ischemia, fix valvular lesions if applicable).
- Avoid nondihydropyridine CCBs.
- Avoid beta-blockers in patients with acutely decompensated HF.
- Note that you may need to hold ACEIs, ARBs, and mineralocorticoid receptor antagonists in patients with acute kidney injury in addition to HF.
  › Reintroduce HF treatment agents slowly.

LONG-TERM MANAGEMENT OF HEART FAILURE WITH REDUCED EJECTION FRACTION[13]

- Address the cause of CHF (e.g., revascularize for ischemia, fix valvular lesions if applicable).
- For EF less than 40%, provide triple therapy: ACEI (or ARB), beta-blocker, and mineralocorticoid receptor antagonists.
- If the patient is unable to tolerate ACEIs or ARBs due to renal function, consider hydralazine or nitroglycerin for afterload reduction.
- Repeat echocardiogram after maximal medical management.
- If the patient continues to have moderate symptoms (NYHA Class II or III), consider:
  › sacubitril-valsartan, or ivabradine in the context of sinus rhythm and a heart rate greater than 70
  › SGLT2 inhibitor in all patients (with or without diabetes)
  › cardiac resynchronization therapy with or without a defibrillator if EF is less than or equal to 35% and the patient meets QRS and/or LBBB criteria (see CCS guidelines algorithm)
- If the patient has severe symptoms and requires continuing inotropic support, consider palliative care versus consulting an HF specialist regarding advanced mechanical circulatory support and possible workup for heart transplantation.

LONG-TERM MANAGEMENT OF HEART FAILURE WITH PRESERVED EJECTION FRACTION

HFpEF has fewer evidence-based treatment options than HFrEF.[13]

- Focus on treating reversible causes (e.g., type 2 diabetes, hypertension, valvular heart disease).
- Manage symptoms and volume status with diuretics.
- Some studies suggest using spironolactone and sacubitril/valsartan for HFpEF to decrease hospital admissions, but this has not proven statistically significant in trials and is not included in recognized treatment guidelines.

CONTINUING FOLLOW-UP

HF is a chronic condition that requires regular reassessment and follow-up; many patients are best managed at a dedicated heart function clinic.

Syncope

These notes are in addition to the **general guide for all consultations** on page 1, and the **starting points for cardiology consultations** at the beginning of this chapter.

Identification

Key information in the identification statement includes the patient's age, gender, and pertinent cardiac risk factors, and whether the patient has known structural heart disease (e.g., previous low EF).

Reason for Referral

The referral may seek to confirm syncopal episodes (acute or recurrent) and/or clarify appropriate management.

History of Present Illness

Clarify the number, frequency, duration of episodes.

Assess the effect of position on episodes: Does the patient experience syncope while supine, sitting, or standing?
› **Supine or recumbent:** more likely arrhythmia
› **Prolonged standing:** more likely vasovagal
› **Supine to standing:** more likely orthostatic

Identify provoking factors: Ask about exercise (during or immediately after); eating (postprandial syncope); urination, defecation, coughing, or swallowing; emotional stress, fear, or pain; and abrupt neck movements.

Determine the disposition of the patient preceding, during, and after episodes:
› **Preceding:** Check for nausea and vomiting, feeling cold or clammy, visual auras or blurry vision, palpitations, shortness of breath, and chest pain.
› **During:** Check for witnessed episodes, tonic-clonic movements, automatisms, bladder or bowel incontinence, and tongue biting.
› **After:** Ask about recovery time, and check for confusion, fatigue, injury, and incontinence.

Past Medical History

Check for:
- structural heart disease (e.g., CAD with or without prior MI, valvular heart disease, CHD, cardiomyopathies, prior cardiac surgery)
- neurologic conditions (e.g., seizure disorders, migraines, Parkinson disease, stroke)
- diabetes mellitus (ask for latest HbA_{1C} result)
- substance abuse (e.g., alcohol, illicit drugs, narcotics)

Medications

Check for:
- diuretics, antihypertensives (relevant to orthostasis), atrioventricular nodal blockers (orthostasis)

- QT-prolonging drugs (e.g., antiarrhythmics, antifungals, quinolones, macrolides, antipsychotics, antidepressants), which confer increased risk of torsade de pointes and polymorphic VT

Allergies
Follow the **general guide for all consultations** and the **starting points for cardiology consultations.**

Family History
Check for[14,15]:
- sudden cardiac death (ask about drownings and single-operator vehicle accidents)
- familial cardiomyopathy (e.g., hypertrophic cardiomyopathy, arrhythmogenic RV cardiomyopathy) or channelopathies (e.g., long/short QT, Brugada syndrome, catecholaminergic polymorphic VT)
- predisposition to syncope, seizure disorders, or migraines

Social History
Ask about:
- alcohol use, drug use, smoking
- occupation
- travel or residence in regions where Lyme disease is endemic; tick bites

Physical Exam
Vital signs: Obtain the patient's:
› BP, heart rate, respiration rate, temperature, oxygen saturation level, and glucose level
› orthostatic BP
› bilateral BP (relevant to aortic dissection)
› pulse pressure (narrow pulse pressure can indicate severe aortic stenosis)
Cardiovascular:
› Perform a carotid sinus massage.
› Look for features of aortic stenosis (e.g., parvus et tardus carotid pulse, paradoxical or single S2, soft or absent S2, midsystolic ejection click, harsh crescendo-decrescendo right upper sternal border murmur).
› Look for features of hypertrophic cardiomyopathy (e.g., sustained apical impulse; crescendo-decrescendo murmur at the left sternal third and fourth intercostal space; louder on standing or the Valsalva maneuver).

Neurological:
> Check the cranial nerve, motor nerves (bulk, tone, power), reflexes, and sensory nerves.
> Assess gait for features of parkinsonism.
> Consider a tilt table test (to confirm vasovagal syncope).

Investigations

LABORATORY INVESTIGATIONS
CBC with differential
Electrolytes, urea, creatinine, glucose
Troponin, BNP, lactate
Endocrine tests: thyrotropin (TSH), HbA_{1C}

OTHER INVESTIGATIONS
12-lead ECG: This assesses for:
> atrioventricular blocks (first, second, third degree)
> bundle branch blocks
> AF and/or atrial flutter (for tachy-brady syndrome, conversion pause, etc.)
> Wolff-Parkinson-White syndrome
> arrhythmogenic RV cardiomyopathy epsilon waves
> Brugada syndrome
> long QT syndrome
> LVH (hypertrophic cardiomyopathy)

Exercise stress test: Order this to assess for suspected exercise-induced arrhythmia.

EEG: Order this on clinical suspicion of seizures.

IMAGING
Transthoracic echocardiogram: If indicated, order this to evaluate for structural or valvular heart disease.

CT of the head: If indicated, order this to evaluate for focal neurologic deficits or suspected seizure activity.

Impression and Plan

GENERAL APPROACH
• Begin by stating the patient profile and listing pertinent risk factors.
• Consider the following differential:
> reflex syncope (i.e., neurocardiogenic)
> orthostatic syncope
> cardiac arrhythmias
> structural cardiopulmonary disease (e.g., aortic stenosis, hypertrophic cardiomyopathy, PE)

RISK STRATIFICATION AND MANAGEMENT
Use risk stratification to clarify management plans.

Hemodynamically Unstable Patients
Provide resuscitation orders including 2 large bore IVs, fluid resuscitation, oxygen, glucose, atropine, isoproterenol, transcutaneous pacing, and transvenous pacing.

- **High-risk patients:** Admit for inpatient monitoring with or without a prolonged monitoring device if no arrhythmia was found during admission.[16,17,18]
- **Patients with significant arrhythmias:** Admit for PPM or ICD.[16,17,18]

Stable Patients
- **Low-risk patients:** Provide outpatient follow-up with or without a Holter monitor or other noninvasive novel cardiac monitoring device.[15,17]
- **Intermediate-risk patients:** Make decisions based on the individual case; consider prolonged ambulatory monitoring for arrhythmia (e.g., event monitor, loop recorder) on suspicion of higher risk.[15,17]

Vasovagal and Situational Syncope
- Counsel the patient to avoid triggers and wear support stockings.
- Stop offending medications.[14,15]

Orthostatic Hypotension
- Counsel the patient to increase fluid intake and wear support stockings.
- Prescribe midodrine and/or fludrocortisone.[14,15]

References
1. Campeau L. Grading of angina pectoris. Circulation. 1976;54:5223. doi: 10.1161/circ.54.3.947585
2. Dolgin, M, Fox A, Gorlin R, et al. Nomenclature and criteria for diagnosis of diseases of the heart and great vessels. 9th ed. Boston: Lippincott Williams and Wilkins; 1994. 334 p.
3. Antman E, Cohen M, Bernink P, et al. The TIMI risk score for unstable angina/non–ST elevation MI: a method for prognostication and therapeutic decision making. JAMA. 2000 Aug 16;284(7):835-42. doi: 10.001/jama.284.7.835
4. Tang E, Wong C, Herbison P. Global Registry of Acute Coronary Events (GRACE) hospital discharge risk score accurately predicts long-term mortality post acute coronary syndrome. Am Heart J. 2007 Jan 1;153(1):29-35. doi: 10.1016/j.ahj.2006.10.004
5. Wilson P, D'Agostino R, Levy D, et al. Prediction of coronary heart disease using risk factor categories. Circulation. 1998;97(18):1837-47. doi: 10.1161/01.cir.97.18.1837
6. Kirchhof P, Cam A, Goette A, et al. Early rhythm-control therapy in patients with atrial fibrillation. N Engl J Med. 2020;383(14):1305-16. doi: 10.1056/NEJMoa2019422
7. AFFIRM writing group. A comparison of rate control and rhythm control in patients with atrial fibrillation. N Engl J Med. 2002; 347(23):1825-33. doi: 10.1056/NEJMoa021328

8. Van Gelder I, Groenveld H, Crijns H, et al. Lenient versus strict rate control in patients with atrial fibrillation. N Engl J Med. 2010; 362(15):1363-73. doi: 10.1056/NEJMoa 1001337

9. Amsterdam E, Wenger N, Brindis R, et al. 2014 AHA/ACC guideline for the management of patients with non–ST-elevation acute coronary syndromes. J Am Coll Cardiol. 2014;64(24); e139-e228. doi: 10.1016/j.jacc.2014.09.017

10. Fitchett D, Theroux P, Brophy J, et al. Assessment and management of acute coronary syndromes (ACS): a Canadian perspective on current guideline-recommended treatment—part 1: non-ST-segment elevation ACS. Can J Cardiol. 2011;27(supp A); S387-S401. doi: 10.1016/j.cjca.2011.08.110

11. Fitchett D, Theroux P, Brophy J, et al. Assessment and management of acute coronary syndromes (ACS): a Canadian perspective on current guideline-recommended treatment—part 2: ST-segment elevation myocardial infarction. Can J Cardiol. 2011; 27(supp A); S402-S412. doi: 10.1016/j.cjca.2011.08.107

12. Hui D. Approach to internal medicine a resource book for clinical practice. New York: Springer; 2016. 459 p.

13. Ezekowitz J, O'Meara E, McDonald M, et al. 2017 comprehensive update of the Canadian Cardiovascular Society guidelines for the management of heart failure. Can J Cardiol. 2017;33(11);1342-1433. doi: 10.1016/j.cjca.2017.08.022

14. Brignole M, Moya A, de Lange F, et al. 2018 ESC guidelines for the diagnosis and management of syncope. European Heart Journal. 2018;39(21):1883-1948. doi: 10.1093/eurheartj/ehy037

15. Puppala V, Dickinson O, Benditt D. Syncope: classification and risk stratification. 2014;63(3):171-77. doi: 10.1016/j.jjcc.2013.03.019

16. Sandhu R, Raj S, Thiruganasambandamoorthy V, et al. Focused clinical practice update: Canadian Cardiovascular Society clinical practice update on the assessment and management of syncope. Can J Cardiol. 2020;36(8):1167-77. doi: 10.1016/j.cjca.2019.12.023

17. Sheldon R, Morillo C, Krahn A, et al. Standardized approaches to the investigation of syncope: Canadian Cardiovascular Society position paper. Can J Cardiol. 2011;27(2):246-53. doi: 10.1016/j.cjca.2010.11.002

18. Shen W, Sheldon R, Benditt D, et al. 2017 ACC/AHA/HRS guideline for the evaluation and management of patients with syncope: a report of the American College of Cardiology/American Heart Association Task Force on Clinical Practice Guidelines, and the Heart Rhythm Society. J Am Coll Cardiol. 2017;70(5):e39-110. doi: 10.1016/j.jacc.2017.03.002

4

Critical Care Medicine

Dr. Jing Ye (Carol) Bao
Dr. Keir Martyn
Dr. Amanallah
    Montazeripouragha
Dr. Matthew Renwick
Dr. Amanda Bettle

REVIEWERS
Dr. Cheryl L. Holmes
Dr. Constantin Shuster
Dr. Daniel Ovakim

Starting Points: Critical Care Consultations

These notes are in addition to the **general guide for all consultations** on page 1.

Critical care consultations often occur without a detailed awareness of the patient's medical history, and the focus must be on rapidly stabilizing the patient through airway, breathing, and circulatory support, followed by identification of disease process and appropriate treatment.[1] Reassess often, don't hesitate to ask for help, and complete a thorough consultation after the patient is stabilized. Patients may not be able to provide their own history, so be sure to ask questions of bystanders, paramedics, and family members whenever possible. For hospitalized patients, read the nursing notes for important clues (e.g., vomiting leading to acute shortness of breath indicating aspiration).

Identification

Key information in the identification statement includes the patient's age, past medical history relevant to the current presentation, current status, and advanced directives. *For example:* "81-year-old female living independently, full code, with bioprosthetic aortic valve repair presenting with 3 days of fever, chills, and hypotension requiring vasopressor support and breathing spontaneously. Advanced directives indicate transfer to advanced level of care including intubation, ventilation, and vasopressor support but no CPR."

Reason for Referral

An example of a reason for referral is undifferentiated shock needing ICU admission.

History of Present Illness

This history is the key part of the consultation. It should establish a clear timeline of events leading to hospitalization and the course of the presentation so far, focusing on pertinent positives and negatives that will guide treatment decisions.[1] It needs to be updated for each person who witnessed or participated in the care of the patient.

Clarify the circumstances of presentation: For example, did the patient arrive independently at the ED? Were they brought by paramedics? (For inpatient consultations, establish details of the hospital stay.)

Document the source of information: Some of these cases result in legal proceedings, so take notes on where information comes from (e.g., "according to bystanders" or "as stated in the EHS record" or "according to the sister").

Determine the baseline functional status of the patient, if known, and the functional status of the patient on arrival.

Clarify the presenting symptoms and pertinent details: The following list is not exhaustive:

> - **Trauma:** mechanism and extent of injury, others dead at scene
> - **Hypovolemic shock:** active hemorrhage, fluid loss from diarrhea and/or vomiting
> - **Cardiogenic shock:** ischemic chest pain, ECG changes, CAD risk factors (prior ACS, smoking, dyslipidemia, family history of premature CAD)
> - **Obstructive shock:** trauma, active malignancy, recent cardiac surgery, PE risk factors
> - **Distributive shock:** infective symptoms (localized to source), immunocompromise (e.g., HIV status), anaphylaxis history (e.g., for suspected anaphylaxis: wheezing, pruritus, hives)
> - **Altered mental status:** pertinent neuroimaging in the context of TBI
> - **Arrhythmia**
> - **Respiratory distress**

Document prehospital events, the patient's course in the ED, and interventions thus far:

> - For cardiac arrest, provide comments on the type of arrest, whether it was witnessed, how much downtime it involved, the duration of CPR,

the amount of cycles or medications given, and the time elapsed until the return of spontaneous circulation.
> List fluids, blood products, and/or antibiotics administered.
> Note airway interventions and the difficulty of intubation, if applicable.
> Note whether vasopressors or other infusions were initiated prior to ICU transfer.

Past Medical History

Assess for chronic diseases: What chronic diseases does the patient have? What is their severity? How, and how well, are they managed?
> When you write your consult, you will need to list these in order of relevance to the presentation. *For example:* "Long-term intermittent hemodialysis MWF for renal failure secondary to diabetic nephropathy"; or "HF with reduced EF secondary to ischemia (EF 25% two months ago) and 3 hospital admissions in the past 12 months, managed with diuresis (never any BiPAP or endotracheal intubation)."

Determine the course of treatment and outcome for any previous ICU admissions.

Call the patient's family doctor and other specialists for additional information.

Past Surgical History

Identify anything relevant to the current presentation (e.g., sepsis from an intraabdominal source with complex bowel surgery history).

Medications

- Look for information on medications from online health records (if available) or from the patient or family.
- Group medications by indication.
- Look for recent changes to prescribed medications and adherence, especially regarding steroids or other immunosuppressive medications.
- Ask about medications that lower BP: opioids, sedatives, antihypertensives, and anxiolytics.
- Ask about OTC medications, herbal medications, and supplements.
- Check for neurological medications, including:
  > sedatives (e.g., propofol infusions, midazolam)
  > analgesia (e.g., opioids, ketamine)
  > neuromuscular blockade (determine time of last dose)

Allergies

- Determine known allergies and reactions.

- If the reason for admission is anaphylaxis, clearly establish the course of previous episodes (e.g., the need for continuous epinephrine infusion).

Family History

Determine relevant history according to the presentation (e.g., a family history of hypertrophic cardiomyopathy or congenital arrhythmia in a patient younger than 50 with cardiac arrest).

Social History

If the patient is unresponsive, obtain collateral information from family members, bystanders, and allied health-care workers.
- Check for and review previous psychiatry consultations, if available.
- Ask about:
  › occupation, economic status, housing situation
  › alcohol use, recreational drug use, smoking
    » Clarify the quantities involved and previous withdrawals.
    » For opioid use disorder, quantify use and route of administration to assess the need for maintenance opioid therapy.
  › sexual and travel history
- Depending on the frailty and comorbidities of the patient, establish a brief functional history using ADLS and IADLs.

Code Status

Identify advanced directives, code status, and substitute decision makers, if applicable.

Physical Examination

Airway, breathing, circulation (ABCs): Ensure the patient is hemodynamically stable, and provide airway protection, as needed.

General appearance: Does the patient look sick or not sick? Awake or obtunded?

Neurological:
  › Assess the patient's level of consciousness (LOC) with a GCS score (break it into components: e.g., E3V3M4), or the Alert-Voice-Pain-Unresponsive (AVPU) scale.
  › Conduct a basic screening exam, including assessing the pupils and checking for nuchal rigidity.
  › Check for monitors or lines (e.g., external ventricular drains, lumbar drains).

Cardiovascular:
  › Check heart rate and rhythm, BP, and warm versus cold extremities.
  › Conduct a brief exam for murmurs and muffled heart sounds, and for lines (arterial line, central venous catheter, IVs).

› Check for cardiovascular medications, including vasopressors (e.g., norepinephrine), inotropes, and antiarrhythmics (e.g., amiodarone).
› Assess JVP:
  » Elevated neck veins suggest obstructive or cardiogenic shock.
  » Flat neck veins occur in distributive and hypovolemic shock.
› Document your findings: *For example:* "90 bpm sinus tachycardia, warm peripheries with flat JVP, no murmurs auscultated, right radial arterial line and left IJ CVC in situ running norepinephrine at 8 mcg/min."

Point-of-care US (POCUS): This is a useful adjunct to physical examination:
› to assess LV function in the setting of shock, or for the presence of pericardial effusion
› to help determine fluid status in assessing the inferior vena cava and lungs (e.g., widespread B-lines indicating pulmonary edema)

Respiratory:
› Check the patient's respiratory rate and oxygen saturation.
› Inspect for tracheal deviation.
› Auscultate the lungs (note clear lungs, wheezes, or crackles).
› Check ventilator settings, if applicable.
  » Note time intubated, size of tube, confirmed placement or not.
  » Ventilator settings include mode, tidal volume, FIO_2, PEEP, and plateau pressures (e.g., volume control mode, tidal volume 550 mL, respiratory rate 16, FIO_2 50%, and PEEP of 9 with plateau pressure 20).
  » Note settings for bilevel positive air pressure (BiPAP) or CPAP settings.
  » If intubation is anticipated, perform an airway assessment (C-spine stability, mouth opening, Mallampati score).

Renal:
› Determine fluid inputs versus renal output.
› Determine IV fluid type and rate.
› Note the presence of Foley catheters or renal replacement therapy (note fluid goal rate).

GI: Conduct a brief exam for distension, peritoneal signs, nasogastric tubes, and abdominal drains.

Recent surgical sites: Inspect and palpate these.

Hematological: Check coagulation studies and transfused blood products.

Endocrine: Check blood glucose level and insulin given.

Dermatological: Focus on manifestations of systemic disease; petechiae or purpura may indicate *Neisseria meningitidis* or *Haemophilus influenzae*.

Investigations

Check for previous troponin and BNP results, and previous ECG findings.

LABORATORY INVESTIGATIONS

Baseline investigations in all critically ill patients: CBC with differential, extended electrolytes, creatinine, urea, glucose, liver enzymes, bilirubin, and coagulation studies (INR, PTT, and fibrinogen)

Lactate and lactate trend

Blood gas: venous blood gas or ABG, with interpretation (check for trends)

Mixed venous oxygen saturation:
› This provides information on oxygen delivery and use.

Specific entities:
› **Troponin:** Pursue this in patients with suspected cardiac involvement (urgently in suspected ACS).
› **Osmolal gap:** This helps identify toxic alcohol ingestion.

MICROBIOLOGY

Blood cultures: Provide specimens from 2 peripheral sites and in-situ lines in suspected infectious etiology.

Sputum culture: Pursue this in suspected pulmonary etiology.

Urine culture and urinalysis

COVID-19 nasopharyngeal swab: Order this on suspicion of SARS-CoV-2 for intubated patients.

IMAGING

Do not send patients outside the ED for imaging until their airway, ventilation, and circulation have stabilized.

Chest x-ray: This is indicated for all critically ill patients.

Additional imaging: Pursue this as needed. Examples include:
› CT pulmonary angiogram for suspected PE (Wells score ≥ 4.5)[2]
› CT of the abdomen and pelvis for suspected intraabdominal sepsis
› CT of the head in depressed LOC or suspected intracranial process

OTHER INVESTIGATIONS

12-lead ECG: Pursue this in all critically ill patients (it is especially useful in the setting of possible ACS, overdose, and postarrest care).

LP: Pursue this in the context of altered LOC.
› Send the specimen for Gram stain, microscopy, bacterial culture, fungal culture, CBC, glucose, and protein.
› Note that a CT of the head is needed before LP if the patient is older than 60 or immunocompromised, or has CNS disease, focal neurological deficits, or papilledema.

Thoracentesis or paracentesis: Pursue this if pleural effusions or ascites are present.

Impression and Plan[1]

Start with a summary:
› Rework the identification statement as indicated by your consultation.
› Summarize relevant past medical history.
› Provide a brief description of presenting events and the patient's course in hospital, and the reason for ICU consultation.
› Provide your impression of the cause and needed immediate management.

List issues by clinical priority:
› List the chief complaint, secondary diagnoses, and chronic conditions.
› Under each issue: identify the probable diagnosis or contributing diagnoses, and provide a short list of differential diagnoses; list investigations and procedures needed to rule diagnoses in or out; and provide a management plan. *For example:* "Issue #1: Massive PE with extensive central clot burden. Unprovoked. Hypotensive 80/35, troponin T 4.1, and RV dilation. Plan for emergency catheter directed thrombolysis and MAP goal > 65 mmHg."

Identify needed subspecialty consultations: List these for each issue.

Anticipate the need for additional lines or intubation: These may include:
› arterial lines for continuous BP monitoring and ABG draws
› central venous catheters for prolonged vasopressor use and repeated draws
› mechanical ventilation for oxygenation or ventilation, or to protect the airway

Describe relevant critical care best practices: These include advanced directives; a description of updates given to the patient's family, or the last discussion with the family; identification of a substitute decision maker; sedation goals (use the Richmond Agitation-Sedation Scale); analgesia; GI ulcer prophylaxis if the patient is intubated; routine DVT prophylaxis with LMWH, if no contraindication; and directions for holding or restarting home medications, for diet, and for disposition following ICU stay.

Ensure immunizations are updated before transfer from ICU.

Update the patient's family doctor or primary care provider.

Communicate the plan: Ensure the bedside nurse is aware of the plan and clearly communicate the reassessment tasks to the incoming team.

Poisoning

These notes are in addition to the **general guide for all consultations** on page 1, and the **starting points for critical care consultations** at the beginning of this chapter.

Poisonings are a time-sensitive medical emergency. Focus first on stabilizing the patient (airway, breathing, circulation, and administration of antidote if indicated), then focus on diagnosis, preventing further absorption or enhancing elimination, and frequent reassessment. Pursue a thorough toxicology consultation after the patient is stable.

Identification

Key information in the identification statement includes the patient's age, gender, pertinent medical history, overdose type, and current status.

Reason for Referral

The referral may seek to confirm poisoning and/or clarify appropriate management.

History of Present Illness

Clarify the details of substance use: Determine the name and amount of each substance involved, routes of administration, and when the substance use occurred, or when the patient was last seen well.

Clarify the circumstances of exposure: Ask about location, surrounding events, and intent.

Clarify symptoms: Establish the time of symptom onset, and the nature and severity of symptoms.[3]

Look for constellations of symptoms: These may indicate a toxidrome associated with a particular class of poisoning, which would clarify treatment options, expected course, and outcomes (e.g., cholinergic toxidromes feature salivation, lacrimation, urination, defection, GI upset, emesis).

Clarify management the patient has received:
> Ask about first-aid measures and steps in the ED to assess and stabilize the patient.
> Check for information about initial vital signs, airway status (intubated or not), and circulatory status (hypotensive, vasopressor support, abnormal ECG).

Identify reversal or decontamination agents given: Determine the patient's response.[3]

Clarify allied health services involved: These could include, for example, poison control or a toxicologist.

Past Medical History

Ask about prior overdoses and treatment course: For example, has the patient repeatedly come to the ED for overdoses? Have they had a previous admission to ICU with mechanical ventilation?

Highlight significant comorbidities that affect care.

Ask about psychiatric evaluations: In particular, ask about depression, borderline personality disorder, and suicide attempts.

Call the patient's family doctor or primary care provider for a complete history.

Past Surgical History

This requires less detail than the patient's past medical history, unless it involves something immediately relevant to the current presentation.

Medications

- Document your source of information for medications (e.g., a provincial database, the patient, or family members).
- Ask about current prescription medications (group them by indication); and OTC medications, herbal medications, and supplements.

Allergies

Follow the **general guide for all consultations** and the **starting points for critical care consultations**.

Family History

Ask about depression and/or suicide.

Social History

- For unresponsive patients, obtain collateral information from family members, bystanders, and allied health-care workers, and from previous psychiatric consultations.
- Ask about:
  › occupation, economic status, housing situation
  › unstable social relationships
  › alcohol use, recreational drug use, smoking (clarify the quantities involved and previous withdrawals)

Code Status

Identify advanced directives, code status, and substitute decision makers, if applicable.

Physical Examination

Airway, breathing, circulation (ABCs): Assess the patient's hemodynamic status and need for airway protection.

General appearance:
› Does the patient look sick or not sick?
› Assess the patient's LOC with a GCS score (break it into components: e.g., E3V3M4).
› Characterize the physiological state as stimulated, depressed, discordant, or normal.

Neurological:
› Conduct a brief exam, noting: pinpoint pupils versus mydriasis; dyskinesia; dystonia; fasciculations; clonus; rigidity; and core temperature.
› Clarify current sedative use.

Cardiovascular: Conduct a brief exam:
› Assess heart rate and rhythm, BP, and warm versus cold extremities.
› Look for lines, including arterial lines, cental venous catheters, and IVs.

POCUS: Assess volume status.

Respiratory:
› Assess respiratory rate and pattern (bradypnea, Kussmaul respiration, hyperventilation) and oxygen saturation.
› Auscultate for abnormal lung sounds.
› In mechanically ventilated patients, check the settings (mode, rate, FIO_2, peak and plateau pressures).
  » Reassess settings with the results of chest x-ray and ABG trend.

Renal:
› Determine fluid inputs versus renal output.
› Assess for acute kidney injury (compare current creatinine to baseline).
› Determine IV fluid type and rate.

GI: Conduct a brief exam and ask about diet.

Hematological: Assess for coagulopathy (e.g., ecchymoses, hemarthrosis, petechiae, wet purpura over mucosa, prolonged bleeding from puncture sites).

Investigations

LABORATORY INVESTIGATIONS

Follow the **starting points for critical care consultations** on baseline laboratory investigations.

Osmolal gap (OG): OG = 2 x Na^+ + BUN + Glucose + 1.25 x Ethanol
› Memory aid: "Two salts and a sticky BUN, and a bottle of wine."
› OG normal ranges are from -14 to + 10 mOsm/L.
› OG is increased in ethylene glycol, isopropyl alcohol, glycerol, mannitol, methanol, and sorbitol toxicity.[4]

Anion gap (AG): $AG = Na^+ - (HCO_3^- + Cl^-)$
› Normal AG is < 10 mmol/L.
› AG is increased in salicylate, carbon monoxide, cyanide, toluene, methanol, ethylene glycol, iron, and paraldehyde toxicity.

Acetaminophen, salicylate, and ethanol levels: Order these in all intentional overdoses with altered LOC.

Urine drug screen: This indicates presence or absence of a limited number of substances.

Specific drug levels: Measuring digoxin, lithium, carbamazepine, phenytoin, theophylline, and valproic acid can help guide management.[5]

Volatile alcohol levels: These are rarely available when needed, though order them if indicated.

IMAGING

Chest x-ray: In all patients, use this to assess for aspiration, acute lung injury from heroin or salicylates, and pneumothorax, and to confirm endotracheal tube (ETT) placement in intubated patients.

OTHER INVESTIGATIONS

12-lead ECG: This is useful in all patients (especially to assess QRS and QTc intervals), and especially in cases of antidepressant and antipsychotic ingestion. For example, in your plan, you might state: "Na+ channel blockade seen in TCA toxicity causes QRS widening which requires sodium bicarbonate to narrow QRS <120 msec and prevent seizures."

Impression and Plan[4]

Document the stability and current status of the patient, and expected trajectory.

Organize issues in order of acuity, and include workup and management for each issue: *For example:* "Issue #1: Acetaminophen ingestion. Witnessed 8 hours prior with initial level 2000 µmol/L. Liver function tests within normal limits and clinically asymptomatic. Started on N-acetylcysteine infusion, will reassess at 21 hours and discontinue when serum acetaminophen levels undetectable, AST normal, INR < 1.5, creatinine at baseline, and patient is clinically well."

Contact a poison control centre: Do this early in the process of admission and management.

Consider decontamination:
› For patients presenting within 1 to 4 hours of GI exposure to a toxin, consider decontamination with activated charcoal, or whole bowel irrigation with polyethylene glycol electrolyte solution.
› Discuss decontamination with poison control before ordering.

Be aware of the indications for overdoses with specific antidotes: For example, use naloxone for opioids, cyproheptadine for serotonin syndrome, and fomepizole for toxic alcohols.

Consider which drugs may be removed by dialysis:
› Examples include lithium, ethylene glycol, methanol, and valproate.
› If indicated, contact a nephrology specialist early.

Consider enhanced elimination with serum and urinary alkalinization: Use this for substances that are weak acids and whose excretion is primarily renal (e.g., salicylate, phenobarbital, methotrexate).

Provide referrals, as indicated, and communicate if services are called:
› **Suspected poisoning:** Call poison control for assistance in management and epidemiologic recording.
› **Intentional overdose:** Arrange a psychiatric evaluation once the patient is responsive. Strongly consider involving social work and/or addictions teams.

Follow critical care best practices: Follow the starting points on critical care consultations, and:
› Consider drug interactions of home medications with the offending agent.
› State if the patient is certified under your jurisdiction's mental health act.
› Monitor the patient for severe withdrawal reactions (benzodiazepines, baclofen) and consider restarting home medications early.

Communicate the plan: Ensure allied health-care providers are aware of the plan, and clearly communicate reassessment tasks to the incoming team.

Update the patient's family doctor or primary care provider.

Respiratory Failure

These notes are in addition to the **general guide for all consultations** on page 1, and the **starting points for critical care consultations** at the beginning of this chapter.

Identification

Key information in the identification statement includes the patient's age, gender, functional status, relevant past medical history, and current status.

Reason for Referral

The referral may seek to clarify failure in ventilation versus oxygenation, or failure that involves both, and acute versus chronic failure.

History of Present Illness

Establish the patient's baseline respiratory function: Was the patient previously healthy? Is the patient on home oxygen for end-stage COPD?

Determine management the patient has received in the ED or ward: Did the patient receive resuscitation or airway support? If on a ward, what was the initial reason for admission?

Clarify associated symptoms: Ask about hemoptysis, cough, crackles, wheeze, chest pain, and fever.

Ask about a history of trauma and/or chest or spine deformities.

Ask about recent surgery.

Assess for inhalation injury: Has the patient had a recent inhalation injury? Does the patient have a history of working near toxic chemicals or organic solvents?

Ask about recent vomiting: Does the patient have aspiration risk factors? Was aspiration witnessed?

Identify potential causes of respiratory failure and/or exacerbating factors: These include:
> **CNS:** decreased drive to breathe due to narcotic, sedative, tumour, brainstem stroke, metabolic alkalosis, CNS infection, hypothyroidism
> **Peripheral nervous system:** Guillain-Barré syndrome; spinal cord injury; myasthenia gravis; botulism; abnormal magnesium and/or phosphate levels; dermatomyositis and/or polymyositis; muscular dystrophy
> **Airway:** COPD, asthma, bronchiectasis, CF
> **Alveoli:** pneumonia, atelectasis, pulmonary edema (cardiogenic, noncardiogenic), interstitial lung disease
> **Blood vessels:** PE, cardiac shunt, pulmonary AVM
> **Pleura:** fibrosis, effusion
> **Chest wall:** obesity, kyphosis, scoliosis

Identify potential causes of cellular hypoxia: Ask about exposure to carbon monoxide, methemoglobinemia, and cyanide.

Past Medical History

Determine any previous admissions or conditions (e.g., COPD, CHF, obstructive sleep apnea), the management these involved, and whether any resulted in escalation to ICU.

Past Surgical History
This is relevant in the context of postoperative pain, residual anesthesia, and atelectasis.

Medications
Ask about:
- sedatives (narcotics, benzodiazepines)
- transfusions (relevant to transfusion-associated circulatory overload and transfusion-related acute lung injury)
- baseline respiratory medications, and any recent escalation in dose or frequency
- drugs that may induce lung disease (nitrofurantoin, amiodarone, chemo, procainamide, hydralazine)

Allergies
Follow the **general guide for all consultations** and the **starting points for critical care consultations.**

Family History
Check for respiratory diseases such as early onset COPD (α_1-antitrypsin deficiency).

Social History
Ask about:
- alcohol use, recreational drug use, smoking
- previous episodes of withdrawal and/or current risk of withdrawal (this can increase the risk of aspiration)
- occupation

Code Status
Identify advanced directives, code status, and substitute decision makers, if applicable.

Physical Examination
Findings that could alter management are particularly important, including altered mentation and facial trauma or deformities that could contraindicate noninvasive positive-pressure ventilation.

General appearance

Airway, breathing, circulation (ABCs): Assess airway status and hemodynamic stability, and note signs of:
> **Increased work of breathing:** respiration rate greater than 35 breaths per minute, diaphoresis, tripod position, accessory muscle use, abdominal paradox, inability to speak in full sentences
> **Hypoxemia:** altered LOC, tachypnea, cyanosis (central, peripheral)
> **Hypercapnia:** headache, asterixis, warm extremities, coma

Airway (for intubation): Determine Mallampati score, and assess for neck stability, neck obstruction (e.g., from obesity), and adequate mouth opening.

Body habitus:
> Assess for obesity, asymmetric or deformed chest wall, and kyphoscoliosis.
> If already intubated, determine the size of the tube and whether its placement is already confirmed by chest x-ray.

Cardiorespiratory: Note findings that suggest a specific etiology for acute respiratory failure, including:
> elevated JVP, peripheral edema, S3 in CHF
> fever, productive cough, pleuritic chest pain in pneumonia
> fatigable bulbar and ocular weaknesses in myasthenia gravis

POCUS: Use this to determine volume status; assess the lungs (A-lines and B-lines); identify pleural effusion; and obtain cardiac views.

Investigations

LABORATORY INVESTIGATIONS

CBC, electrolytes, thyrotropin (TSH)

ABG: This confirms the type of respiratory failure.
> Note that the trend in ABG is more important than a single ABG. Elevated $PaCO_2$ can be a very late sign of deterioration, thus a "normal" $PaCO_2$ can be falsely reassuring, especially in the presence of increased respiratory rate.
> Assess the ratio of PaO_2 to FIO_2: < 300 is a mild oxygenation defect; < 200, a moderate oxygenation defect; < 100, a severe oxygenation defect.

MICROBIOLOGY

• Pursue an infectious workup as needed (see Sepsis in this chapter).
• Note that some specimens require bronchoscopy.

IMAGING

Do not send patients outside the ED for imaging until their airway, ventilation, and circulation have stabilized.

Chest x-ray: This identifies the underlying cause of respiratory failure and confirms ETT placement.

CT of the chest: Consider this in most contexts to better delineate lung pathology and rule out PE.

Impression and Plan[6]

• It is important to differentiate failure of oxygenation, failure of ventilation, and cardiogenic causes of respiratory failure (fluid overload).

- Describe the current status and expected trajectory of the patient. *For example:* "Not improving on BiPAP and may need intubation shortly."
- Indicate the type of respiratory failure:
  › type 1 respiratory failure (hypoxemia): $PaO_2 < 60$ mmHg
  › type 2 respiratory failure (hypercapnia): $PaCO_2 > 50$ mmHg and $PaO_2 < 60$ mmHg
  › mixed

INVASIVE VERSUS NONINVASIVE VENTILATION

The choice depends on the underlying cause and severity of the respiratory failure.

Noninvasive Positive Pressure Ventilation (NIPPV)

- NIPPV is contraindicated if the patient is unable to protect their airway (i.e., due to altered LOC), and in the context of vomiting, significant secretions, poor mask fit (e.g., due to trauma), multiorgan failure, hemodynamic instability, or severe acidosis (pH < 7.1).
- NIPPV can be used in COPD, cardiogenic pulmonary edema, immunocompromised patients, and obesity hypoventilation syndrome.
- Use CPAP if the primary problem is hypoxia (CHF).
- Use BiPAP if the primary problem is hypoventilation (COPD).
- If the patient requires transport or shows signs of deterioration (increased work of breathing, tachycardia, altered mentation, worsening ABG parameters), do not delay intubation.

Endotracheal Intubation and Ventilation

- Be aware that hypotension (etiology is multifactorial) is common after intubation; also consider the hemodynamic effects of induction agents (e.g., ketamine versus propofol).
  › If hypotension is persistent and life-threatening, consider air-trapping lesions or pneumothorax as a cause.
- In cases of high peak inspiratory pressure (> 35 cm H_2O), check the plateau pressure (Pplat).
  › **High Pplat:** This indicates decreased lung or chest wall compliance (pneumothorax, pulmonary edema, pneumonia, atelectasis).
  › **Low Pplat:** This indicates increased airway resistance (bronchospasm, mucus plug, kinked tubing).

MANAGEMENT OF HYPOXEMIA

- The target for PaO_2 is 55–80 mmHg, and for oxygen saturation is 88% to 92%.
- Improve oxygenation by increasing FIO_2 or PEEP.

- Consider starting with FIO_2 at 1.0, and wean FIO_2 as tolerated to a target FIO_2 of less than 0.6. If oxygenation is still suboptimal, increase PEEP until FIO_2 is less than 0.6, or Pplat is > 30 cm H_2O (above this pressure increases the risk of barotrauma).
- If raising PEEP resulted in no change or in worsened oxygenation, or if it raised $PaCO_2$, it means the lung is not recruitable and is overdistended, therefore decrease PEEP.

MANAGEMENT OF HYPERCAPNIA
- Improve ventilation by increasing tidal volume (V_T), respiration rate, or inspiratory pressure.
  › **VT:** The target is ≤ 6 mL/kg ideal body weight for lung-protective ventilation.
  › **Respiration rate:** Decrease inspiratory time, if needed.
  › **Inspiratory pressure:** The target is Pplat < 30 cm H_2O.
- Permissive hypercapnia may be needed in ARDS to ventilate patients with low V_T (in cases where pH < 7.15, increase the respiration rate).

MANAGEMENT OF SEVERE OBSTRUCTIVE ASTHMA OR COPD WITH HYPERCAPNIA
- Decreasing the respiration rate is the best way to increase expiratory time, which in the long run will improve ventilation.
- Expect hypercapnia and respiratory acidosis.
- Do not treat with bicarbonate because this will worsen acidosis.

MANAGEMENT OF ACUTE RESPIRATORY DISTRESS SYNDROME[7]
- Set a lower V_T target of 4–8 mL/kg ideal body weight and set lower inspiratory pressures (Pplat < 30 cm H_2O).
- Consider prone positioning for more than 12 hours/day in severe ARDS (PaO_2 or FIO_2 < 100).
- Consider higher PEEP and using recruitment manoeuvres in cases of moderate to severe ARDS.

Sepsis
These notes are in addition to the **general guide for all consultations** on page 1, and the **starting points for critical care consultations** at the beginning of this chapter.

Identification
Key information in the identification statement includes advanced directives, relevant comorbidities, and presentation.

Reason for Referral

An example of a reason for referral is worsening hypotension due to septic shock, with details about the reason for admission or circumstances leading to septic shock.

History of Present Illness

Determine the timing of blood cultures and antimicrobials: When were blood cultures last drawn? When were antimicrobials initiated?

Assess for general infectious symptoms: Ask about fevers, fatigue, chills, sweats, and rigors.

Assess for current symptoms suggestive of shock: Ask about altered mental status, hyperventilation, and reduced urine output.

Assess for localizing symptoms that may point to an infectious source:
› Check for symptoms related to the head, ears, eyes, nose, and throat, and skin and soft tissue infections.
› Check for cardiovascular, respiratory, GI, GU, and musculoskeletal symptoms.

Pay attention to other contributing or potential causes of shock: These include MI (cardiogenic) or massive PE (obstructive).

Check for current and recent lines and tubes.

Ask about recent surgery or hospitalization.

Ask about recent travel and sick contacts.

Past Medical History

- Determine the patient's infectious history to date, including previous positive cultures and their susceptibilities.
- Identify conditions that may cause immune compromise or predispose the patient to infections.

Past Surgical History

Ask about:
- recent surgeries (these may be sites of infection)
- implanted hardware, such as valves, joints, ventriculoperitoneal shunts, pacemakers, and vascular grafts

Medications

Ask about:
- past antimicrobial management
- immunocompromising medications

Allergies

Pay particular attention to antimicrobial allergies.

Family History
Look for predisposing factors for infection (e.g., primary immunodeficiency).

Social History
Follow the **general guide for all consultations** and the **starting points for critical care consultations.**

Code Status
Identify advanced directives, code status, and substitute decision makers, if applicable.

Physical Examination
Focus on identifying signs that point to an infectious source.

CNS: headache, decreased LOC, lowered GCS score, nuchal rigidity

Head, ears, eyes, nose, throat: swollen lymph nodes, erythematous tympanic membranes, pharyngeal exudates

Cardiovascular: mottled, warm and flushed skin; weak pulse; tachycardia; new murmurs; mechanical clicks indicating prosthetic valve; pedal edema

Pulmonary: tachypnea, diminished lung sounds, wheezes, crackles, dullness on percussion, purulent sputum

GI: ascites; distension; hepatosplenomegaly; signs of peritonitis such as abdominal tenderness and guarding

GU: costovertebral angle tenderness; suprapubic or adnexal tenderness

Musculoskeletal: exposed bone; crepitus; hot and swollen joints; pain out of proportion to visual inspection

Skin and soft tissue: ulcers; petechiae; bullae; tender localized erythema; purpura; purulent surgical sites
› Remember to inspect the patient's back.

Lines and tubes: associated purulence, tenderness, and/or surrounding erythema

Investigations
LABORATORY INVESTIGATIONS
Baseline labs: Order CBC with differential, extended electrolytes, urea, creatinine, CK, urinalysis, and glucose.

Venous blood gas and lactate: These are critical as guides to resuscitation.

Liver function and coagulation studies: Order AST, ALT, ALP, bilirubin, INR, and PTT.

D-dimer and fibrinogen: Pursue this in suspected DIC.

Troponin, BNP: Pursue this in the context of chest pain or abnormal ECG.

Central venous oxygen saturation: This can be useful in undifferentiated shock.

Corticotropin (ACTH) stimulation testing: Consider this in suspected adrenal insufficiency (undifferentiated distributive shock).

MICROBIOLOGY

Cultures: Order blood cultures (peripheral and in-situ lines), urine culture, and sputum culture.

Special tests: Consider tests for urine legionella antigen, viral PCR, and mycobacterial and fungal cultures.

Nasopharyngeal swabs: Test for COVID-19 and other viruses.

IMAGING

Chest x-ray: Pursue this for all patients.

CT or US: Pursue this for any suspected source of infection.

OTHER INVESTIGATIONS

12-lead ECG

LP: Pursue this in altered LOC.

Thoracentesis or paracentesis: Pursue this if pleural effusions or ascites are present.

Transesophageal echocardiogram: Pursue this for suspected endocarditis or sepsis-induced cardiomyopathy.

Impression and Plan

Begin with an identification statement and diagnosis, then describe: the source and treatment of the infection; initial management; further treatment; and additional considerations.

IDENTIFICATION AND DIAGNOSIS

Briefly summarize the patient's identifying information and presentation, and key findings indicating a diagnosis of sepsis and/or septic shock.[8]

- **Sepsis:** life-threatening organ dysfunction caused by dysregulated host response to infection
- **Sepsis clinically diagnosed with having both:**
  › suspected or documented infection based on history, physical examination, and investigations
  › at least 2 out of 3 qSOFA criteria (respiration rate at 22/minute or higher; systolic BP ≤ 100 mmHg; GCS at 13 or lower)

- **Septic shock:** sepsis with lactate measuring > 2 mmol/L, and a MAP < 65 mmHg, despite adequate fluid resuscitation (patients in this situation need vasopressors)

INFECTIOUS SOURCE, PATHOGENS, TREATMENT

Identify the suspected infectious source, suspected pathogens, whether the current antimicrobial regimen has adequate coverage considering host risk factors, and the plan for source control.

- Always consider easy-to-miss sources, such as necrotizing fasciitis, bacterial meningitis, and bowel ischemia.
- Always consider recent surgical-site infections.

GENERAL PRINCIPLES: INITIAL MANAGEMENT OF SEPSIS AND SEPTIC SHOCK

In the first hour[9]:

- Draw blood cultures, ideally prior to starting antibiotics.
- Start broad-spectrum antibiotics.
- Use balanced crystalloid IV fluids and frequently assess volume status.
- Measure lactate level and target resuscitation to normalize lactate.
- Use vasopressors to support a MAP ≥ 65 mmHg.

FURTHER MANAGEMENT

Consider organizing further management by system.[9,10]

Infectious Diseases Management

- Follow up on blood cultures: redraw every 48 hours until negative for 3 days.
- Ensure other necessary cultures are drawn.
- Continue broad-spectrum antibiotics until cultures and sensitivities can direct narrowing antibiotic choice.
- Address potential removal of existing lines and tubes.
- If relevant, consult surgery to address source control.

Cardiovascular Management

- Consider placement of an arterial line and central venous access.
- In the context of hypotension and/or lactate > 4 mmol/L, rapidly administer 30 mL/kg of crystalloid within the first 3 hours.
- The first-line vasopressor is norepinephrine 0.3–3 mcg/kg/min.
- Resuscitation goals include:
  › MAP ≥ 65 mmHg
  › urine output ≥ 0.5mL/kg/hour (possibly higher if oliguric)
  › lactate < 2 mmol/L or 10% reduction in first 6 hours
- For refractory hypotension, consider:
  › epinephrine or vasopressin
  › hydrocortisone (this is controversial): 50 mg IV every 6 hours
  › dobutamine (only if the patient is bradycardic)

Respiratory Management
See Respiratory Failure in this chapter for mechanical ventilation considerations with sepsis-induced ARDS.

Renal Management
See the **starting points for nephrology consultations** for dialysis criteria.

ADDITIONAL CONSIDERATIONS
- The target for glucose is < 10.0 mol/L.
- Consider infection control precautions.
- Ensure immunizations are up to date.

Traumatic Brain Injury and Elevated Intracranial Pressure

These notes are in addition to the **general guide for all consultations** on page 1, and the **starting points for critical care consultations** at the beginning of this chapter.

Identification
Key information in the identification statement includes the patient's functional status and the presence of pertinent neurological deficits.

Reason for Referral
The referral may seek to confirm TBI or elevated intracranial pressure and/or clarify appropriate management.

History of Present Illness[11]
Clarify the mechanism of injury.
Clarify the mode of transfer to hospital.
Clarify timelines and treatment: Establish the timeline of neurological assessments and treatment initiated in the ED.
Establish the time of the patient's last meal: This is relevant if the patient eventually requires surgery.
Determine CNS symptoms: Ask about seizure, confusion, amnesia (establish timeline), nausea and vomiting, photophobia, phonophobia, headache, and loss of vision or altered vision.
Look for spinal cord compression red flags: See sidebar.
Identify associated pain in the whole body: Use the OPQRST AAA mnemonic and specifically pursue pain from spine fractures, rib fractures, long bone fractures, and skull fractures.

Identify syncopal symptoms: Examples include blackouts, fainting, dizziness, and falls.

Identify signs of abdominal trauma: Ask about abdominal pain, bowel movements (regularity, change, last instance), hematemesis, and hemoptysis.

Identify signs of kidney injury: Ask about hematuria, dysuria, and urinary frequency and urgency.

Identify signs rhabdomyolysis: Ask about urine colour and body ache.

Clarify operative course: This is relevant for patients transferred to ICU for monitoring after a neurosurgical intervention.

||||||||||||||||||||||||||||||||||||||||||||||||||||||||||||||||||||||||||||||||||||||||||||||||||||||||||||||||||||||||||||||||||||||||||||||||||||

SPINAL CORD COMPRESSION RED FLAGS

Saddle anesthesia	Bowel incontinence
Urinary incontinence	

Past Medical History

- Obtain information from the patient and those accompanying the patient, and also by contacting the patient's primary care giver and/or specialist.
- Ask about:
  › **Seizures:** most recent, frequency, duration, antiepileptic history
  › **CNS abnormalities:** brain tumour, vascular abnormality, incidentaloma
  › **Previous cardiac history:**
    » **ACS:** onset, type (e.g., unstable angina, NSTEMI, STEMI)
    » **PCI:** stents and type of stents
    » **CABG:** number of grafts, medical management including anticoagulants
    » **Arrhythmia, CHF**
  › **Hematologic disorders:** bleeding disorders, thrombotic disease
  › **GI and renal disorders**

Past Surgical History

Take a detailed history of neurological, cardiac, abdominal, and renal surgeries.

Medications

Ask about:
- neurological medications (establish dose, route, and last dose), especially antiepileptics
- cardiac medications, including anticoagulants and antiplatelet agents

- diabetes medications, including sodium-glucose cotransporter-2 (SGLT2) inhibitors, glucagon-like peptide 1 (GLP 1) receptor agonists
- steroids

Allergies
Follow the **general guide for all consultations** and the **starting points for critical care consultations.**

Family History
Ask about:
- subarachnoid hemorrhage and other CNS abnormalities (tumour, vascular abnormality)
- CAD in first-degree male relatives younger than 55 and female relatives younger than 65

Social History
Ask about:
- alcohol use, recreational drug use, smoking
- baseline functional status

Code Status
Identify advanced directives, code status, and substitute decision makers, if applicable.

Physical Examination
Airway, breathing, circulation (ABCs): Check respiration rate, oxygen saturation, heart rate, and BP, and assess for skin mottling.

Primary and secondary survey: Look for:
› signs of hypoperfusion
› respiratory distress, abnormal respiratory sounds
› peripheral edema
› JVP position, chest deformities, scars, devices
› heart sounds, murmurs, peripheral pulses

POCUS: Assess volume status.

Neurological: Assess for:
› altered mental status[12]
  » Determine the patient's GCS score (note the time of the assessment) and reassess frequently.
  » In unresponsive patients, determine the Full Outline of UnResponsiveness (FOUR) score.
› scalp lacerations or open wounds
› basilar skull facture (periorbital ecchymosis; CSF otorrhea, rhinorrhea; postauricular ecchymosis)

> spinal cord injury (determine the American Spinal Injury Association score)
> signs of herniation or elevated intracranial pressure, including Cushing triad (hypertension, bradycardia, apnea); anisocoria and ipsilateral cranial nerve (CN) III palsy; coma; and motor decerebrate and decorticate posturing

Investigations

LABORATORY INVESTIGATIONS
CBC, metabolic panel, INR, PTT, troponin
ABG, urine, and serum toxicology screen
CK, serum osmolality

IMAGING
Do not send patients outside the ED for imaging until their airway, ventilation, and circulation have stabilized.
CT scan:
> This assesses for:
  » extradural hematoma (convex, lentiform appearance)
  » subdural hematoma (concave diffuse appearance)
  » midline shift (measure, if present)
  » minor hemorrhages, contusions
> Note that minor hemorrhages, contusions, and early ischemia may not be evident.
Cerebral angiography, MRI, and MRA

OTHER INVESTIGATIONS
ECG: This assesses for MI.
EEG: This assesses for seizure.

ADVANCED INVESTIGATIONS
Radionuclide blood flow scans
ICP monitoring
Brain tissue oxygenation monitoring (PbrO2)
Jugular venous oxygen saturation (SjO2)
Cerebral microdialysis
Somatosensory evoked potentials

Impression and Plan
Describe initial stabilization measures and goals: These typically include:
> airway control and rapid sequence intubation with spinal precautions
> large-bore IV access and a central venous catheter
> hemodynamic monitoring and an arterial catheter

› maintaining euvolemia
› avoiding hypotension (keeping systolic BP > 90 mmHg)
› avoiding hypoxia (the target PaO_2 is > 60 mmHg)
› ventilation to maintain $PaCO_2$ at 35–40 mmHg (consider sedation or paralysis if the patient hyperventilates)
› antibiotics for basal skull fractures
› avoiding fever and maintaining normothermia
› antiepileptic medication (in patients with seizure)
› intracranial pressure monitoring and management, if needed (consider mannitol, hypertonic saline in patients with acute signs of transtentorial herniation)[13]
› an early neurosurgical opinion
› frequent reassessment of GCS score and neurological vitals (do this every hour initially)

Describe the key features of the brain injury: These include the mechanism of injury (e.g., traumatic injury versus systemic causes of secondary injury), severity of the injury, and symptoms (e.g., shock, hypoxemia, hypercapnia, hyperpyrexia, seizure).

Describe reasons for admission: Examples include moderate to severe brain injury; concomitant trauma; hemodynamic and/or respiratory compromise; shock; need for monitoring of intracranial pressure; and organ failure.

Outline general management measures: These include:
› monitoring airway, breathing, and circulation
› cervical spine collar (all patients)
› pain control
› DVT prophylaxis with a sequential compression device or stockings
› prevention of stress gastric ulcers
› nosocomial infection prevention

List long-term considerations: These include:
› early enteral feeding (this may improve the outcome)
› hypoxemia and hypotension (these may worsen the outcome)
› safety measures and fall prevention
› complications, including hydrocephalus; central diabetes insipidus; SIADH; cerebral salt wasting; late pediatric TBI; seizures; motor, sensory, and/or psychological compromise; nosocomial infections (VAP, blood stream infection, UTI); chronic respiratory failure; DVT, PE; CHF
› discharge planning (e.g., rehabilitation medicine consultation, up-to-date immunizations, updating the patient's family doctor)

References

1. Kress J, Hall J. Approach to the patient with critical illness. In: Kasper D, Fauci A, Hauser S , et al, editors. Harrison's principles of internal medicine. 19th ed. New York; McGraw-Hill Education; 2015. p. 1729-36.
2. Van Es N, Kraaijpoel N, Klok F, et al. The original and simplified Wells rules and age-adjusted D-dimer testing to rule out pulmonary embolism: an individual patient data meta-analysis. J Thromb Haemost. 2017;15(4):678-84. doi: 10.1111/jth.13630
3. Mycyk M. Poisoning and drug overdose. In: Kasper D, Fauci A, Hauser S, et al, editors. Harrison's principles of internal medicine. 19th ed. New York; McGraw-Hill Education; 2015. p. 473e1-12.
4. Levine M, Brooks D, Truitt C, et al. Toxicology in the ICU part 1: general overview and approach to treatment. Chest. 2011;140(3):795-806. doi: 10.1378/chest.10-2548
5. Brooks D, Levine M, O'Connor A, et al. Toxicology in the ICU part 2: specific toxins." Chest. 2011;140(4):1072-85. doi: 10.1378/chest.10-2726
6. Hall J, Schmidt G, Kress J. Principles of critical care. 4th ed. New York: McGraw-Hill Education; 2015. 1392 p.
7. Fan E, Del Sorbo L, Goligher E, et al. An official American Thoracic Society/European Society of Intensive Care Medicine/Society of Critical Care Medicine clinical practice guideline: mechanical ventilation in adult patients with acute respiratory distress syndrome. Am J Respir Crit Care Med. 2017;195(9):1253-63. doi: 10.1164/rccm.201703-0548ST
8. Singer M, Deutschman C, Seymour C, et al. The Third International Consensus Definitions for Sepsis and Septic Shock (Sepsis-3). JAMA. 2016;315(8):801-10. doi: 10.1001/jama.2016.0287
9. Levy M, Evans L, Rhodes A. The Surviving Sepsis Campaign bundle: 2018 update. Critical Care Med. 2018;46(6):997-1000. doi: 10.1097/CCM.0000000000003199
10. Rhodes A, Evans L, Alhazzani W, et al. Surviving Sepsis Campaign: International Guidelines for Management of Sepsis and Septic Shock: 2016. Critical Care Med. 2017;45(3):486-552. doi: 10.1097/CCM.0000000000002255
11. Yunen J, Frendl G, Gasperino J, editors. The 5-minute ICU consult. Philadelphia: Lippincott Williams & Wilkins; 2012. 512 p.
12. Kasprowicz M, Burzynska M, Melcer T, et al. A comparison of the Full Outline of UnResponsiveness (FOUR) score and Glasgow Coma Score (GCS) in predictive modelling in traumatic brain injury. Brit J Neurosurg. 2016;30(2):211-20. doi: 10.3109/02688697.2016.1161173
13. Ellenbogen R, Sekhar L, Kitchen N. Principles of neurological surgery e-book. Amsterdam: Elsevier Health Sciences; 2017. 848 p.

5

Dermatology

Dr. Linghong Linda Zhou

REVIEWER
Dr. Sheila Au

Starting Points: Dermatology Consultations

These notes are in addition to the **general guide for all consultations** on page 1.

Identification

Key information in the identification statement includes pertinent past medical history.

Reason for Referral

The referral may seek to confirm a dermatological condition and/or clarify appropriate management.

History of Present Illness

Though it is occasionally true that dermatologists may need only to inspect the skin to diagnose the condition, this is frequently not the case: a detailed history is often very helpful.

QUESTIONS FOR ALL PATIENTS

- What is your skin concern?
- When did it start?
- What parts of the body does it affect?
- How has it evolved?
  › How has it changed, in size, shape, and/or colour?
  › How have individual lesions changed?
  › Has it gotten better or worse? What makes it better or worse?
- How does it affect you?

› Consider following up on specific symptoms (e.g., ask about pruritus, burning, tenderness, bleeding).

• What treatments have you used? Has the treatment helped?

FOCUSED FOLLOW-UP QUESTIONS

These can help narrow the differential diagnosis. They may vary based on the patient's preliminary history and your working differential diagnosis. For example:

• **Atopic dermatitis:** Ask about health-related behaviours, which are important to understand, including:
  › bathing and showering, and using hot versus lukewarm water
  › when and how often the patient moisturizes
  › impact on daily life (e.g., on sleep, memory, concentration)

• **Suspected skin cancer:** Ask about a history of skin cancer (clarify the type of skin cancer, location, patient age at diagnosis, and how it was treated), environmental exposures (e.g., UV radiation, PUVA, tanning beds, ionizing radiation, HPV, smoking), genetic risk factors (skin type, freckling, red hair, genetic syndromes), and immunosuppression (e.g., organ transplantation, leukemia).

REVIEW OF SYSTEMS

This varies based on your working differential diagnosis. For example:

• **Suspected connective tissue disease:** Ask about sun exposure history over the past weeks to months; alopecia; mouth ulcers; Raynaud phenomenon; arthralgias and arthritis; and fatigue.

• **Generalized morbilliform eruption:** The 2 most common causes are drugs and viruses: ask about medication use and infectious symptoms.

Past Medical History

• Start with previous dermatologic conditions, followed by all other pertinent medical conditions.

• In certain conditions, you may need to elicit specific information (e.g., in a patient with suspected herpes zoster, ask about a history of chickenpox and vaccination).

Past Surgical History

• Check for surgeries of dermatological relevance (e.g., prior scars that suggest previous biopsies or excisions for skin cancers).

• For conditions in particular areas of the body (e.g., the red leg), check for surgeries in that area (e.g., varicose vein surgeries if considering venous insufficiency).

Medications

• In addition to systemic medications, it is particularly important to ask about all topical medications.

- In suspected drug eruptions, look up the patient's "drug chart": this provides the clearest temporal relationships between prescribed medications and the onset of eruptions, and typically covers the previous 3 months.

Allergies

Follow the **general guide for all consultations.**

Family History

- Ask about dermatologic conditions in family members.
- Family history may play a role in, and help diagnose, certain dermatologic conditions. For example:
  › In a child with chronic, waxing and waning, pruritic red papules in flexural surfaces, ask about a family history of atopy.
  › In those with multiple café-au-lait macules, ask about a family history of neurofibromatosis.
  › Common conditions (e.g., psoriasis, vitiligo, androgenetic alopecia, autoimmune conditions, and skin cancer) have a strong genetic component.
  › In suspected skin cancer, ask about a family history of skin cancer.

Social History

Social history is particularly helpful in some disorders:
- **Certain chronic, severe, or treatment-resistant skin conditions:**
  › Examples include severe scabies infection or treatment-resistant seborrheic dermatitis.
  › Consider risk factors for both hereditary and acquired immunosuppression.
- **Suspected contact dermatitis:** A complete "skin exposure history" is vital:
  › Ask about occupational exposures, home exposures, and hobbies.
  › Keep in mind that patients can develop sensitivity to chronic contacts (sensitivities do not necessarily come from new exposures).

Physical Examination

See the **quick review of key terms** in this section.
Full body skin examination:
  › Perform this for new patients with undiagnosed skin conditions, for new eruptions on the body, and for concerns about malignancy.
  › Be thorough and systematic every time, so as not to miss any areas (e.g., examine each patient from head to toe): even if the eruption is on one part of the body, other findings on other body sites can provide valuable clues to the overall diagnosis.

» **Tip 1:** Before beginning, ensure sufficient lighting, appropriate draping, and patient comfort.

» **Tip 2:** Verbalize what part of the body you'd like to examine next as this helps patients feel more comfortable and also allows them to help you.

» **Tip 3:** Palpation is useful to assess lesions for texture, consistency (e.g., firmness, fluctuance), tenderness, and depth.

» **Tip 4:** The following tools may be helpful: ruler, penlight, magnifying lens, dermatoscope.

Examine the nails, hair, and mucous membranes: These can provide very helpful clues to the skin condition (e.g., proximal nail-fold capillary loop changes in suspected autoimmune rheumatic diseases; nail pitting and oil-drop changes in psoriasis; shallow nail pitting in alopecia areata; Wickham striae in lichen planus; scarring alopecia in discoid lupus erythematosus).

‖‖

PHYSICAL EXAMINATION: QUICK REVIEW OF KEY TERMS IN DERMATOLOGY

In general, pay more attention to the configuration and distribution of primary lesions than secondary lesions, because primary lesions tend to be the most reliable manifestation and characteristic of the disease.

Primary lesions: These arise de novo as a direct result of the disease process (for descriptors of individual lesions, see Figure 5.1 and Table 5.1).

Secondary lesions: These evolve from primary lesions, either by natural evolution of the lesion or as a result of the patient's activities (for descriptors of individual lesions, see Figure 5.1 and Table 5.1).

Configuration: This is the pattern in which lesions are arranged and how they relate to each other.

› Occasionally, a configuration may be characteristic for a disease.

› Configurations can be *grouped, serpiginous, annular, geographic, reticulated,* or *linear.*

› Linear configurations can be *dermatomal, segmental, blaschkoid,* or *sporotrichoid.*

›› Grouped (i.e., herpetiform) vesicles suggest HSV.

›› Serpiginous plaques suggest cutaneous larva migrans.

›› Linearly streaked vesicles suggest contact dermatitis.

›› Sporotrichoid papules or nodules suggest sporotrichosis or other infections.

Distribution: This is the anatomic location of lesions.
> › Many skin conditions have favoured distributions,
>   which can be an important clue.
> › Distribution includes regional preference (e.g., scalp, face,
>   genitalia), distribution pattern (e.g., extensor, flexural),
>   photodistribution, and unilateral versus bilateral distribution.
>> » A seborrheic distribution, including the head, neck,
>>   and upper trunk (areas rich in sebaceous glands), may
>>   indicate seborrheic dermatitis and acne vulgaris.
>> » A solely extensor distribution may point toward a
>>   diagnosis of psoriasis over nummular dermatitis
>>   when primary lesions appear similar.
>> » Lesions following Langer cleavage lines, or natural
>>   skin tension lines, may indicate pityriasis rosea
>>   or erythema dyschromicum perstans.
>> » The presence of photodistribution may indicate
>>   photodermatoses, including polymorphous light
>>   eruption, phototoxic drug reactions, or autoimmune
>>   connective tissue diseases (AI-CTDs).

FIGURE 5.1. PRIMARY SKIN LESIONS

Nonpalpable	Palpable (solid)	Palpable (fluid/pus filled)	Wheal
Macule (< 1 cm)	Papule (< 1 cm)	Vesicle (< 1 cm)	Telangiectases
Patch (> 1 cm)	Plaque (> 1 cm)	Bullae (> 1 cm)	Burrow
	Nodule (↑ depth, > 1 cm)	Cyst (sac with lining)	Comedo
	Tumour (↑ depth, > 2 cm)	Pustule (pus filled)	

Table 5.1. Secondary Skin Lesions

TERM	DESCRIPTION
Scale	Thickened stratum corneum that accumulates when production exceeds shedding Usually white or yellow Flakes easily
Crust	Dried serum and debris Usually darker, often yellow or brown Adherent but reveals a weeping base when removed (can be hemorrhagic)
Lichenification	Epidermal hyperplasia that presents as thickened skin with accentuated skin markings
Fissure	Linear break in the skin that can extend into the dermis Often painful
Atrophy	Depression and/or thinning Epidermal or dermal in location, leading to wrinkling and translucency, as well as possible indentation on palpation
Excoriation	Exogenous injury to part or all of the epidermis, often from scratching due to pruritus Linear or punctate
Erosion	Partial loss of epidermis (or epithelium) Generally nonscarring
Ulceration	Full-thickness loss of epidermis with extension into the dermis or even subcutaneous tissue Possibly scarring

Investigations

The most common investigations in dermatology are skin biopsy and swabs.

Skin biopsy: Clinicopathologic correlation may be the only way to confirm a diagnosis in certain conditions.

› Types of biopsy include: excisional biopsy (removal of entire lesion for study), incisional biopsy (e.g., punch biopsy: removal of a sample of a lesion, from 2–8 mm), and shave biopsy (removal of a superficial sample of a lesion and used only when superficial sampling is considered appropriate).

› Generally, samples are lesional and sent for hematoxylin and eosin (H&E) staining (transported via formalin). A key exception is primary blistering disorders, in which an additional perilesional sample is taken for DIF (transported via Michel's medium).

Swabs: Types include:
- › **Bacterial swab:** This can provide culture and sensitivity for bacteria (and *Candida*, but not deep fungi). An example of its use is in folliculitis (where pustules may need to be deroofed).
- › **Viral swab:** This is most commonly used to detect HSV and VZV. The swab is rubbed against a vesicle or crusted erosion, or a vesicle is deroofed and the contents and base are swabbed.
- › Note that swabs commonly undergo PCR, given its ease and rapidity; Tzanck smears are no longer readily performed.

Other investigations: These include laboratory investigations, microbiology, and imaging, and are considered on a case-by-case basis.

Impression and Plan

Start with a summary of the basics: State the patient's age, sex, pertinent past medical history, and current symptoms, and list pertinent findings from physical examination and investigations.
- › *For example:* "This is a 20-year-old male presenting with pruritic erythematous plaques with thick, silvery scale over the extensor surfaces, scalp, umbilicus, and gluteal cleft. Estimated BSA is approximately 5%."

State the most likely diagnosis and give a differential diagnosis: Also describe any proposed further investigations and the management approach.
- › *For example:* "This presentation is most in keeping with psoriasis, though the differential diagnosis includes nummular dermatitis and tinea corporis. We recommend initiating topical treatment of the eruption, with follow-up in 4 weeks for assessment of response to treatment."

Write topical prescriptions clearly: Remember to include: active ingredient, vehicle (e.g., ointment, cream, lotion, foam), concentration, directions, quantity, and number of refills.
- › *For example:* "Betamethasone valerate 0.1% cream, apply to affected areas on the arms twice a day until improved."
- › Note that, in general, 30 g of topical therapy will cover the average adult body in a 1-time application (see Table 5.2 for more guidelines).

Table 5.2. Quantities for Topical Prescriptions

AREA OF APPLICATION	GRAMS (TWICE DAILY FOR 7–10 DAYS)
Full body	450
Half body	250
Arms and legs	125
Hands and feet	25–30
Face	15–30

Drug (Morbilliform) Eruptions

These notes are in addition to the **general guide for all consultations** on page 1, and the **starting points for dermatology consultations** at the beginning of this chapter.

Identification

Follow **the general guide for all consultations** and the **starting points for dermatology consultations.**

Reason for Referral

The referral may seek assessment of maculopapular rash as a possible drug eruption, with a request to clarify the cause and rule out a severe cutaneous adverse reaction (SCAR).

History of Present Illness

Clarify why the patient has sought care: In an inpatient setting, why was the patient admitted to hospital?

Pursue the main differential diagnosis for morbilliform drug eruptions: The main differential is infection. Ask:

› When did the rash start?

› Where did it start and how has it progressed? (A typical drug eruption starts as papules on the trunk that coalesce into plaques on the trunk, with later involvement of the extremities.)

Assess for SCAR red flags: See sidebar.

Assess for other potential triggers: Examples include infectious symptoms and risk factors in a viral exanthem (e.g., fever, malaise, sore throat, sick contacts, travel).

Conduct a review of systems: Assess for musculoskeletal symptoms (arthralgias, myalgias), pulmonic symptoms (dyspnea, wheezing, stridor), cardiac symptoms (chest pain), GI symptoms (jaundice, abdomen pain), and CNS involvement.

‖‖‖

RED FLAGS FOR SEVERE CUTANEOUS ADVERSE REACTION (SCAR)

Symptoms of drug rash with eosinophilia and systemic symptoms (DRESS), Stevens-Johnson syndrome (SJS), and toxic epidural neurolysis (TEN) are red flags, including:

- fever (exanthematous drug eruptions typically have no fever)
- facial edema or erythema (DRESS)
- mucous membrane involvement (SJS/TEN), including photophobia, "grittiness," mouth pain, erosions and ulcers on the lips, dysuria
- skin tenderness or blistering (SJS/TEN)

Past Medical History

- Start with previous dermatologic conditions, followed by all other pertinent medical conditions.
- Check for medical conditions and patient characteristics that may predispose the patient to morbilliform drug eruptions (e.g., HIV infection, immunosuppression).
- Ask about prior organ or bone marrow transplantation (relevant to GVHD).

Past Surgical History

Follow the **general guide for all consultations** and the **starting points for dermatology consultations**.

Medications

- Ask about prescription, OTC, complementary, and as-needed drugs, including doses and routes.
  › Review all drugs ingested within 3 months prior to the rash onset.
  › Differentiate between new medications and those with prior sensitization.
  › A "drug chart" is essential and should be done for any suspected drug eruption, no matter how many or few medications the patient has taken.
- Ask specifically about high-risk medications such as: aromatic anticonvulsants (phenytoin, carbamazepine, phenobarbital), lamotrigine, NSAIDs, antibiotics (aminopenicillins, cephalosporins, sulfonamides), allopurinol, abacavir, and nevirapine.
  › Consider consulting references on drug reactions (e.g., Pubmed, Litt's Drug Eruption and Reaction Database, IBM Micromedex, pharmaceutical monographs).

- Ask about previous drug allergies and reactions: clarify the medications at issue, the time course, prior sensitizations (see Drug Eruptions in this chapter), and response to rechallenge.

Allergies
Follow the **general guide for all consultations.**

Family History
Ask about:
- underlying dermatologic conditions
- drug allergies, morbilliform eruptions, SCARs
- ethnicity and HLA-associated drug eruptions, such as:
  › Asian descent (HLA-B*1502: carbamazepine)
  › European descent (HLA-A*31:01: carbamazepine)
  › Han Chinese descent (HLA-B*1502: lamotrigine and phenytoin)
  › Han Chinese descent (HLA-B*58:01: allopurinol)

Social History
Ask about alcohol use, IV drug use, and travel and sexual history.

Physical Examination
Vital signs
General impression: Is the patient in acute distress? Does the patient look unwell?
Primary and secondary lesions: Assess their number and distribution.
  › Other relevant characteristics may include: monomorphous versus polymorphous; lesion character by site; and symmetrical versus asymmetrical.
  › Identify lesions as targetoid, vesicles, bullae, pustules, and/or papules.
  › Look for confluent erythema, skin necrosis, purpura, and dusky areas (seen in SJS/TEN).
Face: Check for edema and lymphadenopathy (seen in DRESS).
Mucous membranes: Typically, SJS/TEN presents with: mucous membrane involvement, including the eyes, oral mucosa, and genital mucosa; skin tenderness and sloughing; dusky bullae; and positive Nikolsky sign. Note, however, that early SJS/TEN may resemble a morbilliform drug eruption.

Investigations
Laboratory investigations: Order:
  › CBC with differential and peripheral smear (with particular attention to eosinophils, lymphocytes, platelets)

> creatinine, urea, urinalysis, liver function tests, CK, lipase, CRP, fasting glucose, thyrotropin (TSH), free T_4

Other investigations:
> Order PCR for HHV 6, HHV 7, EBV, and CMV.
> Typically, no other investigations are needed.
> Consider a skin biopsy in some cases: histopathology does not typically distinguish exanthematous drug eruptions from its differential diagnoses of early DRESS or viral exanthems, but may help differentiate it from early SJS/TEN and/or early acute generalized exanthematous pustulosis (AGEP).

Impression and Plan

DIFFERENTIAL DIAGNOSES

Consider morphologic clues: In addition to past medical history, current symptoms, and pertinent investigation findings, consider morphologic clues:
> **Wheals:** urticaria, serum sickness-like eruption, adult-onset Still disease, periodic fever syndromes
> **Confluent erythema:** early DRESS, SJS/TEN, AGEP, pustular psoriasis, viral exanthems
> **Facial edema:** DRESS, AGEP
> **Sterile pustules:** AGEP, pustular psoriasis, DRESS, Sweet syndrome
> **Blisters:** drug-induced autoimmune bullous disorders, erythema multiforme (EM), SJS/TEN, DRESS, Sweet syndrome, PLEVA, cutaneous lupus erythematosus, GVHD, viral exanthems
> **Purpura:** vasculitis, viral exanthems, viral hemorrhagic fevers, other infections (e.g., rickettsial disease, meningococcemia)
> **Mucosal involvement:** EM, SJS/TEN, viral exanthem, GVHD, drug-induced autoimmune bullous disorders, periodic fever syndromes
> **Flu-like symptoms:** viral exanthem, DRESS, SJS/TEN, EM, other infections (e.g., EBV, CMV, acute HIV exanthem, scarlet fever, rickettsial disease, meningococcemia, GVHD, TSS, secondary syphilis, adult Kawasaki disease)

Consult references:
> Examples include Litt's Drug Eruption and Reaction Database, Pubmed, IBM Micromedex, and pharmaceutical monographs.
> Consult a beta-lactam antibiotic cross-allergy chart for cross-reactivity with known allergens.
> **Tip:** Create a drug chart for any suspected drug-induced exanthem to see timelines in the most visual and easy-to-interpret way.

Use scoring systems: These include:
> RegiSCAR or J-SCAR diagnostic criteria for DRESS
> SCORTEN for SJS and TEN prognosis

PLAN

As part of your plan, consider the course of common drug eruptions:

- **Urticaria:** minutes to hours
- **AGEP:** less than 4 days
- **Exanthematous drug eruption:** 4 to 14 days
- **Early SJS/TEN:** 7 to 21 days
- **Fixed drug eruption (generalized):** 1 to 2 weeks
- **DRESS or drug-induced hypersensitivity syndrome:** 15 days to 3 months

Pruritus Secondary to Viral Exanthem

- Supportive care is usually sufficient.
- If the patient is particularly symptomatic with pruritus, consider prescribing topical corticosteroids.

Drug-Induced Pruritus

- Discontinue the culprit drug.
- Consider "treating through" when the suspected drug is of paramount importance to the patient's overall health, the eruption is **not** considered a SCAR (i.e., DRESS, SJS/TEN), and there is no satisfactory substitute drug.
- Supportive measures for a typical morbilliform drug eruption include topical corticosteroids and, much less commonly, systemic corticosteroids. Sedating antihistamines are not recommended; nonsedating antihistamines may be tried but may not be helpful.

Suspected Severe Cutaneous Adverse Reaction

- Consult a dermatologist and consider admission to a ward, ICU, or a burn care unit, depending on the clinical scenario.
- Treatment of SCARs is highly dependent on the specific entity and clinical scenario, but it can include supportive care, skin care, topical steroids, systemic steroids, cyclosporin, and anti-TNF agents.
  › Once stable, consider outpatient referral to a drug eruption or SCAR clinic for further workup (e.g., lymphocyte toxicity testing for DRESS, patch testing for AGEP).
  › In DRESS or SJS/TEN, first-degree family members should be counselled to avoid the culprit drug.

Generalized Pruritus

These notes are in addition to the **general guide for all consultations** on page 1, and the **starting points for dermatology consultations** at the beginning of this chapter.

Identification
Follow the **general guide for all consultations** and the **starting points for dermatology consultations.**

Reason for Referral
The referral may involve assessing for primary dermatoses or for systemic causes of pruritus.

History of Present Illness
Clarify why the patient has sought care: In an inpatient setting, why was the patient admitted to hospital?

Characterize the pruritus:
› When did the pruritus begin?
› Is there anywhere it is most severe?
› How has it progressed?
› Does anything make it better or worse?
› Does the patient scratch or manipulate the skin (i.e., use the hands or use tools)?
› Who has the patient previously seen for this condition? What investigations were done? What prior treatments were tried and how effective were they?
› Is there associated burning or pain? How does it affect the patient's quality of life (e.g., sleep, concentration, memory)?

Assess for risk factors: Ask about:
› **Primary dermatoses:** associated skin lesions (establish the location of the primary lesions and the overall distribution [e.g., papules, wheals])
› **Secondary lesions, in the absence of specific skin disease:** excoriations, erosions, ulcerations, lichenification
› **Sensory or sensorimotor neuropathy:** associated burning, pain, stinging, tingling, paresthesia, hypo- or hyperesthesia, muscle weakness
› **CNS lesions:** motor deficits
› **Malignancies, including hematologic malignancies:** fever, unexplained weight loss, fatigue, night sweats, lymphadenopathy
› **HIV infection:** fever, unexplained weight loss, fatigue, night sweats
› **Liver and kidney disease:** nausea, anorexia, malaise, fatigue, jaundice, weight loss, edema
› **Endocrine disease:** diabetes (polyuria, polydipsia, polyphagia), thyroid disease (fatigue, cold sensitivity, constipation, dry skin, weight loss or gain, puffy face, hoarseness, muscle weakness)
› **Carcinoid syndrome:** flushing, diarrhea

Conduct a review of systems: Assess for:
> **Scabies, lice, other infestations:** close contacts who are similarly pruritic; residing in a nursing home or other close-contact living situation; "burrows" in interdigital spaces, wrists, ankles, nipples, scrotal nodules in men (characteristic for scabies)
>> **Tip:** In general, scabies does not involve the head and neck, except in children and immunocompromised adults.
> **Bullous pemphigoid:** severe pruritus, dermatitis, or urticarial plaques for weeks to months before tense blisters form
> **Contact dermatitis:** skin exposures (consider a skin exposure history if an exogenous source is suspected)
> **Xerosis:** pruritus that is worse with dry, cold weather, and worse with long, hot baths; lack of emollient use
> **Constitutional symptoms:** fever, chills, malaise, night sweats, unintentional weight loss, lymphadenopathy, specific malignancy screening

Past Medical History
Ask about:
- prior dermatologic conditions, especially those that may cause itch (e.g., dermatitis, psoriasis, lichen planus, dermatitis herpetiformis, id reaction)
- kidney disease, liver disease, diabetes mellitus, thyroid disease, HIV infection, and malignancy (especially hematologic)
- celiac disease (which is associated with dermatitis herpetiformis, but may be asymptomatic)
- psychiatric history if relevant (e.g., OCD, delusions of parasitosis, substance abuse)

Past Surgical History
Follow the **general guide for all consultations** and the **starting points for dermatology consultations**.

Medications
Ask about:
- prescription, OTC, complementary, and as-needed drugs, including doses and routes
- topical treatments, including emollients and moisturizers
- drugs that may contribute to pruritus, including NSAIDs and opiates

Allergies
Follow the **general guide for all consultations**.

Family History

Ask about:

- cutaneous conditions (e.g., dermatitides [atopy], psoriasis, lichen planus)
- systemic conditions, including kidney disease, liver disease, diabetes mellitus, thyroid disease, HIV infection, malignancy (especially hematologic), and psychiatric history

Social History

Ask about:

- alcohol use, IV drug use, use of substances (e.g., opioids)
- travel and sexual history
- sick contacts, contact with day cares, crowded living conditions, contact sports, poor nutrition, stress

Physical Examination

Vital signs

General impression: Is the patient in acute distress? Does the patient appear unwell?

Primary and secondary lesions: Assess their number, configuration, and distribution, including:
  › thin, irregular "burrows" or tracks in interdigital spaces and other body folds, including scrotal nodules
  › wheals suggestive of urticarial dermatoses
  › ill-defined or well-defined erythematous plaques with scale or crust (assess plaque characteristics [e.g., fine white scale versus thick yellow greasy scale])
  › vesicles or blisters suggestive of an immunobullous condition
  › jaundice, scleral icterus

Signs of potential scratching: These include:
  › excoriations, erosions, ulcerations
  › lichenification
  › dome-shaped nodules with secondary changes of scale and crust (i.e., prurigo nodules)
  › linear welts (e.g., dermatographism)

Investigations

Order investigations on a case-by-case basis, and consider them especially in the context of pruritus with no primary skin lesions. Depending on the working differential diagnoses, no investigations may be needed.

Laboratory investigations: CBC, renal and liver function tests, fasting glucose, HbA_{1c}, iron panel (iron, ferritin, TIBC), thyrotropin (TSH), ESR or CRP, urinalysis, protein electrophoresis (serum or urine)

Skin biopsy: 2 samples total for H&E staining and DIF (e.g., when assessing for immunobullous disorders)

Age-appropriate malignancy screening: as appropriate (e.g., chest x-ray, abdominal US, serum tumour markers, stool exams for occult blood)

Impression and Plan

DIFFERENTIAL DIAGNOSES

Primary dermatoses: Patients have evident primary lesions: these manifest in a broad range of conditions including eczematous, papulosquamous, urticarial, immunobullous, and connective tissue diseases; photodermatoses; and drug eruptions.

Other: Patients do not have primary lesions, only secondary lesions. Consider:

› **Dermatographism:** Primary lesions may not be seen unless the skin is scratched.

› **Infection and infestations:** This includes scabies and pediculosis.

› **Renal pruritus:** This is particularly relevant in patients with advanced CKD or those requiring dialysis.

› **Liver disease:** This includes both extrahepatic and intrahepatic causes.

› **Diabetes:** This classically presents with genital pruritus or is accompanied by neuropathy.

› **Thyroid disease:** Lesions are more commonly due to hyperthyroidism, but may also be related to hypothyroidism and hypoparathyroidism.

› **HIV infection:** This may predispose patients to conditions such as seborrheic dermatitis, eosinophilic folliculitis, and pruritic papular eruptions.

› **Malignancy and hematologic causes:** These include paraneoplastic syndromes, Hodgkin lymphoma, polycythemia vera, and iron deficiency.

› **Psychiatric causes:** These include OCD, delusions of parasitosis, and substance abuse.

TREATMENT

Treat the underlying condition. For example:

• **Scabies:**

› Prescribe permethrin 5% lotion over the entire body, which the patient should wash off after 8 to 14 hours. The patient should perform this treatment twice: at 0 days and 7 days.

› Prescribe oral ivermectin in recalcitrant cases.

• **Dermatographism:** Prescribe nonsedating second-generation H1 antihistamines (you can titrate these up to 4 times standard dosing).

• **Renal pruritus:** Examples of treatments include topical emollients, topical corticosteroids, phototherapy, and gabapentin.

The Red Face

These notes are in addition to the **general guide for all consultations** on page 1, and the **starting points for dermatology consultations** at the beginning of this chapter.

Identification

Follow the **general guide for all consultations** and the **starting points for dermatology consultations**.

Reason for Referral

The referral will seek assessment for the cause of the red face (e.g., "please assess for autoimmune connective tissue disease") and/or guidance on appropriate management.

History of Present Illness

Clarify why the patient has sought care: In an inpatient setting, why was the patient admitted to hospital?

Characterize the facial eruption:
› Establish the features of the primary lesion (e.g., erythematous papule, plaque) and secondary lesions (e.g., scale, crust, excoriations, erosions).
› Establish the distribution and number of lesions.
› Clarify:
  » when it started
  » how it has progressed
  » whether it comes and goes
  » how it affects the patient (e.g., asymptomatic, pruritus, tenderness, burning, pain)
  » what makes it better or worse
  » who the patient has seen about the condition
  » investigations undertaken
  » treatments tried and their effect

Conduct a review of systems:
› **Rosacea:** This is transient flushing with or without edema and/or pimple-like bumps on the cheeks, forehead, and nose, and with or without ocular involvement (e.g., blepharitis with or without rhinophyma). Common triggers include alcohol, hot or spicy foods and beverages, exercise, and weather (heat, cold, wind).
› **Seborrheic dermatitis:** This features erythematous plaques with yellow, greasy scale, which may be worse with immunosuppression (e.g., HIV infection) and neurologic conditions (e.g., Parkinson disease, MS).
› **Psoriasis:** Facial psoriasis often affects seborrheic sites and can also affect other body sites, including extensor surfaces, the umbilicus,

the gluteal cleft, and nails. It can also lead to joint pain and swelling, enthesitis, dactylitis, and inflammatory back pain.

› **Contact dermatitis:** Consider a skin exposure history with particular attention to distribution of the eruption.

› **Polymorphous light eruption:** This features photosensitivity, acute sun exposure, and seasonal fluctuation (worse every spring with improvement over the rest of the year).

› **Rheumatologic screen:** Examples of rheumatologic-associated skin conditions include dermatomyositis and cutaneous lupus. Ask about oral ulcers, alopecia, arthralgias, myalgias, constitutional symptoms, Raynaud phenomenon, proximal muscle weakness, and organ-specific issues (i.e., respiratory, cardiovascular, renal).

  » **Tip:** Malar rash (butterfly rash) is associated with active SLE. It is generally fixed and infiltrated, and may weep or crust. Rosacea is the most common mimicker, but rosacea is usually chronic and not associated with systemic disease.

› **Infection (erysipelas):** This features tender erythematous dermal plaques, immunocompromised states, and local trauma.

› **Periorificial dermatitis:** This features multiple monomorphous papules and micropustules around the eyes, eyelids, and mouth. It is commonly associated with chronic use of topical corticosteroids, and may sting and burn.

› **Acne:** This features papules, pustules, and comedones, with or without nodules, cysts, and scarring, involving the forehead, nose, chin, and cheeks, and possibly the upper chest and back. It spares the eyelids.

› **Constitutional symptoms:** Examples include fever, chills, malaise, night sweats, and unintentional weight loss. Consider specific malignancy screening.

› **Other cutaneous involvement:** Ask about hair and nail changes (e.g., scarring alopecia, nail-fold telangiectases, nail dystrophy, oral mucosal ulcers).

Past Medical History

Ask about:

• prior dermatologic conditions (e.g., dermatitis, rosacea, psoriasis, AI-CTDs, infection)
• immunosuppression and neurologic conditions (e.g., Parkinson disease, recent infections, autoimmune diseases, arthritis, metabolic syndromes, psychiatric conditions)

Past Surgical History

Follow the **general guide for all consultations** and the **starting points for dermatology consultations.**

Medications

Ask about:

- prescription, OTC, complementary, and as-needed drugs, including doses and routes
- topical treatments (e.g., moisturizers, topical corticosteroids, topical calcineurin inhibitors)
- medications that increase photosensitivity (e.g., methotrexate, tetracycline antibiotics, antifungals)
- other systemic medications such as prednisone

Allergies

Follow the **general guide for all consultations.**

Family History

Ask about:

- cutaneous conditions (e.g., rosacea, dermatitides [including atopy], psoriasis)
- rheumatologic conditions (e.g., AI-CTDs or other autoimmune diseases)

Social History

Ask about:

- alcohol use, IV drug use
- travel and sexual history
- sick contacts, contact with day cares, crowded living conditions, contact sports, poor nutrition, stress

Physical Examination

Vital signs

General impression: Is the patient in acute distress? Does the patient look unwell?

Primary and secondary lesions: Assess:

- › number
- › distribution (e.g., central or diffuse face; photodistribution [sparing or involving the nasolabial folds])
- › presence and characteristics of scale or crust (e.g., thick, yellow, greasy scale in seborrheic dermatitis)
- › presence of comedones (acne vulgaris)

Disease-specific features: Examples include:

- › **Rosacea:** facial edema or erythema, ocular involvement (e.g., blepharitis), rhinophyma
- › **Dermatomyositis:** heliotrope rash, Gottron papules, Gottron sign, nonscarring alopecia, nail-fold changes (e.g., ragged cuticles,

cuticular hypertrophy, nail-fold telangiectases; facial erythema; V-sign, shawl sign, holster sign; flagellate erythema; extracutaneous signs such as proximal muscle weakness, dysphagia)

› **Cutaneous lupus erythematosus:** violaceous facial plaques (acute cutaneous lupus, tumid lupus), discoid plaques (i.e., atrophy, scarring, involvement of the conchal bowls of the ears, scarring alopecia), oral ulcers, Raynaud phenomenon, acrocyanosis, diffuse nonscarring alopecia, livedo reticularis, palmar erythema, nail-fold telangiectases, purpura

Investigations

Order investigations on a case-by-case basis. Depending on the working differential diagnoses, no investigations may be needed.

Suspected Autoimmune Connective Tissue Disease

Laboratory investigations: Consider these in most cases, including CBC with differential; creatinine, urea; urinalysis and/or urine albumin-to-creatinine ratio; ALT; ANA; extractable nuclear antigen; C3 and/or C4; and CRP.

Other investigations: Also consider CK; EMG; imaging (MRI or US); pulmonary function test with carbon monoxide diffusion; CT of the chest; ECG; echocardiogram and/or Holter monitor; barium swallow and/or manometry; and antiphospholipid antibody profile.

Skin biopsy: In suspected cutaneous lupus, provide 2 samples total for H&E staining and DIF.

Age-appropriate malignancy screening

Suspected infection

Culture and sensitivity

Blood cultures (2)

Impression and Plan

DIFFERENTIAL DIAGNOSES

Consider morphologic and other clues:

- **Central face with no scale:** rosacea (erythrotelangiectatic type)
- **Central face with scale:** seborrheic dermatitis
- **Erythematous plaques with scale:** seborrheic dermatitis, atopic dermatitis, contact dermatitis, psoriasis
- **Papulopustules:** acne vulgaris, rosacea (papulopustular type), periorificial dermatitis
- **Photodistributed violaceous papules and plaques, with or without scale:** cutaneous lupus erythematosus, dermatomyositis
- **Tender erythematous plaques in an acutely unwell patient:** erysipelas

TREATMENT

Treat the underlying condition. For example:

- **Seborrheic dermatitis:** Prescribe a combination of a mild topical corticosteroid and a topical antifungal cream or shampoo.
- **Rosacea:** Counsel trigger avoidance, gentle facial skin care, and protection from sunlight, and prescribe topical agents (e.g., azelaic acid, metronidazole, ivermectin, sodium sulfacetamide, erythromycin, clindamycin) and/or systemic agents (e.g., doxycycline, minocycline, tetracycline, azithromycin, isotretinoin).
- **Cutaneous lupus erythematosus:** Counsel protection from sunlight and smoking cessation, and prescribe topical or intralesional corticosteroids, topical calcineurin inhibitors, antimalarials (e.g., hydroxychloroquine), and/or other systemic agents (e.g., systemic corticosteroids, steroid-sparing immunosuppressants).

The Red Leg

These notes are in addition to the **general guide for all consultations** on page 1, and the **starting points for dermatology consultations** at the beginning of this chapter.

Identification

Follow the **general guide for all consultations** and the **starting points for dermatology consultations**.

Reason for Referral

The referral will seek assessment for the cause of the red leg (e.g., "the patient has bilateral, tender, red legs: please assess for cellulitis") and/or guidance on appropriate management.

History of Present Illness

Clarify why the patient has sought care: In an inpatient setting, why was the patient admitted to hospital?

Characterize the eruption on the legs:
  › What did the patient notice (e.g., papules, plaques, patches, vesicles, bullae)?
  › Was the redness bilateral or unilateral? (Stasis dermatitis is often bilateral; cellulitis is rarely bilateral.)
  › When and where did it start and how has it progressed?
  › How does it affect the patient? (Dermatitis is pruritic; cellulitis and acute lipodermatosclerosis are tender and burning.)
  › What makes it better?

> What makes it worse (e.g., water exposure; hot showers; dry weather; aggravating contacts; prolonged standing; rubbing or scratching)?
> Who has the patient previously seen for this condition? What investigations were done? What prior treatments were tried and how effective were they?

Assess for risk factors of working diagnoses:
> **Diagnosis of prior conditions:** Examples include stasis dermatitis, atopic dermatitis, asteatotic dermatitis, contact dermatitis, psoriasis, lichen planus, lichen simplex, tinea infections, cellulitis, panniculitis, vasculitis, necrobiosis lipoidica, and pretibial myxedema.
> **Prior dermatology visits:** Ask about skin biopsies and patch testing.
> **Stasis dermatitis:** Ask about varicose veins, medial leg ulcers, chronic swelling, aggravating topical medications (superimposed allergic contact dermatitis), and symptoms that are worse with heat and prolonged standing.
> **Other eczematous and papulosquamous conditions:** Ask about personal or family history of atopy, aggravating topical or systemic medications, prior allergens, and chronic rubbing and/or scratching (itch-scratch-itch cycle).
> **Infection:** Ask about fever, malaise, local trauma, ulcers and/or wounds, venous insufficiency, impaired lymphatics, chronic leg edema, tinea pedis, lymphadenopathy, MRSA risks (e.g., IV drug use; incarceration; men who have sex with men; work in health care or prolonged hospital stay), close contacts with similar findings and/or pruritus, and salt or fresh water exposures (e.g., from water sports).

Conduct a review of systems:
> **Venous stasis or insufficiency:** Ask about varicose veins; chronic leg swelling; venous leg ulcers; history of thrombosis and/or cellulitis; and aching that is worse with prolonged standing and exposure to hot water, better with leg elevation and use of compression socks or stockings.
> **Asteatotic dermatitis:** Ask about a "dry riverbed" appearance in superficial fissuring of the skin; pruritic, red patches, typically on the lower extremities; and common triggers (low humidity, excessive bathing, poor moisturization).
> **Psoriasis:** Ask about red, scaly papules and plaques in extensor distribution; characteristic nail changes; inflammatory joint pain; triggers, including recent infections (e.g., strep throat), hypercalcemia, beta-blockers, lithium, NSAIDs, steroids, anti-TNFs, and stress; and associated comorbidities (e.g., metabolic syndrome).
> **Infectious:** Ask about immune-system compromise, constitutional symptoms, pain, fever, lymphadenopathy, and previous episodes.

> **Panniculitis (including acute lipodermatosclerosis):** Ask about constitutional symptoms, infectious symptoms (e.g., cough; GI symptoms such as abdominal pain; nausea and vomiting; diarrhea; constipation), new medications, pregnancy, TB contacts, and travel history.
> **Vasculitis:** Ask about constitutional symptoms, recent URTI, ENT symptoms (e.g., sore throat; nasal, sinus, or ear pain; dyspnea; wheezing; hemoptysis), abdominal pain, diarrhea, and neurologic symptoms (e.g., foot or wrist drop).
> **Pretibial myxedema:** Screen for symptoms of hyperthyroidism (Graves disease): palpitations, tremors, weight loss, and hyperhidrosis.
> **Necrobiosis lipoidica:** Ask about long-standing erythematous plaques on the legs (these are typical), which may be associated with diabetes mellitus and thyroid disease, and may ulcerate with minor trauma.

Past Medical History
Ask about:
- **Atopy:** dermatitis, asthma, allergic rhinitis
- **Other cutaneous dermatoses or risk factors:** psoriasis, ichthyosis, hypercalcemia, HBV, HCV, GVHD, organ transplantation, hypothyroidism
- **Venous stasis:** venous insufficiency, varicose veins, DVT, lymphedema, obesity
- **Infection:** prior cellulitis (clarify when it occurred, the organism involved, treatment received), immune-system compromise (e.g., diabetes, tinea, HIV infection)
- **Panniculitis:** sarcoidosis, inflammatory bowel disease, Behçet syndrome, neoplasms, pregnancy, recent infections (and medications)
- **Vasculitis:** inflammatory disorders, infections, malignancy, drugs (e.g., penicillin, sulfa drugs, allopurinol, phenytoin)
- **Necrobiosis lipoidica:** diabetes, dyslipidemia, thyroid disease, hypertension, obesity
- **Pretibial myxedema:** hyperthyroidism (e.g., Graves disease)
- **Systemic causes of pruritus:** kidney or liver disease; endocrine disorders (e.g., diabetes or thyroid disease, hematologic malignancies)

Past Surgical History
Follow the **general guide for all consultations** and the **starting points for dermatology consultations.**

Medications
- Ask about prescription, OTC, complementary, and as-needed drugs, including doses and routes.

- As indicated by the differential diagnoses, consider specifically asking about moisturizers, topical or systemic corticosteroids, retinoid use, diuretics, beta-blockers, lithium, TNF-α inhibitors, gold, quinine, quinidine, ACEIs, NSAIDs, OCs, and antibiotics.

Allergies
Follow the **general guide for all consultations.**

Family History
Ask about:
- underlying dermatologic conditions, including atopy, psoriasis, and ichthyosis
- diabetes, thyroid disorders, venous and arterial disorders, and lymphedema

Social History
- Ask about:
  > smoking, alcohol use, IV drug use, and cocaine use (relevant to levamisole-induced vasculitis)
  > living conditions (sick contacts, fomites, prolonged exposure to cold weather)
  > occupation (e.g., Does it involve prolonged standing? Does it provide insurance for medications and compression stockings?)
- If contact dermatitis is suspected, take a skin exposure history (keep in mind that chronic topical exposures may be culprits, not just new exposures).

Physical Examination
Vital signs
General impression: Note any acute distress.
Skin: Note the primary lesions, any secondary lesions, and their distribution and configuration. For example:
  > **Eczematous and papulosquamous:** erythematous papules and plaques with scale, lichenification, fissures, excoriations; localized swelling or blistering; a distribution predominantly involving flexural areas, as opposed to a diffuse distribution, or a distribution suggesting an exogenous cause (e.g., linear); ill-defined versus well-defined
  > **Venous stasis or insufficiency:** bilateral involvement, circumferential tender erythema of the calf, hyperpigmentation (hemosiderin deposits), varicosities, atrophie blanche, ulcers in the "gaiter" area, lipodermatosclerosis ("inverted champagne bottle" shape of the leg)
  > **Cellulitis:** unilateral, lymphatic streaking; edematous plaques (tight, shiny skin); secondary yellow crust (impetiginization); purulence; pain

> **Panniculitis:** tender, firm, deep discrete erythematous nodules; minimal to no secondary changes
> **Pretibial myxedema:** erythematous, indurated plaques or nodules; peau d'orange texture; bilateral distribution on pretibial shins
> **Necrobiosis lipoidica:** erythematous plaques with a central, shiny, atrophic, yellow hue and telangiectases; ulceration
> **Small-vessel vasculitis or vasculopathy:** purpura (nonblanchable papules and patches), livedo reticularis, ulcers, bilateral distribution, and other involvement (especially gravity-dependent areas)

Palpation: Assess for lymphadenopathy, bilateral lower extremity pulses, tenderness, warmth, edema, crepitus, and fluctuance.

Investigations

GENERAL APPROACH

- Order investigations on a case-by-case basis.
- In many cases, no investigations are necessary.
- Note that venous insufficiency is very common and is a clinical diagnosis.

LABORATORY INVESTIGATIONS

Infection: Order CBC, creatinine, urea, urinalysis, and CRP.

Vasculitis: Order CBC, creatinine, urea, urinalysis, throat swab. Consider CRP, ANA, extractable nuclear antigen, antineutrophil cytoplasmic antibodies, C3, and C4.

Other: Consider a fasting glucose, HbA_{1c}, thyrotropin (TSH), α_1-antitrypsin levels, and antistreptolysin O titer.

MICROBIOLOGY

Consider blood cultures (2) and tissue culture.

IMAGING

Consider ABI (this is abnormal in arterial insufficiency).

SKIN BIOPSY

Pursue this to confirm a diagnosis of, for example, vasculitis or panniculitis.

PATCH TESTING

Pursue this in suspected allergic contact dermatitis.

Impression and Plan

DIFFERENTIAL DIAGNOSIS

Consider morphologic and other clues to reach a diagnosis:
- **Ill-defined erythematous plaques with scale, and with or without hyperpigmentation:** eczematous (e.g., venous stasis or insufficiency

[hyperpigmentation]); atopic dermatitis (predominantly in flexures); asteatotic dermatitis (cracked "dry riverbed" appearance); contact dermatitis; lichen simplex chronicus

- **Well-demarcated erythematous plaques, usually with thick silvery scale:** psoriasis
- **Ill-defined, erythematous, warm, tender plaques, with systemic signs and symptoms (fever, elevated WBC, elevated CRP) and risk factors:** cellulitis, other infections
- **Multiple, erythematous, tender nodules with or without ulceration:** panniculitis
- **Purpuric lesions:** vasculitis, cellulitis, other infections (e.g., meningococcemia, rickettsial), calciphylaxis (retiform purpura)
- **Other:** pretibial myxedema, necrobiosis lipoidica, necrotizing fasciitis (see chapter 10: Infectious Diseases)

TREATMENT

Treat the underlying condition. For example, in venous (stasis) dermatitis, consider weight management, calf-muscle pump strengthening, leg elevation, topical corticosteroids, and compression socks or stockings.

6

Endocrinology and Metabolism

Dr. Ahsen Chaudhry
Dr. Jusung Hwang
Dr. Alexa Clark
Dr. Sadiq Juma Al Lawati

REVIEWER
Dr. Jordanna Kapeluto

Starting Points: Endocrinology Consultations

These notes are in addition to the **general guide for all consultations** on page 1.

Identification
Follow the general guide for all consultations.

Reason for Referral
The referral may seek to confirm an endocrine disorder and/or clarify appropriate management.

History of Present Illness
Clarify why the patient has sought care: In an inpatient setting, why was the patient admitted to hospital?

Clarify the course of events: What major treatments and procedures has the patient had?

Characterize the presenting symptoms: Apply the mnemonic OPQRST AAA to identify clinical symptoms and signs of hormone deficiency, excess, or axis dysregulation.

Identify possible causes: Ask about risk factors, pertinent positives and negatives, and precipitating events.

Determine the consequences of the presenting illness: How does it affect the patient's functioning and comorbidities? What impacts might it have on the development of future conditions (e.g., long-standing diabetes mellitus resulting in impaired vision)?

Perform a full endocrine review of systems:

› **General:** Ask about fevers; chills; recent weight change (quantify amount, rate of loss or gain, and intentional versus unintentional); heat or cold intolerance; changes in clothing, glove, and shoe size; fatigue; and changes in mood, anxiety, and sleep patterns.

› **Head, ears, eyes, nose, throat:** Ask about headache; vision changes (diplopia, decreased acuity, visual field defects, decreased nighttime vision); use of glasses or contact lenses; lumps or masses in the neck; and recent URTI symptoms (rhinorrhea, sore throat, otalgia).

› **Cardiovascular:** Ask about angina; dyspnea on exertion; palpitations; orthopnea; paroxysmal nocturnal dyspnea; peripheral edema; extremity claudication; easy bruising or bleeding; and wounds or ulcers in the extremities.

› **Respiratory:** Ask about dyspnea, cough, sputum, hemoptysis, and wheezing.

› **Abdominal, GI:** Ask about appetite changes; dysphagia; changes in bowel habits; abdominal pain; jaundice; and pruritus.

› **GU:** Ask about polyuria, nocturia, hematuria, incontinence, frothy urine, UTI symptoms, renal colic, and changes in menstruation.

› **Neurological:** Ask about changes or loss in sensation; weakness; paralysis; tremors; and seizures.

Past Medical History

Clarify the patient's endocrine history:

› Identify endocrine comorbidities.

› In patients with a history of hormone excess or deficiency, determine the level of the defect (e.g., primary versus secondary versus tertiary), the date and result of any hormone axis testing (e.g., cosyntropin [ACTH] stimulation test for adrenal insufficiency), and dosages of relevant medications.

Clarify comorbidities: The most important are cardiovascular, renal, GI, and autoimmune conditions, and malignancies.

Past Surgical History

Ask about:

• thyroid or abdominal surgery
• neurosurgical interventions
• organ transplantation history

Medications

- Ask about current medications:
  - › For insulin, determine types, doses, timing, and recent adjustments.
  - › For hormone replacement regimens, determine doses, patient weight, and recent adjustments.
- When interpreting hormone assays, stimulation, or inhibition tests, search for concomitant use of medications that will interfere with the assay or test.
- Pay particular attention to immunosuppressants and steroids: establish dose, route of administration, and duration.

Allergies

Follow the **general guide for all consultations.**

Family History

Ask about:
- endocrine diseases
- autoimmune disorders
- malignancies
- features of MEN syndrome (if the patient has a tumour associated with MEN syndrome), including pituitary tumours, pancreatic or neuroendocrine tumours, pheochromocytoma, parathyroid hyperplasia, hypercalcemia, medullary thyroid carcinoma, mucosal neuroma

Social History

Ask about:
- ethnic background
- alcohol use, recreational drug use, smoking
- occupation
- factors affecting the patient's ability to adhere to, or pay for, medications (e.g., financial situation and drug coverage)

Physical Examination

Vital signs: Obtain the patient's temperature, heart rate, BP, orthostatic vitals, and oxygen saturation.

Body size: Determine the patient's weight, height, BMI, and body habitus.

General impression: Assess for level of consciousness, orientation, and signs of distress, anxiety, and diaphoresis.

Head, ears, nose, throat: Perform a thyroid examination (including an examination for Graves ophthalmopathy), and assess for the presence of mucosal neuromas and/or marfanoid features (associated with MEN-2B).

Cardiovascular and respiratory: Perform a standard examination with focused attention for evidence of HF, arrhythmias, and right-sided murmurs (on suspicion of carcinoid syndrome).

Abdominal: Perform a standard abdominal examination.

Integumentary: Look for changes in skin pigmentation, skin tags, abdominal striae, and acanthosis nigricans.

Neurological: Perform a standard screening exam with focused attention for visual field deficits, peripheral neuropathy, mononeuropathy, and tremors.

Investigations

Obtain the patient's most recent capillary blood glucose (CBG) level.

LABORATORY INVESTIGATIONS

CBC and differential

Electrolytes, Mg, Ca, PO_4, urea, creatinine

Liver enzymes and liver function tests

HbA_{1c}

Urinalysis, urine microscopy, urine albumin-to-creatinine ratio

ECG

Other: investigations relevant to the clinical context and question

Impression and Plan

Start with a summary:

› Update the patient's identification and describe the presenting issues and history.

› Include pertinent positives and negatives, signs, symptoms, and investigations.

› Provide provisional diagnoses.

Provide supporting evidence: Describe clinical signs and symptoms, and biochemical abnormalities that correspond to abnormalities in a hormonal axis (describe the level of the defect).

Organize the issues: Order them by acuity; impact on hemodynamic stability, level of consciousness, and hospitalization; and the need for inpatient management (e.g., insulin therapy in a new diabetic ketoacidosis) versus outpatient management (e.g., thyroid hormone dose adjustment in an otherwise stable patient with hypothyroidism).

Provide an organized plan: For each issue, address the probable etiologies, next steps in investigation, and your management approach.

Collaborate with allied health-care providers: These could include dietitians, nurse educators, and social workers to help with nonpharmacological therapies.

Outline a plan for outpatient or long-term follow-up: Describe blood-work monitoring, any further screening required, and how to adjust or titrate medication doses.

Adrenal Insufficiency

These notes are in addition to the **general guide for all consultations** on page 1, and the **starting points for endocrinology consultations** at the beginning of this chapter.

Identification

Follow the **general guide for all consultations**.

Reason for Referral

The referral may seek a workup for, or management of, adrenal insufficiency (AI).

History of Present Illness

Clarify why the patient has sought care: In an inpatient setting, why was the patient admitted to hospital?

Characterize the AI: It can present acutely, for example as shock (warm, with vasodilation) or as adrenal crisis.

› Determine the presence of hemodynamic instability, and the need for ICU admission or pressor requirements.

› Identify other causes or critical illness contributing to hemodynamic instability or shock.

Identify symptoms of chronic AI: These vary depending on primary AI (loss of glucocorticoids and mineralocorticoids) versus secondary AI (loss of glucocorticoids). Ask about:

› **General symptoms:** fatigue, weakness, weight loss, anorexia; nausea, vomiting, abdominal pain; arthralgia, myalgia; hyponatremia

› **Symptoms of primary AI:** skin darkening, easy tanning (hyperpigmentation arises from increased corticotropin [ACTH]), salt craving, symptomatic hypotension or orthostasis

› **Symptoms of secondary AI:** features of pituitary adenoma (see Pituitary Adenoma in this chapter)

Determine the most recent cortisol levels: Examples include random cortisol, morning cortisol, and corticotropin (ACTH) values.

Identify possible or precipitating causes of new-onset AI: These include:

> exogenous glucocorticoid withdrawal (ask about a history of glucocorticoid use and dose changes)
> underlying autoimmune disorders (primary hypothyroidism, hypoparathyroidism, type 1 diabetes, primary ovarian insufficiency, celiac disease)
> medications (opioids, ketoconazole, fluconazole, phenytoin, rifampin, etomidate, mifepristone)
> history of adrenalectomy, pituitary surgery, radiation
> head or abdominal trauma
> infiltrative disorders (ask about risk factors for TB or fungal infection; sarcoidosis; lymphoma)
> metastatic disease (ask about underlying cancer, most prominently lung, renal cell, melanoma)
> bilateral adrenal hemorrhage (ask about coagulopathy, anticoagulation, sepsis, meningococcemia, DIC)
> other conditions associated with AI (autoimmune polyglandular syndrome, classic congenital adrenal hyperplasia, triple A syndrome, x-linked adrenoleukodystrophy)

Clarify precipitating causes of adrenal crisis in known AI:
> glucocorticoid omission or subtherapeutic dose
> acute illness
> volume depletion
> physiological stress (e.g., trauma, surgery)

Past Medical History
Ask about:
- a history of AI (clarify etiology, previous admissions, ICU stay, use of steroid supplementation)
- underlying autoimmune disorders
- malignancy

Past Surgical History
Ask about adrenalectomy, pituitary surgery, and radiation.

Medications
Ask about:
- glucocorticoids (clarify type, dose, length of use, plan for steroid dose taper, indication)
- anticoagulants
- immunosuppressants
- OCs, opioids, ketoconazole, fluconazole, phenytoin, rifampin, etomidate, mifepristone

Allergies
Follow the **general guide for all consultations**.

Family History
Ask about autoimmune disorders.

Social History
Follow the **general guide for all consultations** and the **starting points for endocrinology consultations**.

Physical Examination
General appearance: body habitus, level of consciousness
Vital signs:
> Assess for the presence of shock and current pressor requirements.
> Include orthostatic vitals.

Ears: calcification of the auricular cartilages
Other: signs of primary versus secondary AI
> **Primary:** increased pigmentation (extensor surfaces, palmar creases, dental-gingival margins, lips), vitiligo (associated with autoimmune adrenalitis)
> **Secondary:** visual field defects (see Pituitary Adenoma in this chapter)

Investigations

LABORATORY INVESTIGATIONS
CBC and differential, MCV
Metabolic panel: electrolytes, glucose, Mg, Ca, PO_4, urea, creatinine, liver enzymes, and liver function tests
> Assess for hyponatremia and hypoglycemia.
> Primary AI produces hyperkalemia and metabolic acidosis (from mineralocorticoid deficiency).

INR, PTT
Thyrotropin (TSH), free T_4, free T_3
Morning cortisol (screening test)
> A value < 80 nmol/L suggests AI; a value > 500 nmol/L often rules it out.
> If the value is 80–500 nmol/L in suspected AI, proceed to a cosyntropin stimulation test.
> Report if the patient was on steroid supplementation prior to the test.
> Note that oral-contraceptive use and low serum albumin (e.g., nephrotic syndrome) can affect test accuracy.

Corticotropin (ACTH) level: In the presence of low cortisol, high ACTH suggests primary AI, and low or inappropriately normal ACTH suggests secondary AI.

Cosyntropin (ACTH) stimulation:
› Pursue this as a confirmatory test.
› Record the baseline ACTH level and cortisol before and 60 minutes after cosyntropin administration (250 mcg IV/IM).
› Normal response is a rise in cortisol to > 500 nmol/L at 30 to 60 minutes.
› In cases of recent secondary AI, the adrenal glands may still be capable of responding to cosyntropin stimulation. A low-dose (1 mcg) cosyntropin stimulation test or insulin-induced hypoglycemia test (gold standard for AI) may be used instead.

Plasma renin activity and aldosterone level

Additional workup: Pursue additional investigations as directed by signs of possible precipitating causes of adrenal crisis (e.g., ischemia, infection, inflammation, trauma).

IMAGING

Abdominal CT, dedicated adrenal protocol

CT or MRI of the head: Pursue this for a suspected secondary cause.

Impression and Plan

SUMMARY

In your summary of the case, state if AI is present, the level of the defect (primary versus secondary), evidence for etiology or precipitating cause, and degree of illness (e.g., presence of shock, adrenal crisis).

MANAGEMENT OF ADRENAL CRISIS

• Secure airway, breathing, and circulation (ABCs) and involve ICU.
• Provide fluid resuscitation and pressor support as needed.
• Provide hydrocortisone 100 mg IV every 8 hours, or 50 mg IV every 6 hours.
• Identify and treat the precipitating causes.
• Treat other causes of shock.
• Search for concomitant hypothyroidism (see Thyroid Disorders in this chapter).

MANAGEMENT OF CHRONIC ADRENAL INSUFFICIENCY

Glucocorticoid Supplementation

• Prescribe hydrocortisone: 10–12 mg/m^2/day orally, which typically equates to 15–25 mg/day in 2 to 3 divided doses (e.g., 10 mg at time of waking and 5 mg at 14:00 hours) or oral prednisone 5 mg daily.[1]
• Adjust the dose to achieve a clinical response of no signs or symptoms of cortisol deficiency or excess.
• Evaluate for long-term complications of corticosteroid use.

Mineralocorticoid Supplementation
- This is only for primary AI.
- Prescribe fludrocortisone: 0.05–0.2 mg orally every morning.
- Adjust the dose to achieve normal BP and normal serum sodium and potassium levels.

Adrenal Androgen Supplementation
- Consider this in the nonacute setting for women.
- Prescribe dehydroepiandrosterone: 25–50 mg orally every day.
- Discontinue this therapy if the patient shows no effects after 6 months.

Adrenal Crisis Prevention
- In states of illness, corticosteroid dose must be increased.
- Educate and provide the patient with "sick day" rules regarding temporary corticosteroid dose increase.[1]
- Discuss obtaining a steroid emergency card or medical alert bracelet.
- For minor stress (e.g., cold, flu, minor procedure, fever), the patient should take 2 to 3 times the basal dose for 2 to 3 days; when beginning to improve, they should wean back to their normal dose over 3 to 5 days.
- For moderate to high stress (e.g., serious illness, major procedure), provide hydrocortisone 100 mg IV every 8 hours, or 50 mg IV every 6 hours for 24 hours; if the patient improves, begin to wean.
- For nausea and vomiting, administer hydrocortisone 100 mg IM in the community if the patient cannot tolerate oral medications.
- Patients on chronic steroid therapy taking > 5 mg of prednisone (or other equivalent steroid dose) for more than 3 weeks should be considered for stress dosing as above.

Diabetes Mellitus

These notes are in addition to the **general guide for all consultations** on page 1, and the **starting points for endocrinology consultations** at the beginning of this chapter.

Identification

Key information in the identification statement includes relevant comorbidities, type of diabetes, and recent HbA_{1c} results.

Reason for Referral

The referral may seek to confirm diabetes and/or clarify management of diabetic ketoacidosis (DKA) and/or hyperglycemic hyperosmolar syndrome (HHS).

History of Present Illness

Clarify why the patient has sought care: In an inpatient setting, why was the patient admitted to hospital?

For patients with DKA or HHS, determine:
> › precipitating factors, including infection, inflammation (e.g., pancreatitis), ischemic events (MI, stroke), noncompliance with medication, recent medication changes, intoxication, initial presentation of diabetes, surgery, and pregnancy
> › initial glucose, anion gap, β-hydroxybutyrate, and bicarbonate levels
> › management for DKA or HHS so far, including whether the patient has been transitioned to subcutaneous insulin

For patients not experiencing DKA or HHS, identify:
> › recent or ongoing illness and/or inflammatory disorders (recognize their role in acutely affecting glycemic control and insulin requirements.

Clarify in-hospital glucose and insulin requirements: This is usually provided as:
> › a table of CBGs and insulin or oral antihyperglycemics (see Table 6.1)
> › a summary of glucose and infusion settings and/or the total daily amount of insulin if the patient is on an insulin infusion

For steroid-exacerbated hyperglycemia, determine:
> › the type, timing, and dosage of any glucocorticoids
> › in postoperative patients: the diabetic medication adjustments made preoperatively, insulin requirements intraoperatively, and pressor or insulin infusion requirements
> › in postoperative renal-transplant patients: the graft function (because insulin requirements will increase as renal clearance increases)

Clarify the patient's diet in hospital: Is the patient receiving enteral feeds or TPN? If yes, what is the composition?

Table 6.1. Example of an In-Hospital Glucose Log Demonstrating a Single Day for a Patient on Basal-Bolus Insulin

	BEFORE BREAKFAST	BEFORE LUNCH	BEFORE DINNER	BEFORE BEDTIME	03:00
CBG	11.1	7.8	13.9	7.9	8.9
Glargine				15	
Lispro (nutritional)	4	4	4		
Lispro (sliding scale)	2		3		

Abbreviation: CBG: capillary blood glucose

Assess for indications to initiate insulin therapy: Ask about the
presence of symptomatic hyperglycemia (polyuria, polydipsia,
blurred vision) and/or metabolic decompensation (significant
hyperglycemia, unintentional weight loss, and DKA or HHS).

Ask about previous episodes: Has the patient had hypoglycemic
episodes before? If yes, ask about symptoms, including:

› **Neuroglycopenia:** fatigue, confusion, anxiety, blurred vision, headache
› **Adrenergic symptoms:** sweating, tremors, tachycardia, palpitations

Past Medical History

Ask about diabetes history:

› Establish the type of diabetes the patient has and the date of
  diagnosis.
› Who provides management (endocrinologist, internist, or family
  doctor)?
› What is the patient's most recent HbA_{1c} result and prior HbA_{1c}
  result?
› Does the patient use insulin and/or oral antihyperglycemics (OAHs)?
› Does the patient check their CBG at home? If yes, what are the usual
  fasting and postprandial readings?
› In type 1 diabetes, determine the insulin sensitivity factor,
  carbohydrate ratio, and use of an insulin pump.
› Does the patient have a history of DKA or HHS?
› Does the patient have a history of severe hypoglycemia leading to
  hospitalization, seizure, and/or decreased level of consciousness?
› Does the patient have intact hypoglycemic awareness, and recognize
  when the symptoms of hypoglycemia (e.g., sweating, tremors,
  palpitations, nausea, hunger, headache, dizziness, blurry vision, or
  drowsiness) are occurring?

Identify macrovascular complications: These include CAD, stroke or
TIA, peripheral vascular disease, and amputations.

Identify microvascular complications: These include:

› **Retinopathy:** When did the patient last see an ophthalmologist or
  optometrist? Has the patient had treatment for diabetic retinopathy?
› **Neuropathy:** Does the patient have a history of feet ulcers or infections?
› **Nephropathy:** Ask about renal function, recent urine albumin-to-
  creatinine ratio, and dialysis received or planned.

Check for other features of metabolic syndrome: These include
hypertension, dyslipidemia, hypertriglyceridemia, and visceral
obesity and/or increased waist circumference.

Ask about disorders that contribute to diabetes development: These
include pancreatitis, cystic fibrosis, hemochromatosis, acromegaly,
Cushing syndrome, hyperthyroidism, and pheochromocytoma.[2]

Clarify pregnancy status and history: Is the patient currently pregnant, or is there history of pregnancy complicated by gestational diabetes?

Past Surgical History

Ask about:

- a history of pancreatic surgery or resection
- transplant history (determine the organ, date, and use of steroids and immunosuppressants)

Medications

Ask about:

- **Oral antihyperglycemics (OAHs):** Determine the dose, recent adjustments, use of other drug classes in the past, and any associated intolerances.
- **Insulin:** Determine the types, regimen (e.g., basal-bolus versus basal only), dose, timing, and recent adjustments, and whether the patient uses a custom correction scale.
- **Glucocorticoids:** Determine the type, dose, duration, timing, indication, and plan for tapering.
- **Other drugs that affect glycemic control:** These include calcineurin inhibitors (tacrolimus, cyclosporine), beta-blockers, epinephrine or norepinephrine, fluoroquinolones, antipsychotics, and antidepressants.[3]

Allergies

Follow the **general guide for all consultations.**

Family History

Ask about:

- diabetes in any family member (clarify type and age of onset)
- multiple family members with diabetes with onset at a young age and/or who are not obese (evidence of autosomal dominant inheritance of diabetes suggests monogenic diabetes, such as mature onset diabetes of the young [MODY])

Social History

Ask about:

- average weekly exercise duration and intensity
- diet composition

Physical Examination

Weight, height, body habitus

Level of consciousness, Kussmaul breathing, volume status

Integumentary: acanthosis nigricans, insulin injection sites, presence
of lipohypertrophy
Peripheral vascular: temperature, pulses, capillary refill
Feet: ulcers, infections, trauma, Charcot foot (diabetic foot exam)
Peripheral neurological: sensation, proprioception, vibration, ankle
reflex, 10 g monofilament test (if available)

Investigations

FOR ALL PATIENTS
CBC and differential
Electrolytes, Mg, Ca, PO_4, creatinine (eGFR), urea
HbA_{1c}, lipid panel
Urine albumin-to-creatinine:
› Check for the most recent result (note that it can be falsely elevated in
acute illness).

IN DIABETIC KETOACIDOSIS OR HYPERGLYCEMIC HYPEROSMOLAR SYNDROME
Additional initial investigations: Order serum osmolality;
β-hydroxybutyrate; urinalysis; liver function tests; lipase; lactate;
venous blood gas or ABG; troponin; ECG; blood cultures; chest
x-ray; β-HCG (in females of reproductive age); CBG; anion gap
(use the measured *uncorrected* sodium to calculate anion gap);
serum glucose; osmolality.
› **Findings in DKA:** anion gap > 12, β-hydroxybutyrate > 2, HCO_3
< 18, blood glucose > 15, pH < 7.3
› **Findings in HHS:** possible minimal ketone elevation, but usually
more profound hyperglycemia (> 50 mmol/L) and elevated serum
osmolality
Investigations to monitor treatment of DKA and HHS:
› Order CBG every hour while the patient is on insulin infusion; and
electrolytes, anion gap, serum glucose, and serum osmolality every
2 hours until the anion gap is closed.
› *If it is unclear whether patient has type 1 versus type 2 diabetes,*
check a fasting c-peptide level with a fasting serum glucose and
consider pancreatic autoantibody testing (e.g., antiglutamate
decarboxylase-65, antiislet cell antibodies).
Genetic testing: Consider this in the context of young-onset diabetes,
no evidence of metabolic syndrome, family history of multiple
members with diabetes and autosomal dominant pattern of
inheritance, and negative antibody testing.

Impression and Plan

SUMMARY

In your summary of the case, state the type of diabetes, include the most-recent HbA_{1c} result, and describe known microvascular and macrovascular complications.

PRINCIPLES OF DIABETIC KETOACIDOSIS AND HYPERGLYCEMIC HYPEROSMOLAR SYNDROME MANAGEMENT

Most institutions have their own DKA and HHS preprinted order sets that you can use.

Provide volume resuscitation: Patients usually have a 5–7 L fluid deficit on presentation that needs repletion; however, maintain caution in states of CHF and CKD.

Close the anion gap: Use insulin infusion (typically starting at 0.1 U/kg/hr).

Provide potassium maintenance:
› Maintain potassium at > 3.3 meq using potassium in IV fluids (start supplementation if potassium is < 5.3 meq while on insulin infusion).
› Consider slowing down or briefly holding insulin infusion if there is concern for severe hypokalemia.

Provide glucose maintenance:
› Avoid rapidly decreasing glucose (this risks hypoglycemia and cerebral edema).
› Aim to maintain glucose > 10 mmol/L until resolution of DKA or HHS.

Search for and treat precipitating causes.

Assess for suitability of transition to subcutaneous insulin:
› Patients ready for transition have a closed anion gap, are alert (normal level of consciousness), and are able to take food by mouth.
› Overlap infusion and long-acting subcutaneous insulin by at least 2 hours before stopping infusion.

PRINCIPLES OF INPATIENT DIABETES MANAGEMENT

- If the patient has type 1 diabetes and is newly started on insulin, estimate the total daily dose as 0.3–0.5 units/kg, with 50% administered as basal and the rest split between meals as bolus insulin.
- For type 2 diabetes, strategies to improve glycemic control include increasing the dose of the current OAH, adding other classes of OAHs, or adding insulin (on a basal-only or basal-bolus regimen).
- In patients with cardiovascular disease, suggest the use of sodium-glucose cotransporter-2 (SGLT2) inhibitors or glucagon-like peptide 1 receptor (GLP-1) agonists if there are no contraindications.
- In hospital, the target for preprandial glucose is 5–8 mmol/L and for random glucose is < 10 mmol/L in noncritically ill patients. In

critical care settings, aim to maintain glucose within 6–10 mmol/L (hypoglycemia has high morbidity).[4]

- On admission, if the patient is hemodynamically unstable, or has renal impairment, it is common practice to hold OAHs (particularly metformin, sulfonylureas, SGLT2 inhibitors).
  › If continuing or restarting OAHs, ensure that the doses are appropriate for the patient's renal function.
- For insulin administration, aim to establish a basal-bolus regimen in hospital rather than relying on a sliding scale alone.
- Management of specific causes of hyperglycemia includes:
  › **Steroid-induced hyperglycemia:** This is mainly due to increased insulin resistance and gluconeogenesis, so consider insulin with steroid administration: the choice depends on the steroid type (e.g., NPH insulin is reasonable for prednisone as it has similar duration of action).
  › **TPN-associated hyperglycemia:** Consider giving regular insulin in the TPN bag.

CONSIDERATIONS FOR LONG-TERM OR OUTPATIENT MANAGEMENT

Identify an HbA$_{1c}$ target: For most patients it is less than 7%, but consider higher targets in elderly and/or frail patients, and patients at high risk for hypoglycemia.[5]

Discuss follow-up screening for microvascular complications: Refer to Diabetes Canada guidelines.

Provide diabetes education: For inpatients, do this before discharge. Information should cover:
  › insulin use if the patient will have an insulin prescription
  › driving guidelines[6]
  › nonpharmacological management, including exercise, diet, and weight loss (refer to Diabetes Canada guidelines)[7]

Pituitary Adenoma

These notes are in addition to the **general guide for all consultations** on page 1, and the **starting points for endocrinology consultations** at the beginning of this chapter.

Identification

Key information in the identification statement includes the patient's main presenting symptoms (e.g., headache, diplopia, vision loss, nausea, vomiting, shock).

Reason for Referral

The referral may seek a workup for, or management of, pituitary adenoma (or suprasellar lesion).

History of Present Illness

Determine how the pituitary adenoma was identified: Options include:
> MRI or CT of the head or sella
> ophthalmology assessment
> neurosurgical assessment

Ask about adenoma mass effect symptoms: These include visual field defects (bitemporal hemianopia or quadrantanopia); headache (including "thunderclap" headache, suggestive of apoplexy); altered visual acuity; stalk compression leading to hyperprolactinemia; diplopia; nausea and vomiting (apoplexy); cranial nerve (CN) III, IV, and/or VI palsy; and rhinorrhea.

Ask about symptoms of hormone deficiency: These include:
> **Adrenal insufficiency:** shock (rare), hemodynamic instability (rare), symptoms of hypotension, weight loss, nausea, vomiting, fatigue (see Adrenal Insufficiency in this chapter)
> **Hypothyroidism:** weight gain, cold intolerance, constipation, fatigue, mood and/or sleep changes, decreased appetite, menstrual changes (see Thyroid Disorders in this chapter)
> **Hypogonadism:** infertility, oligo- or amenorrhea, decreased morning erections, loss of muscle mass
> **Growth hormone (GH) deficiency:** fatigue, loss of muscle mass
> **Diabetes insipidus:** polydipsia, polyuria, hypernatremia (this may not be present if patient has adequate fluid intake)

Ask about symptoms of hormone excess: These include:
> **Hyperprolactinemia:** oligo- or amenorrhea (establish the date of menarche, usual cycle length, last menstrual period), infertility, galactorrhea
> **Cushing disease:** labile mood, psychosis, skin thinning, easy bruising, changes in facial features ("moon facies"), weight gain, hirsutism, acne, dysmenorrhea, proximal muscle weakness
> **Acromegaly:** increase in hand and/or foot size (changes in the fit of rings and shoes), coarsening of facial features, macrognathia (large or protruding jaw), macroglossia (large tongue), increased gap between teeth, sleep apnea, carpal tunnel symptoms, hypertension
> **Hyperthyroidism:** weight loss, heat intolerance, tremor, increased sweating, palpitations, HF symptoms, menstrual changes (see Thyroid Disorders in this chapter)

Past Medical History
Ask about:
- malignancy (particularly breast, lung, renal cell, lymphoma)
- infiltrative diseases (tuberculosis, sarcoidosis, Langerhans cell histiocytosis, hemochromatosis)
- radiation to the head and/or neck
- recent hemorrhage or shock (these are risk factors for pituitary apoplexy)
- current pregnancy or postpartum status

Past Surgical History
Ask about a history of intracranial surgery.

Medications
Ask about:
- medications that can cause hyperprolactinemia, including SSRIs, antidopaminergic medications (e.g., antipsychotics, metoclopramide, domperidone, methyldopa), TCAs, and opioids
- glucocorticoid use (this is associated with secondary and tertiary adrenal insufficiency)
- chronic opiate use (associated with secondary and tertiary adrenal insufficiency, and hypothalamic hypogonadism)
- immune checkpoint inhibitors (associated with hypophysitis)

Allergies
Follow the **general guide for all consultations**.

Family History
Ask about features of MEN-1 syndrome: pituitary adenomas, hypercalcemia (parathyroid hyperplasia or adenoma), pancreatic islet cell tumours, and neuroendocrine tumours.

Social History
Ask about the patient's desire for fertility (this is important in the context of hypogonadism treatment).

Physical Examination
See Thyroid Disorders in this chapter for findings of hyper- and hypothyroidism.
Vital signs: orthostatic vital signs, weight and height, overall stability
Head, ears, eyes, nose, throat:
> Assess visual fields by confrontation (the classic defect is bitemporal hemianopia or quadrantanopia).

> Perform a cranial nerve exam for CN II/III, IV, and VI palsies.
> Assess for signs that suggest elevated corticotropin (ACTH) and/or cortisol (acne, hirsutism, supraclavicular fat pad, plethoric facies).
> Assess for signs that suggest elevated GH (frontal-skull bossing, macroglossia, prognathism [pronounced mandible]).

Chest, cardiovascular: Assess for signs that suggest:
> elevated prolactin (galactorrhea, gynecomastia, and/or breast tenderness)
> elevated GH (cardiomegaly, signs of HF, peripheral edema)

Abdominal: Assess for signs that suggest:
> elevated corticotropin (ACTH) and/or cortisol (central obesity, wide violaceous striae [> 1 cm])
> elevated GH (hepatosplenomegaly)

Dermatological, neurological, musculoskeletal:
> Look for tremors, bruises, and poor wound healing.
> Assess proximal muscle strength and deep tendon reflexes.
> Assess for elevated corticotropin (ACTH) (hyperpigmentation: notably at palmar creases, buccal mucosa, and prior surgical scars).
> Assess for elevated GH (skin tags, acanthosis nigricans).

Investigations

LABORATORY INVESTIGATIONS

CBC and differential

Electrolytes, Mg, Ca, PO_4, creatinine (eGFR), urea

Pituitary panel: Pursue the following tests as a first evaluation of a pituitary mass.
  » **Adrenal:** morning or random cortisol, corticotropin (ACTH)
  » **Thyroid:** thyrotropin (TSH), free T_4, free T_3
  » **Gonadal:** LH; FSH; estradiol and progesterone (women); total testosterone (men)
  » **GH:** fasting glucose, IGF-1
  » **ADH:** urine output; serum electrolytes and osmolality; urine osmolality
  » **Prolactin:** prolactin and/or macroprolactin

For clinical suspicion of Cushing disease: Conduct an initial screen with a 24-hour urine free cortisol, 1 mg dexamethasone suppression test, or midnight salivary cortisol.

For corticotropin (ACTH) deficiency: See Adrenal Insufficiency in this chapter.

For clinical suspicion of diabetes insipidus: Clinical suspicion would arise, for example, in a patient with polyuria and low urine osmolality. Confirm the diagnosis with a water deprivation test and desmopressin challenge.

IMAGING
CT of the head
MRI pituitary protocol

Impression and Plan

SUMMARY

In your summary of the case, describe whether the adenoma is:
- functioning versus nonfunctioning (no signs of excess hormone production)
- a microadenoma versus macroadenoma (> 1 cm)
- causing hemodynamic instability, visual deficits, or hormone deficiency

MANAGEMENT

Macroadenoma

- Refer the patient to an ophthalmologist for formal visual field testing (e.g., Goldmann visual field test) and to a neurosurgeon, particularly when there is mass effect and/or visual field or optic apparatus compromise.
- Monitor the progression of the tumour with serial MRI.

Hormone Deficiencies[8]

- A nonfunctioning adenoma affects hormones in the following order: GH, LH, FSH, thyrotropin (TSH), corticotropin (ACTH), prolactin, and posterior pituitary hormones (mnemonic: Go Look For The Adenoma Please). When all pituitary hormones are affected, it is termed *panhypopituitarism*.
- Secondary (central) adrenal insufficiency and hypothyroidism must be treated (see Adrenal Insufficiency and Thyroid Disorders in this chapter).
- Administer desmopressin replacement in patients with central diabetes insipidus.
- Hypogonadotropic hypogonadism can be treated with estrogen, progesterone (female), and testosterone (male), but if the patient desires fertility, gonadotropin stimulation will be required for treatment.

Prolactinoma

- Exclude other causes of hyperprolactinemia: stalk compression, pregnancy, medications, hypothyroidism, lactation, CKD, chest wall pathology, stress, and hook effect.
- Begin with medical therapy using dopamine agonists: cabergoline (more effective and better tolerated) or bromocriptine (or rarely quinagolide).

- Refer the patient to a neurosurgeon if acute visual field defects are present. Note, however, that prolactinomas are typically sensitive to dopamine agonist therapy, and transsphenoidal surgery is usually considered when a tumour is refractory to medical therapy.

Cushing Disease
- Pituitary tumours that produce corticotropin (ACTH) cause Cushing disease.
- After establishing hypercortisolemia, localize the source as the pituitary gland with a high-dose dexamethasone suppression test and/or inferior petrosal sinus sampling.
- Refer the patient to a neurosurgeon for transsphenoidal surgery. The patient may require steroid replacement therapy postoperatively.

Thyroid Disorders

These notes are in addition to the **general guide for all consultations** on page 1, and the **starting points for endocrinology consultations** at the beginning of this chapter.

Identification
Follow the **general guide for all consultations**.

Reason for Referral
The referral may seek a workup for, or management of, thyroid disorder, or tests for abnormal thyroid function.

History of Present Illness
Identify the pattern of thyroid function test abnormality: See Table 6.2.

Establish the time course and development of symptoms:
> **Symptoms of hyperthyroidism:** increased anxiety, restlessness, agitation; insomnia; heat intolerance; sweating; hair loss or thinning; palpitations; dyspnea on exertion; weight loss; hyperdefecation; increased appetite; polydipsia; polyuria; nocturia; oligo- or amenorrhea
>> **"Apathetic thyrotoxicosis":** weakness and asthenia (sometimes these are the only presenting symptoms in older patients)
> **Symptoms of hypothyroidism:** increased fatigue; depressed mood; decline in cognitive function and/or memory; cold intolerance; dry skin; increased hair loss; myalgias; carpal tunnel syndrome; weight gain; constipation; decreased appetite; menorrhagia

Symptoms of specific thyroid disorders include:
> **Graves disease with ophthalmopathy:** eye irritation, eye pain with movement, diplopia
> **Subacute thyroiditis:** recent URTI symptoms, unilateral or bilateral neck pain
> **Acute bacterial (suppurative) thyroiditis:** fever, painful neck, dysphagia, dysphonia
> **Pituitary adenoma** (see Pituitary Adenoma in this chapter)

Identify intercurrent illness and inflammatory states: This is especially important if you suspect nonthyroidal illness syndrome (NTIS).

Ask about:
> enlarged neck, neck mass, or neck nodule
> recent pregnancy and delivery (this is associated with postpartum thyroiditis)
> pregnancy status and plans for pregnancy in the near future (this has treatment implications)
> recent use of iodine-containing medications, or recent contrast CT scans

Clarify current management: If the patient has known thyroid disorder, ask who provides the patient with care, the frequency of thyroid function tests, date of the last test, and dose adjustment.

Past Medical History
Ask about:
- cardiovascular history (CAD, CHF, arrhythmias)
- history of malignancy, radiation exposure to the head and neck, fractures, osteoporosis

Past Surgical History
Ask about:
- a history of neck or thyroid surgery
- neurosurgical interventions

Medications
Ask about:
- thyroid hormone replacement, if relevant
  > Determine the dosage, recent adjustments, and timing with meals.
  > For weight-based dosing, ask about the patient's weight.
- recent or ongoing use of amiodarone, lithium, interferon alpha, alemtuzumab, natural therapies, herbal supplements, thyroid hormone extracts
- drugs that affect thyroid function tests (e.g., dopamine, octreotide, OCs, heparin, biotin)[9]

- drugs that impair thyroid hormone absorption (e.g., calcium, iron supplements)
- prior treatment with immune checkpoint inhibitors

Allergies

Follow the **general guide for all consultations.**

Family History

Ask about thyroid disorders and thyroid malignancy.

Social History

Assess for risk factors for iodine deficiency (e.g., poor access to nutrition, recently moved from a developing country).

Physical Examination

Vital signs: Watch in particular for signs of hemodynamic instability.

General impression: Assess for level of consciousness:
› Patients with hyperthyroidism may exhibit hyperactivity and rapid speech.
› Patients with hypothyroidism may exhibit lethargy, slowed speech, and slow movements.

Thyroid: Perform a focused thyroid exam: assess for goitre, nodules, bruit, and retrosternal goitre (percuss for dullness over the sternum; look for Pemberton sign).

Signs of hyperthyroidism:
› Assess for tachycardia, systolic hypertension, warm and moist skin, diaphoresis, tremor, proximal muscle weakness, hyperreflexia, and stare with lid retraction and lid lag.
› Assess for Graves disease, including signs of ophthalmopathy (exophthalmos, periorbital edema, diplopia, conjunctival injection), pretibial myxedema, diffusely enlarged thyroid, and thyroid acropachy.
› Signs of "thyroid storm" include tachycardia, hypertension, hyperthermia, altered level of consciousness, delirium, and shock.

Signs of hypothyroidism:
› Assess for slow speech, bradycardia, diastolic hypertension, dry and thick skin, cool extremities, periorbital edema, hair loss (including the outer third of eyebrows), peripheral edema, delayed deep tendon reflexes, myopathy (weakness), and myoedema.
› Signs of myxedema coma include hypotension, bradypnea, hypothermia, and decreased level of consciousness.

Investigations

LABORATORY INVESTIGATIONS

CBC and differential, MCV

Electrolytes, Mg, Ca, PO_4, urea, creatinine (eGFR)

Liver enzymes and liver function tests

Thyrotropin (TSH), free T_4, free T_3

Hypothyroidism

Antithyroid peroxidase antibody (anti-TPO antibody): This can be elevated in any autoimmune thyroid disorder; however, it is more specific for autoimmune hypothyroidism.

Hyperthyroidism

Thyroid receptor antibody (TRAb): This is specific for Graves disease.

OTHER INVESTIGATIONS

ECG: Assess for arrhythmias such as AF.

IMAGING

Hyperthyroidism

Radioactive iodine (RAI) uptake scan: In patients who have had recent iodine administration, which can interfere with RAI uptake scan, consider a technetium-99 scan.
  › Interpretation: Graves disease exhibits diffusely increased uptake; multinodular toxic goiter or toxic adenoma exhibits single or multiple foci of increased uptake ("hot nodules"); thyroiditis exhibits decreased or absent uptake.

Other Indications

Thyroid ultrasound: Pursue this to characterize nodules found on physical examination.

Pituitary disease: See Pituitary Adenoma in this chapter.

Table 6.2. Patterns of Abnormality in Thyroid Function Tests[10]

	↑ THYROTROPIN (TSH)	NORMAL THYROTROPIN (TSH)	↓ THYROTROPIN (TSH)
↑ FT$_4$ and FT$_3$	Central hyperthyroidism or thyroid hormone resistance		Primary hyperthyroidism
Normal FT$_4$ and FT$_3$	Subclinical hypothyroidism	Euthyroid	Subclinical hyperthyroidism NTIS
↓ FT$_4$ and FT$_3$	Primary hypothyroidism	Central hypothyroidism NTIS	
Normal or ↑ FT$_4$, ↓ FT$_3$	NTIS (recovery phase)	NTIS	

Abbreviations: FT$_3$: free T$_3$; FT$_4$: free T$_4$; NTIS: nonthyroidal illness syndrome; TSH: thyroid-stimulating hormone (thyrotropin)

Impression and Plan

After summarizing the case, present your provisional diagnosis with reference to the clinical and biochemical pattern of thyroid abnormality, and use information from your history, exam, and investigations to outline probable etiologies.

HYPERTHYROIDISM MANAGEMENT

- For Graves disease, multinodular toxic goitre, and toxic adenoma, treatment options include medications (methimazole/propylthiouracil, beta-blockers for symptom control), RAI, or surgery.
- Consider cholestyramine 4 g orally 4 times per day in combination with methimazole to more rapidly lower serum T_4 and T_3.
- In Graves disease, assess the severity of Graves ophthalmopathy (GO) before recommending an RAI uptake scan (RAI can worsen it). Glucocorticoids can be used to reduce progression in patients undergoing an RAI uptake scan. In severe GO disease, refer the patient to an ophthalmologist.
- Management of thyroiditis is supportive, with monitoring of thyroid indices every 4 to 6 weeks until they are normal.
- *Note:* Pregnancy status and near-future plans of pregnancy are important considerations in management of hyperthyroidism.

Thyroid Storm

- Suspect thyroid storm in patients with biochemical hyperthyroidism, and with altered level of consciousness, fevers, and/or hemodynamic instability.
- The Burch-Wartofsky score is useful in estimating the likelihood of thyroid storm (a score greater than 25 supports the diagnosis).[11]
- Involve ICU and secure the patient's ABCs.
- Treatment includes:
  › thionamide (propylthiouracil 200 mg orally every 4 hours is preferred over methimazole because propylthiouracil, not methimazole, blocks peripheral conversion of T_4 to T_3), *followed by:*
    » iodine solution (Lugol iodine solution 10 drops every 8 hours, given at least 1 hour after the loading dose of propylthiouracil)
    » propranolol (60–80 mg orally every 4 hours)
    » glucocorticoids (to inhibit peripheral conversion of T_4 to T_3)

HYPOTHYROIDISM MANAGEMENT

- In patients who need permanent thyroid hormone replacement, the starting maintenance dose of levothyroxine is estimated at 1.6 mcg/kg/day.

- In cases where CAD is a concern, or in elderly patients, consider starting levothyroxine at a low dose (50 mcg/day, or half of estimated maintenance dose) and titrating it up slowly.
- *Do not treat* NTIS with thyroid hormone replacement.
  › Suspect NTIS in patients with compatible thyroid function test results and who have another active illness or are hospitalized.
  › If thyrotropin (TSH) is > 20 mlU/L, it is unlikely to be NTIS.

Myxedema Coma

- Suspect myxedema coma in patients with a history or biochemical evidence of hypothyroidism, and who have: decreased heart rate, respiration rate, BP, temperature, CBG, and level of consciousness; hyponatremia; and generalized nonpitting edema. Often, these patients have longstanding untreated hypothyroidism and/or exposure to an acute stressful trigger (e.g., infection, surgery).
- Involve ICU and secure the patient's ABCs.
- Treatment includes prompt glucocorticoids first, and IV levothyroxine if the oral route is not possible or in suspected bowel edema.

MONITORING THERAPY AND DOSE TITRATION

- After initiating therapy, thyrotropin (TSH) levels take weeks to respond, so test thyroid function every 4 to 6 weeks.
- Levothyroxine doses should be adjusted every 4 to 6 weeks until thyrotropin (TSH) levels are stable in the normal range (in primary hypothyroidism) and/or until free T_4 is in mid–normal range (central hypothyroidism). Once a maintenance dose is established, advise patients to get thyroid function tests annually.

References

1. Bornstein S, Allolio B, Arlt W, et al. Diagnosis and treatment of primary adrenal insufficiency: an Endocrine Society clinical practice guideline. Journal of Clinical Endocrinology & Metabolism. 2016;101(2):364-89. doi: 10.1210/jc.2015-1710
2. American Diabetes Association. Diagnosis and classification of diabetes mellitus. Diabetes Care. 2010;33(suppl 1):S62-9. doi: 10.2337/dc10-S062
3. Thomas Z, Bandali F, McCowen K, et al. Drug-induced endocrine disorders in the intensive care unit. Crit Care Med. 2010;38:S219-30. doi:10.1097/CCM.0b013d3181dda0f2
4. Diabetes Canada Clinical Practice Guidelines Expert Committee. Diabetes Canada 2018 clinical practice guidelines for the prevention and management of diabetes in Canada [Internet]. Toronto: Canadian Diabetes Society; 2018 [updated in parts (2020, 2021); cited 2022 Jan 10]. Available from: http://guidelines.diabetes.ca/cpg
5. Imran S, Agarwal G, Bajaj H, et al. Diabetes Canada 2018 clinical practice guidelines for the prevention and management of diabetes in Canada: targets for glycemic control [Internet]. Toronto: Canadian Diabetes Society; 2018 [cited 2022 Jan 10]. Available from: http://guidelines.diabetes.ca/cpg/chapter8

6. Houlden R, Berard L, Lakoff J, et al. Diabetes Canada 2018 clinical practice guidelines for the prevention and management of diabetes in Canada: diabetes and driving [Internet]. Toronto: Canadian Diabetes Society; 2018 [cited 2022 Jan 10]. Available from: http://guidelines.diabetes.ca/cpg/chapter21

7. Wharton S, Pedersen S, Lau D, et al. Diabetes Canada 2018 clinical practice guidelines for the prevention and management of diabetes in Canada: weight management in diabetes. Toronto: Canadian Diabetes Society; 2018 [cited 2022 Jan 10]. Available from: http://guidelines.diabetes.ca/cpg/chapter17

8. Fleseriu M, Hashim I, Karavitaki N, et al. Hormonal replacement in hypopituitarism in adults: an Endocrine Society clinical practice guideline. Journal of Clinical Endocrinology & Metabolism. 2016;101(11):3888-921. doi: 10.1210/jc.2016-2118

9. Favresse J, Burlacu M-C, Maiter D, et al. Interferences with thyroid function immunoassays: clinical implications and detection algorithm. Endocrine Reviews. 2018;39(5):830-50. doi: 10.1210/er.2018-00119

10. Gurnell M, Halsall D, Chatterjee V. What should be done when thyroid function tests do not make sense? Clin Endocrinol (Oxf). 2011;74(6):673-8. doi: 10.1111/j.1365-2265.2011.04023.x

11. Burch H, Wartofsky L. Life-threatening thyrotoxicosis. Thyroid storm. Endocrinol Metab Clin North Am. 1993;22(2):263-77. PMID: 8325286

7

Gastroenterology

Dr. Amrit Jhajj
Dr. Ciarán Galts
Dr. Eric Sonke
Dr. Harjot Bedi
Dr. Sepehr Nassiri
Dr. Marcel Tomaszewski

REVIEWERS
Dr. Rohit Pai
Dr. Dustin Loomes

Starting Points: Gastroenterology Consultations

These notes are in addition to the **general guide for all consultations** on page 1.

Identification

Follow the **general guide for all consultations**.

Reason for Referral

The referral may seek to confirm a gastroenterological disorder and/or clarify appropriate management.

History of Present Illness

The questions you ask for this history heavily depend on the reason for referral and acuity of the patient. For instance, a severely cirrhotic patient with reduced level of consciousness may not be able to provide a history as well as a patient with mild GI bleeding who is otherwise well.

Characterize the presenting symptoms: Apply the mnemonic OPQRST AAA.

Conduct a review of GI systems: Ask about:
› **Typical bowel habits:** frequency, quality, other issues, character on Bristol stool chart
› **Changes in bowel habits:**

» Has the patient had constipation or diarrhea? (*If diarrhea, do they have any travel history or exposure to sick contacts?*)

» Ask about changes in the frequency of bowel movements, nocturnal bowel movements, stool character based on the Bristol stool chart, hematochezia, presence of mucus, steatorrhea, and tenesmus.

» Ask questions based on the working differential diagnosis (osmotic, secretory, inflammatory).

› **Abdominal pain:** Clarify the location:
  » general versus localized
  » epigastric (this suggests GERD, or a gastric or hepatobiliary cause)
  » right upper quadrant (hepatobiliary)
  » right lower quadrant (appendicitis, Crohn ileitis)
  » left lower quadrant (diverticulitis)
  » suprapubic (GU)

› **Symptoms of inflammatory bowel disease (IBD):** arthralgias, rash, ophthalmologic issues (e.g., uveitis), oral ulcers

› **Other symptoms:** dysphagia, odynophagia, early satiety, frequent aspiration, nausea, vomiting, heartburn, poor nutritional status, weight loss, drenching night sweats

Past Medical History

Identify GI-related diseases:

› Examples include cirrhosis, previous GI bleeds, GERD, and IBD (clarify subtype).

› For each, clarify the year of diagnosis, course of the disease, disease-related complications, endoscopic procedures, and specialists the patients has seen.

› You will need to include a note on this in your impression and plan. *For example:* "Idiopathic pancreatitis diagnosed in 2016, with complete workup done at that time, followed by Dr. XYZ, with 6 admissions for pancreatitis since that time, none requiring ICU and with no known complications."

Clarify other pertinent medical conditions: Cardiovascular, oncologic, and cognitive conditions are especially important (e.g., conditions requiring anticoagulation such as AF are important in GI bleeding).

Past Surgical History

Ask about abdominal surgeries and when they took place (e.g., bowel resection, appendectomy, caesarian section).

Medications

Ask about:
- current medications, doses, and routes of administration
- recent medication changes

- immunosuppressant treatments
- previous treatments for IBD
- medications relevant to GI bleeding and liver disease (NSAIDs, including acetylsalicylic acid; steroids; anticoagulants and antiplatelets)
- medications relevant to encephalopathy (lactulose compliance, other sedating medications)
- other important medications (antibiotics; laxatives; acid suppressants including PPIs, H2 receptor antagonists)

Allergies
Follow the **general guide for all consultations.**

Family History
Ask about:
- IBD
- malignancies (esophageal, gastric, pancreatic, hepatocellular carcinoma [HCC], colorectal cancer)
- autoimmune diseases

Social History
Ask about:
- alcohol use (always ask about prior and current use)
- drug use, particularly IV street drugs (relevant to HCV and HIV)
- smoking
- occupation, housing situation, what city they live in if not local, level of independence
- other significant social history (e.g., recently widowed, recently lost housing)

Code Status
Identify advanced directives, code status, and substitute decision makers, if applicable.

Physical Examination
Vital signs: Obtain the patient's temperature, orthostatic BP, heart and respiratory rate, and oxygenation status.
Weight
General impression: Assess the patient for GCS score, alertness and orientation, signs of distress, signs of bleeding, jaundice, pallor, and other striking features (e.g., bloody emesis at bedside).
Abdominal:
  › **Inspection:** Check for scars, distension, bulging flanks, caput medusa, ostomy, and obvious masses.

› **Auscultation:** Assess bowel sounds.
› **Percussion:** Check for peritonitis, shifting dullness, hepatomegaly, and splenomegaly (Castell sign, Nixon sign, Traube space).
› **Palpation:** Check for tenderness (note location), rebound, guarding, McBurney sign, Murphy sign, pulsating mass (AAA), masses, and ascites.
› **DRE:** Assess stool colour and rectal tone, and check for palpable masses, perianal findings, fistula, hemorrhoids, and prolapse.
Cardiovascular, respiratory: Perform a standard exam, with attention to signs of volume overload, which can occur in cirrhosis.
Neurological: Check for asterixis and assess the distribution of weakness (if any).
Dermatological: Check for spider angiomata (upper trunk).
Ophthalmological: Check for scleral icterus.

Investigations

LABORATORY INVESTIGATIONS
Review previous blood work (CBC, renal function, electrolytes, hepatitis serologies) and previous endoscopic procedures (note dates and findings).
Liver: INR, bilirubin, liver enzymes, platelets, albumin
GI bleeding: hemoglobin, platelets, INR, PTT, BUN-to-creatinine ratio
IBD: WBC, CRP, fecal calprotectin, albumin
Pancreas: lipase, urea, Ca, triglycerides

IMAGING
Check previous or current:
- US or CT for pertinent comments (e.g., on cirrhosis, splenomegaly, ascites)
- MRI of the pelvis for fistulizing Crohn disease

Impression and Plan
Start with a summary: Include the most likely diagnosis.
Prioritize the patient's issues as appropriate: Common first issues are GI bleeding, reduced level of consciousness (likely hepatic encephalopathy), decompensated cirrhosis, IBD flare, and pancreatitis.
› Use scoring systems as appropriate (see the presentations in this chapter).
› Provide a differential diagnosis (e.g., the etiology of upper GI bleeding).
List and describe the rest of the patient's GI and non-GI issues.

Discuss DVT prophylaxis.

Provide the patient's code status.

Dysphagia

These notes are in addition to the **general guide for all consultations** on page 1, and the **starting points for gastroenterology consultations** at the beginning of this chapter.

Identification

Follow the **general guide for all consultations**.

Reason for Referral

- Examples of reason for referral include patient concerns about "painful swallowing," "difficulty swallowing," or "food sticking."
- In some cases, the referral may ask you to assess whether a PEG tube is appropriate.

History of Present Illness

Ask about food bolus obstruction:
> This is characterized by acute onset dysphagia while eating (typically meat).
> Symptoms include choking, refusal to eat, hypersalivation, retrosternal fullness, and regurgitation of undigested food.

Clarify symptoms of oropharyngeal versus esophageal dysphagia:
> Ask the patient to point to the area of obstruction: if retrosternal, the problem is likely esophageal; if suprasternal, it could be oropharyngeal or referred pain from the esophagus.
> Oropharyngeal dysphagia involves difficulty initiating the swallow, and coughing, choking, nasal regurgitation, dysarthria, and dysphonia. It is associated with an increased risk of aspiration.
> Esophageal dysphagia involves food sticking shortly after swallowing.

Clarify symptoms of structural versus motility disorder: Does the patient have difficulty with solids, liquids, or both?
> Structural disorders involve difficulty with solids more than liquids (may progress to liquids).
> Motility disorders (scleroderma) involve difficulty with solids and liquids.

Clarify the timeline:
> Symptoms with rapid progression over weeks to months are concerning for malignancy, especially in the context of weight loss.

> Slowly progressive symptoms suggest peptic stricture or achalasia.
> Intermittent symptoms suggest eosinophilic esophagitis (EOE),
  esophageal ring, or spasm.
> Adaptive behaviours such as chewing more carefully, longer mealtimes,
  drinking more water during meals, and changes in the positioning of
  the head and neck during swallowing suggest chronicity.

Assess for red flags: See sidebar.

Ask about other associated symptoms and patterns: These include:
> heartburn (this suggests peptic stricture or a motility disorder)
> weight loss, anorexia, and anemia (malignancy)
> regurgitation of bland and undigested food with or without
  noncardiac chest pain (achalasia)
> regurgitation involving an acidic or sour taste (GERD)
> halitosis (Zenker diverticulum, advanced achalasia, or long-term
  obstruction)
> odynophagia (infectious cause [*Candida*, CMV, HSV], pill, caustic
  injury)

Establish what foods are most difficult: This is useful for counselling
the patient.

|||||||||||||||||||||||||||||||||||||||||||||||||||||||||||||||||||||||||||||||||||||||||||||||||||||||||||||||||||||||||||||||||

RED FLAGS IN DYSPHAGIA

Older than 50	Bleeding and/or anemia
Odynophagia	Vomiting
Weight loss	

Past Medical History

Ask about:
- **Previous upper endoscopies:**
  > Establish the dates and findings, including relevant pathology.
- **History of malignancy:**
  > Establish the date of diagnosis; stage and type of malignancy;
    treatment and dates of treatment (e.g., radiation, chemotherapy,
    surgery); and any follow-up planned.
- **Risk factors for esophageal adenocarcinoma or peptic stricture:**
  GERD, Barrett esophagus, obesity, hiatal hernia
- **Risk factors for squamous cell carcinoma:** history of esophageal
  caustic injury, achalasia, radiation esophagitis, HPV infection,
  Plummer-Vinson syndrome
- **Risk factors for EOE:** history of food allergies, environmental allergies,
  seasonal allergies, asthma, eczema

- **Neurological disorders:** myasthenia gravis, Parkinson disease, MS, muscular dystrophy, stroke, dementia
- **Stricture from a previous caustic injury or radiation**
- **Autoimmune disorders:** scleroderma, Sjögren syndrome, mixed connective tissue disease
- **Immunosuppression:** diabetes mellitus, HIV/AIDS, BMT, solid organ transplant (these are risk factors for infectious esophagitis)
- **Crohn disease** (esophageal involvement)
- **Thyroid disease** (compression from goiter)
- **Chagas disease**

Past Surgical History
Ask about surgeries involving the larynx, esophagus, stomach, or spine.

Medications
Ask about:
- medications associated with pill esophagitis, including bisphosphonates (Alendronate), acetylsalicylic acid, NSAIDs, antibiotics (tetracycline, doxycycline, clindamycin), vitamin C, potassium chloride, iron compounds, and quinidine
- fluid intake when taking pills
- immunosuppressants, PPIs

Allergies
Follow the **general guide for all consultations.**

Family History
Ask about malignancies, EOE, and autoimmune disorders.

Social History
Ask about:
- alcohol use, smoking
- socioeconomic status (lower status may increase the risk of esophageal squamous cell carcinoma)

Physical Examination
Airway, breathing, circulation (ABCs)
Vital signs
General impression: Can the patient manage their secretions? Are they in respiratory distress?
Signs of malnourishment: Assess for loss of subcutaneous fat, muscle wasting, and peripheral edema.

Head, ears, nose, throat: Assess for conjunctival pallor; lymphadenopathy; halitosis; oral thrush and/or ulcers; and visible and/or palpable masses.

Neurological: Perform a screening neurological exam focusing on cranial nerves and upper motor neuron signs.

Integumentary: Assess for features of CREST syndrome (calcinosis, Raynaud phenomenon, esophageal dysmotility, sclerodactyly, telangiectasia).

Abdominal: Check for umbilical lymphadenopathy and masses.

Investigations

LABORATORY INVESTIGATIONS

CBC with differential

Creatinine (eGFR)

Electrolytes (Na, K, Cl, HCO_3), extended electrolytes (Ca, Mg, PO_4)

Other nutritional markers: Examples include iron studies, vitamin B_{12}, and albumin.

Thyrotropin (TSH)

Infectious workup: Pursue this in immunosuppressed patients.

IMAGING

Chest x-ray:
› Look for aspiration.
› A small or absent gastric bubble with or without widening of the mediastinum suggests achalasia.

OTHER INVESTIGATIONS

Pursue other investigations based on the differential diagnosis, current guidelines, and expert opinion.

Gastroscopy: Pursue this in patients with red-flag symptoms.

Fiberoptic nasopharyngeal laryngoscopy

Barium swallow: Pursue this for suspected structural lesions.

Esophageal manometry or 24-hour pH impedance test: Pursue this for suspected motility disorders.

Swallowing assessment: Consider assessment by a speech-language pathologist or occupational therapist.

Modified barium swallow: Use this to assess the oropharyngeal phase of swallowing.

Impression and Plan

Start with a summary: Include your working diagnosis and differential diagnoses.

Consider next steps: These could include further investigations, treatments, and patient counselling.

Provide information on PEG tube insertion, as indicated: If you are being asked to assess the patient for PEG tube insertion, make sure you assess whether the measure is appropriate, the patient's nutritional status, and the patient's goals of care.

Discuss DVT prophylaxis.

Provide the patient's code status.

Elevated Liver Enzymes

These notes are in addition to the **general guide for all consultations** on page 1, and the **starting points for gastroenterology consultations** at the beginning of this chapter.

Identification

Key information in the identification statement includes relevant GI-related medical history.

Reason for Referral

The referral may seek to confirm a liver enzyme abnormality and/or clarify appropriate management.

⎯⎯

DIFFERENTIAL DIAGNOSIS FOR ELEVATED LIVER ENZYMES

Hepatocellular injury: predominantly AST and/or ALT elevation

    Infection: HAV, HBV, HCV, HDV, HEV, EBV, CMV, HSV, VZV

    Autoimmune: autoimmune hepatitis

    Nonalcoholic fatty liver disease (NAFLD)

    Alcohol use, medications (acetaminophen, statins, others)

    Vascular: ischemic ("shock liver"), Budd-Chiari syndrome, congestive, sinusoidal obstructive syndrome

    Hereditary: hemochromatosis, Wilson disease, α_1-antitrypsin deficiency

Cholestasis: predominantly direct bilirubin, ALP, and GGT elevation

    Tumour-obstructing biliary tree (pancreatic, cholangiocarcinoma)

Primary sclerosing cholangitis
Cirrhosis
Hepatitis
Medications (sex hormones, others)
TPN
Primary biliary cholangitis
Sepsis, postoperative
Choledocholithiasis
Infiltrative pattern: predominantly ALP and GGT elevation
Malignancy: HCC, metastases, lymphoma
Granuloma: TB, sarcoid, *Histoplasma capsulatum*
Abscess: bacterial, amebic, echinococcus
Amyloid
Other
Isolated indirect hyperbilirubinemia: Crigler-Najjar
syndrome, Gilbert syndrome, hemolysis
Pregnancy: acute fatty liver of pregnancy, HELLP syndrome
Celiac disease
Non-GI sources: bone (ALP without GGT), muscle
(transaminase), cardiac (transaminase, with troponin)

History of Present Illness
- Symptoms may vary, from no symptoms to manifestations of acute fulminant liver failure.
- Ask about:
  › right upper quadrant pain
  › fatigue, malaise
  › lethargy
  › anorexia
  › jaundice, acholic stools, dark urine
  › abdominal distention (ascites)

Past Medical History
See Differential Diagnosis for Elevated Liver Enzymes in this section, which lists conditions to ask about.

Medications
Ask about:
- herbal and OTC medications (these frequently cause liver injury)
- medications commonly involved in liver injury, including acetaminophen, NSAIDs, amiodarone, labetalol, statins, phenytoin,

valproic acids, carbamazepine, diltiazem, fluoroquinolones, amoxicillin-clavulanate, sulfonamides, trimethoprim-sulfamethoxazole, tetracycline, propylthiouracil, indinavir, allopurinol
> Consider consulting the online reference on drug-induced liver injury, LiverTox.[1]

Family History
Ask about:
- hemochromatosis
- α_1-antitrypsin deficiency
- Wilson disease

Social History
Ask about:
- alcohol use, IV drug use, multiple sexual partners
- recent travel history, with presence of GI issues during or after the trip
- occupational or recreational exposure to hepatotoxins (e.g., industrial chemicals, mushroom picking)

Physical Examination
Vital signs:
> Hemodynamic instability may indicate sepsis.
> Fever may be present with viral infections or sepsis.

General impression: Check for:
> altered mental status, weakness, and asterixis
> jaundice (this suggests a primary liver etiology)
> hypervolemia (high JVP suggests CHF or hepatic congestion)

Abdominal: Assess for:
> right upper quadrant tenderness
> ascites (bulging flanks, positive fluid wave test, shifting dullness)
> stigmata of liver disease (hepatomegaly, splenomegaly, spider angiomata, palmar erythema, clubbing, Dupuytren contracture, leukonychia, Terry nails, gynecomastia, loss of chest hair in men, testicular atrophy, caput medusa, hemorrhoids)

Investigations
LABORATORY INVESTIGATIONS
CBC, LDH, haptoglobin
Electrolytes (Na, K, Cl, HCO_3), extended electrolytes (Ca, Mg, PO_4)
Creatinine (eGFR), urea
Liver enzymes (AST, ALT, ALP, GGT) and liver function (albumin, bilirubin, INR, PTT)
Lipase

Lactate, ABG
Serum drug screen: acetaminophen and alcohol level
Pregnancy test (if female)
Blood cultures
HAV, HBV, HCV serologies
› Consider HDV if HBV is positive.
› Consider HEV in pregnant patients.
HIV, EBV, CMV, HSV
**ANA, anti-smooth muscle antibodies, antimitochondrial antibodies,
antibodies to liver/kidney microsomes[2]**
Quantitative immunoglobulin (IgG), CRP
Ferritin, iron studies
Ceruloplasmin
α1-antitrypsin level
AFP level
CK, thyrotropin (TSH)

IMAGING
Abdominal US with Doppler: Use this to:
› further characterize liver parenchyma
› assess for stones or sludge in the biliary tract, biliary duct dilation,
and portal vein thrombus
› rule out Budd-Chiari syndrome
Abdominal CT, triphasic liver protocol: This assesses for the
presence of liver lesions, infectious cysts, and signs of tumour.
Magnetic resonance cholangiopancreatography (MRCP):
This assesses for biliary strictures, cholangiocarcinoma, and
choledocholithiasis.

Impression and Plan

SUMMARY
• Include the most likely diagnosis and differential diagnoses based on
the pattern of enzyme elevation.
• Indicate whether acute liver failure is present (encephalopathy, INR
higher than 1.5, with elevated liver enzymes).

TREATMENT
• Treatment is highly dependent on etiology (see Differential Diagnosis
for Elevated Liver Enzymes in this section).
• Secure ABCs, and provide oxygen support and IV hydration, as indicated.
Underlying Etiologies
HBV: antiviral therapy (this may be required)

HCV: antiviral therapy (this cures HCV)
Alcohol: abstinence, nutritional support
Autoimmune hepatitis: steroids, azathioprine
Acetaminophen: N-acetylcysteine (NAC)
NAFLD: weight loss
Budd-Chiari syndrome: anticoagulation[3]
Wilson disease: D-penicillamine, trientine[4]
Hemochromatosis: phlebotomy[5]
Biliary obstruction: ERCP
Primary biliary cirrhosis: ursodiol
HELLP syndrome: delivery

Cirrhosis Complications

Hepatic encephalopathy: Continue lactulose with or without rifaximin.[6]

Ascites: Provide diuretics, restrict the patient's salt and water intake, and pursue diagnostic or therapeutic paracentesis to rule out spontaneous bacterial peritonitis.

Varices: Pursue EGD to rule out varices and provide a nonselective beta-blocker if varices are present.

Hepatorenal syndrome: Closely monitor kidney function and fluid status.[7]

Hepatocellular carcinoma: Screen for this in all patients with cirrhosis with a liver US or triphasic CT scan of liver.

Acute Liver Failure, Decompensated Cirrhosis

- Use the Model for End Stage Liver Disease with sodium (MELD-Na) to assess severity.
- Consider referral of patients with MELD-Na scores greater than 15 for liver transplantation.

OTHER NOTES
- Discuss DVT prophylaxis.
- Provide the patient's code status.

Gastrointestinal Bleeding

These notes are in addition to the **general guide for all consultations** on page 1, and the **starting points for gastroenterology consultations** at the beginning of this chapter.

Identification

Follow the **general guide for all consultations.**

Reason for Referral

The referral may seek to confirm GI bleeding and/or clarify appropriate management. It may mention objective findings of GI bleeding (hematemesis, hematochezia, melena), and describe the patient's hemoglobin trend and hemodynamic stability.

History of Present Illness

Characterize the bleed[8]: Clarify:
› hematemesis versus hemoptysis versus epistaxis versus coffee-grounds emesis
› melena (tarry black) versus hematochezia (bright red)
› blood mixed in the stool versus outside the stool

Ask about associated symptoms:
› bowel movement urgency or tenesmus
› dysphagia or odynophagia
› pain (apply the mnemonic OPQRST AAA)
› postprandial pain, GERD, retching
› symptomatic anemia (fatigue, dyspnea, angina, palpitations)

Assess for upper GI bleeding (in the context of melena or coffee-grounds emesis): Ask about a history or symptoms of:
› **Peptic ulcer disease:** NSAID use, alcohol use, history of *Helicobacter pylori*, abdominal pain relieved by meals, GERD
› **Variceal bleeding:** liver disease, encephalopathy, alcohol use
› **Mallory-Weiss tear:** recent vomiting, hematemesis
› **Pseudo GI bleeding:** iron pills, bismuth, blueberries
› **Dieulafoy lesion:** previous upper GI bleeding of unclear etiology
› **Non-GI source:** epistaxis, hemoptysis

Assess for lower GI bleeding (in the context of hematochezia): Ask about a history or symptoms of:
› **Diverticular bleeding:** painless, large-volume bleeding, history of diverticulosis
› **Hemorrhoids:** painful or painless; sensation of "something down there"; nonsevere bleeding; irregular bowel habits
› **Ischemic colitis:** history of peripheral vascular disease, CAD, recent painful bowel movement followed by blood
› **Angiodysplasia/Heyde syndrome:** aortic stenosis
› **Postpolypectomy bleeding:** recent colonoscopy
› **Colitis:** infections, IBD, radiation

Assess for both upper and lower GI bleeding:
> **Malignancy:** Ask about constitutional symptoms.
> **Aortoenteric fistula:**
>> This involves both upper and lower GI bleeding.
>> It is life-threatening.
>> Ask about a recent angiogram or vascular procedure.

Conduct a GI review of systems: Ask about:
> typical bowel habits (frequency, quality, colour, odour, stool character on Bristol chart, changes)
> diet, nutritional status

Past Medical History

Ask about previous endoscopic procedures: Establish the dates and findings.

Identify GI-related diseases:
> Examples include previous GI bleeds, liver disease, GERD, IBD (clarify subtype), and diverticulosis.
> For each, clarify the year of diagnosis, course of the disease, disease-related complications, and gastroenterologists the patient has seen.

Clarify comorbidities: Ask about chronic kidney disease, aortic stenosis, and cardiac conditions.

Clarify other pertinent medical conditions: Examples include VTE for which anticoagulation would be used.

Past Surgical History

Follow the **general guide for all consultations** and the **starting points for gastroenterology consultations.**

Medications

Ask about:
- antiplatelets, anticoagulants, NSAIDs
- current medications (clarify doses and routes of administration)

Allergies

Follow the **general guide for all consultations.**

Family History

Ask about:
- colon adenocarcinoma
- IBD

Social History

Ask about:
- alcohol use, IV drug use

- recent travel history with GI issues during or after the trip

Physical Examination

Vital signs: orthostatic vitals, tachycardia, oxygen saturation

General impression: mentation, distress, body habitus, paleness or jaundice

Head, neck: blood in nares or mouth

Abdominal:
> Look for epigastric tenderness, and stigmata of chronic liver disease or portal hypertension.
> Perform a DRE, assessing for melena, hematochezia, fissures, hemorrhoids, and anorectal pathology.

Other: volume status

Investigations

LABORATORY INVESTIGATIONS

CBC, group and screen, cross match: Thrombocytopenia may suggest cirrhosis.

Creatinine (eGFR), urea

Electrolytes (Na, K, Cl, HCO$_3$)

BUN-to-creatinine ratio: A ratio > 30:1 is a strong indicator of upper GI bleeding.

Liver enzymes (AST, ALT, ALP, GGT) and liver function (albumin, bilirubin, INR, PTT)

Helicobacter pylori: Consider testing for this.

IMAGING

Chest x-ray: This assesses for aspiration and pneumomediastinum.

Abdominal x-ray: Pursue this on concern for perforation and bleeding in duodenal ulcer, or severe diverticulitis with microperforations.

Abdominal CT: Pursue this in suspected peritonitis that is not detected on plain films.

Impression and Plan

SUMMARY

- Include the most likely diagnosis and differential diagnoses.
- For upper GI bleeding, provide a Glasgow-Blatchford Bleeding Score (this identifies low-risk patients who may be appropriate for outpatient management).[9]
- For lower GI bleeding, provide an Oakland Score (this determines if outpatient management is feasible for low-risk patients).[10]

Differential Diagnoses
- See History of Present Illness in this section for a breakdown.
- Consider where the bleed is coming from and why.
- In bright red blood from the rectum:
  › Always consider upper GI bleeding: remember that it can present with fresh blood in stools.
  › In patients younger than 40, common causes include colitis, hemorrhoids, and colonic ulcer.
  › In patients older than 40, common causes include colon adenocarcinoma, diverticulosis, and angiodysplasia.

TREATMENT
Secure ABCs, and provide oxygen support and IV hydration in a monitored setting, as indicated.

Blood Transfusion
The target for hemoglobin is > 70 g/L (or > 80 g/L in known CAD, or based on clinical judgement in massive bleeding).

Anticoagulation
Order anticoagulation reversal agents in patients with an INR greater than 2.5 and significant bleeding:
- **Vitamin K:** 10 units IV
- **FFP:** 2–4 units IV
- **Massive transfusion protocol (1:1:1):**
  » Pursue this in patients requiring 3 or more units of packed RBCs over 1 hour, or in hemodynamically unstable patients requiring any 4 blood components over 30 minutes.

Significant Bleeding
- In significant bleeding, administer pantoprazole: 80 mg IV, then 8 mg/hour.
  › In known cirrhosis, or in patients at high risk of cirrhosis, add octreotide (50 mcg IV bolus, then 50 mcg/hour) and ceftriaxone (2 g).
- Consider the need for urgent cessation of bleeding, including:
  › surgery in hyperacute or uncontrollable bleeding
  › interventional radiology in stable patients with significant active bleeding and/or a previous failed endoscopy
  › endoscopy in hemodynamically stable patients, or patients in a heavily monitored setting such as the ICU (consider optimal preparation)

OTHER NOTES
- Hold DVT prophylaxis and any anticoagulation.
- Provide the patient's code status.

Pancreatitis

These notes are in addition to the **general guide for all consultations** on page 1, and the **starting points for gastroenterology consultations** at the beginning of this chapter.

Identification

Follow the **general guide for all consultations.**

Reason for Referral

The referral typically seeks guidance on the management of pancreatitis and/or its complications.

History of Present Illness

Characterize the abdominal pain: Patterns include:

› constant pain that is epigastric and/or localized to upper quadrants (90% of cases)
› band-like pain that radiates to the back (50%)
› pain that peaks 10 to 20 minutes after meals (common)
› moderate-severe pain and unbearable pain (typical)
› no pain (10%)

Clarify other symptoms: Ask about:

› nausea and vomiting (90% of cases)
› anorexia (this indicates course and severity)
› fever and jaundice (this suggests concurrent cholangitis)
› weight loss and steatorrhea (this suggests chronic pancreatitis)

Assess for clues to etiology: Ask about a history and symptoms of:

› **Gallstones (40% of cases):** history of biliary colic
› **Excessive alcohol intake (30% of cases)**
› **Hypertriglyceridemia:** xanthomas, known history
› **ERCP:** recently performed
› **Trauma:** blunt or penetrating
› **Drugs:** new medications (see Medications in this section)
› **Malignancy:** constitutional symptoms, jaundice, acholic stools, dark urine
› **Hypercalcemia:** moans, groans, stones, psychiatric overtones
› **Autoimmune disease:** obstructive uropathy, CKD, parotitis
› **Infection or ischemia:** shock, bypass, fevers
› **Sphincter of Oddi dysfunction:** recurrent postprandial pain and intermittent jaundice
› **Scorpion sting:** Trinidadian scorpions

Clarify the time of onset: This is important if a patient becomes unstable.
> Early deterioration (less than 1 week from onset) suggests SIRS and/or organ failure.
> Late deterioration (more than 1 week from onset) suggests local complications.

Past Medical History
Ask about:
- a history of pancreatitis (establish the date of diagnosis, cause, and complications)
- high-yield entities, which include cholelithiasis, recent ERCP, and diagnosed or suspected alcohol use disorder
- lower-yield entities, including malignancy (consider the possibility of metastasis), vasculitis (SLE, polyarteritis nodosa), chronic infection (HIV, TB), and autoimmune disorders (autoimmune hepatitis)

Past Surgical History
Ask about recent abdominal surgeries.

Medications
- Ask about prescriptions for pancreatic enzymes (isozyme), which suggests underlying chronic pancreatitis.
- Drugs cause 1% of pancreatitis cases.
- Focus on new agents or dose changes.
- Drugs implicated in pancreatitis include[11]:
  > **Antimicrobials:** dapsone, isoniazid, trimethoprim-sulfamethoxazole, metronidazole, tetracycline, lamivudine, nelfinavir, pentamidine
  > **Antiinflammatories:** azathioprine, mesalamine, steroids, sulindac
  > **Cardiovascular medications:** enalapril, losartan, furosemide, hydrochlorothiazide, statins, bezafibrate, amiodarone, procainamide
  > **Cytotoxic medications:** mercaptopurine, cytarabine, ifosfamide
  > **Endocrine medications:** methimazole, clomiphene, estrogen, dipeptidyl peptidase 4 inhibitors, glucagonlike peptide 1 agonists
  > **Other:** codeine, omeprazole, valproic acid

Allergies
Follow the **general guide for all consultations**.

Family History
Consider an inherited cause when the patient is younger than 30,[12] or has a significant family history of idiopathic pancreatitis.

Social History
- Focus on alcohol use: the risk of acute pancreatitis increases with the dose and duration of alcohol use.
- Tobacco smoking increases the risk of chronic pancreatitis.
- Heavy cannabis use may be associated with pancreatitis.[11]

Physical Examination
Vital signs: These often indicate severity or complications.
› Obtain and assess qSOFA criteria, including GCS score, respiration rate, and systolic BP.[13]
› Reduced oxygen saturation suggests ARDS or aspiration.
› Low-grade fever suggests inflammation, *not infection.*

Abdominal:
› **Inspection:** Signs of retroperitoneal hemorrhage are rarely present, but may include bruising over the flanks (Grey Turner sign) or periumbilical area (Cullen sign).
› **Auscultation:** Loss of bowel sounds suggests ileus.
› **Palpation and percussion:**
  » Look for epigastric guarding or tenderness.
  » Check for a palpable gallbladder (Courvoisier sign).
  » A tense and distended abdomen suggests tense ascites versus abdominal compartment syndrome.
› **Murphy sign:** A positive sign suggests cholecystitis.

Other: Assess volume status and check for jaundice (jaundice suggests an obstructive cause).

Investigations
LABORATORY INVESTIGATIONS
CBC

Electrolytes (Na, K, Cl, HCO_3), extended electrolytes (Ca, Mg, PO_4)

Creatinine (eGFR), urea

Liver enzymes (AST, ALT, ALP, GGT) and liver function (albumin, bilirubin, INR, PTT)

Triglycerides, LDH

Blood cultures: Obtain 2 samples from 2 different sites.

IgG subclasses: Consider this for IgG4 disease.

Genetic testing: Consider this for hereditary pancreatitis.

CRP: Use this (not lipase) to monitor response.

Interpretation
- **ALT:** A finding > 150 U/L has a 95% PPV for gallstone etiology.[14]
- **Lipase:**
  › Note that lipase is preferred over amylase.

› Lipase 3 times greater than ULN suggests acute pancreatitis
  (sensitivity 99%, specificity 99%).[15]
› Lipase > 10 000 U/L has 80% PPV for biliary etiology and 99% NPV
  for alcohol.[15]
› Note that lipase can be normal in chronic pancreatitis (burned out
  pancreas).

IMAGING

Abdominal US: Pursue this to rule out biliary pathology.

Abdominal CT with contrast:
› This is not often indicated at first presentation.
› It is useful to rule out complications in patients who are not
  improving after 2 to 3 days.
› It can detect pancreatic cysts, nodules, and calcifications.

MRCP: Consider this when there is no clear cause identified, and
  there is suspicion of pancreatic ductal obstruction (e.g., from biliary
  sludge, anatomic variation, malignancy).

Endoscopic US: Pursue this on suspicion of biliary disease where
  laboratory investigations and imaging are inconclusive (endoscopic
  US has more sensitivity than MRCP).

CT-guided fine-needle aspiration: This is not usually required, but
  it can rule out infected necrosis in patients with a poor response to
  antibiotics.

Impression and Plan

State the cause of the pancreatitis: For example, state the cause as
  excessive alcohol intake or stones.

Note the criteria for acute pancreatitis: The diagnosis of acute
  pancreatitis requires at least 2 of the following:
› characteristic abdominal pain
› lipase levels greater than 3 times ULN
› signs of pancreatic inflammation on imaging

Describe the severity of the pancreatitis:
› Consider using a scoring system (e.g., BISAP,[16] Ranson,[17]
  APACHE-II,[18] Revised Atlanta Criteria[19]).
› In general, you can classify severity this way:
  » **Mild:** no organ failure; no systemic or local complications
  » **Moderate:** organ failure for less than 48 hours and/or complications
  » **Severe:** organ failure for more than 48 hours

TREATMENT

Secure ABCs and provide early IV hydration:
› These patients need fluids.
› Administer 1–2 L bolus, followed by 250–500 mL/hour.

› Ringer lactate may be superior to normal saline.[20]
› Be cautious with hydration in elderly patients, and patients with acute kidney injury, CKD, and/or CHF.

Provide pain control: opiates (meperidine is not superior)

Provide antiemetics as needed.

Provide early enteral feeding:
› **Mild pancreatitis:** Start a low-residue, low-fat diet within 48 hours, with progression as tolerated.[21]
› **Ileus:** Provide nutrition through a nasogastric or nasojejunal tube and allow nothing by mouth.
› **Severe pancreatitis:** Provide enteral feeding within 2 to 3 days and avoid TPN.[22]

Consider antibiotics:
› Antibiotics are appropriate only on suspicion of infected necrosis (air within a peripancreatic fluid collection).
› Don't just treat a fever and elevated WBC count.

Etiology and Complications: Specific Management

Gallstone pancreatitis: ERCP within 24 hours if ongoing obstruction[24]; cholecystectomy

Excessive alcohol intake: cessation, addiction counselling, Clinical Institute Withdrawal Assessment for Alcohol

Hypertriglyceridemia: insulin infusion, fibrates

IgG4 disease, autoimmune pancreatitis: steroid taper

Disrupted duct syndrome: pancreatic stenting

Pseudocyst, pancreatic necrosis: draining (only if symptomatic and mature [present for more than 4 weeks])

Infected necrosis: antibiotics; draining via endoscopy or interventional radiology, as clinical status dictates

Other:
› Watch for ARDS, hypocalcemia, and DIC.

References

1. LiverTox: clinical and research information on drug-induced liver injury [Internet]. Bethesda (MD): National Institute of Diabetes and Digestive and Kidney Diseases; 2012 [cited 2022 Jan 10]. Available from: https://pubmed.ncbi.nlm.nih.gov/31643176/

2. Kerkar N, Chan A. Autoimmune hepatitis, sclerosing cholangitis, and autoimmune sclerosing cholangitis or overlap syndrome. Clin Liver Dis. 2018;22(4):689-702. doi:10.1016/j.cld.2018.06.005

3. Hitawala A, Gupta V. Budd Chiari syndrome [Internet]. Treasure Island (FL): StatPearls Publishing; 2020 [updated 2021 Jun 4; cited 2022 Jan 10]. Available from: https://www.ncbi.nlm.nih.gov/books/NBK558941/#article-18680.s14

4. Aggarwal A, Bhatt M. Advances in treatment of Wilson disease. Tremor Other Hyperkinet Mov (N Y). 2018;8:525. doi:10.7916/D841881D

5. Voloshina N, Osipenko M, Litvinova N, et al. Hemochromatosis - modern condition of the problem. Ter Arkh. 2018;90(3):107-12. doi:10.26442/terarkh2018903107-112

6. Said V, Garcia-Trujillo E. Beyond lactulose: treatment options for hepatic encephalopathy. Gastroenterol Nursing. 2019;42(3):277-85. doi:10.1097/SGA.0000000000000376

7. Mansour D, McPherson S. Management of decompensated cirrhosis. Clin Med. 2018;18(suppl 2):s60-65. doi:10.7861/clinmedicine.18-2-s60

8. Kim B, Li B, Engel A, et al. Diagnosis of gastrointestinal bleeding: a practical guide for clinicians. World J Gastrointest Pathophysiol. 2014;5(4):467-78. doi: 10.429/wjgp.v5.i4.467

9. Monteiro S, Gonçalves T, Magalhães J, et al. Upper gastrointestinal bleeding risk scores: who, when and why? World J Gastrointest Pathophysiol. 2016;7(1):86-96. doi: 10.429/wjgp.v7.i1.86

10. Oakland K, Kothiwale S, Forehand T, et al. External validation of the Oakland score to assess safe hospital discharge among adult patients with acute lower gastrointestinal bleeding in the US. JAMA Netw Open. 2020;3(7):e209630. doi: 10.1001/jamanetworkopen.2020.9630

11. Badalov N, Baradarian R, Iswara K, et al. Drug-induced acute pancreatitis: an evidence-based review. Clinical Gastroenterol Hepatol. 2007;5(6):648-61. doi: 10.1016/j.cgh.2006.11.123

12. Tenner S, Baillie J, DeWitt J, et al. American College of Gastroenterology guideline: management of acute pancreatitis. American J Gastroenterol. 2013;108(9):1400-15. doi: 10.1038/ajg.2013.2218

13. Singer M, Deutschman C, Seymour C, et al. The Third International Consensus Definitions for Sepsis and Septic Shock (Sepsis-3). JAMA. 2016;315(8):801-10. doi: 10.1001/jama.2016.0287

14. Tenner S, Dubner H, Steinberg W. Predicting gallstone pancreatitis with laboratory parameters: a meta-analysis. Am J of Gastroenterol. 1994;89(10):1863-66. PMID: 7942684

15. Cornett D, Spier B, Eggert A, et al. The causes and outcome of acute pancreatitis associated with serum lipase >10,000 U/L. Dig Dis Sci. 2011;56(11):3376-81. doi: 10.1007/s10620-011-1752-5

16. Wu B, Johannes R, Sun X, et al. The early prediction of mortality in acute pancreatitis: a large population-based study. Gut. 2008;57(12):1698-1703. doi: 10.1136/gut.2008.152702

17. Ranson J, Rifkind K, Roses D, et al. Objective early identification of severe acute pancreatitis. Am J Gastroenterol. 1974;61(6):443-51. PMID: 4835417

18. Larvin M, McMahon M. APACHE-II score for assessment and monitoring of acute pancreatitis. Lancet. 1989:2(8656):201-5. doi: 10.1016/s0140-6736(89)90381-4

19. Vege S, Gardner T, Chari S, et al. Low mortality and high morbidity in severe acute pancreatitis without organ failure: a case for revising the Atlanta Classification to include "moderately severe acute pancreatitis." Am J Gastroenterol. 2009;104(3):710-15. doi: 10.1038/ajg.2008.77

20. Wu B, Hwang J, Gardner T, et al. Lactated Ringer's solution reduces systemic inflammation compared with saline in patients with acute pancreatitis. Clin Gastroenterol Hepatol. 2011;9(8):710-1.e1. doi: 10.1016/j.cgh.2011.04.026

21. Vege S, DiMagno M, Forsmark C, et al. Initial medical treatment of acute pancreatitis: American Gastroenterological Association Institute technical review. Gastroenterology. 2018 Mar 1;154(4):1103-39. doi: 10.1053/j.gastro.2018.01.031

22. Yi F, Ge L, Zhao J, et al. Meta-analysis: total parenteral nutrition versus total enteral nutrition in predicted severe acute pancreatitis. Intern Med. 2012;51(6):523-30. doi: 10.2169/internalmedicine.51.6685

23. Al-Omran M, Albalawi Z, Tashkandi M, et al. Enteral versus parenteral nutrition for acute pancreatitis. Cochrane Database Syst Review. 2010(1);CD002837. doi: 10.1002/14651858. CD002837.pub2

24. Fogel E, Sherman S. ERCP for gallstone pancreatitis. N Engl J Med. 2014;370(2):150-57. doi: 10.1056/NEJMct1208450

8

Geriatric Medicine

Dr. Clara Tsui
Dr. Lindsay Schnarr
Dr. Claire Wu

REVIEWER
Dr. Mark Fok

Starting Points: Comprehensive Geriatric Assessments

These notes are in addition to the **general guide for all consultations** on page 1.

Identification

Key information in the identification statement includes the patient's age, living circumstances (living at home, or in an assisted- or independent-living facility, or in a long-term care facility; home supports; living alone or with family), and relevant comorbidities.

Reason for Referral

Common reasons for referral include a comprehensive geriatric assessment (CGA), disposition planning, and assessment of chronic medical issues.

History of Present Illness

Focus on a review of systems with attention to common geriatric problems. Family members are often present and are a useful source of collateral information. Try to let the patient answer questions first, and then have others answer or fill in details.

Assess cognition:
> How do you think your memory is? Have you or your family members noticed any changes?

> Do you misplace things easily? Have you gotten lost while out for a walk or while driving? Have you ever left the stove on or tap running and forgot about it?

Ask about falls:
> Have you had any falls in the last year? How many?
> Are you afraid of falling?
> What were the circumstances around these falls (e.g., tripping, dizziness, loss of balance, or loss of consciousness)?
> Were you injured in these falls?
> Do you use any gait aids (e.g., cane, walker, wheelchair)?

Assess sleep patterns:
> Do you have problems with sleep?
> What time do you go to bed and wake up?
> How many times do you get up at night? Are you getting up to urinate?
> Do you have any unusual movements or behaviours during sleep?
> Do you snore, choke, or gasp for air? Do you nap during the day?

Ask about continence:
> Have you had any leakage of urine in the past 3 months? Do you wear a pad or a brief?
> Do you have any issues with constipation? Do you have loose stools or diarrhea?
> Have you had any accidents where you soil yourself?

Assess mood: Screen for depression and screen for elder abuse.

Assess nutrition:
> How is your appetite? How many meals do you eat per day?
> Have you noticed any weight loss?

Ask about polypharmacy:
> Do you take more than 5 medications?

Assess for pain: Ask about issues with pain, discomfort, and soreness. If the patient has issues, conduct a pain history by applying the mnemonic OPQRST AAA, and clarify treatments tried.

Past Medical History

- Review all past medical history.
- Start with relevant geriatric issues, including:
    > **Dementia or MCI:** Determine the diagnosis, if known (e.g., AD, Lewy body dementia); the patient's cognitive assessment score via Montreal Cognitive Assessment (MoCA), MMSE, or Rowland Universal Dementia Assessment Scale (RUDAS); the date of diagnosis; specialists involved; and medications.
    > **Fractures or head injuries:** Determine dates and interventions.
    > **Parkinson disease:** Determine the date of diagnosis, specialists involved, and medications.

> **Osteoporosis or osteopenia:** Determine BMD score and medications.

Past Surgical History

Ask about:

- joint replacements, fracture repairs
- incontinence-related interventions (pessary, bladder suspension, transurethral resection of the prostate)

Medications

Ask about:

- all medications, including OTC medications
- recent medication changes
- supplements, and natural or herbal medications
- delivery method, including whether the medications are blister packed or in bottles, and who administers the medications (e.g., self or caregiver)
- issues with remembering to take medications

Allergies

Ask about medications that have caused side effects, but not true anaphylaxis (e.g., dizziness, hypotension, nausea).

Family History

Ask about dementia, Parkinson disease, and osteoporosis.

Social History

A detailed social history is an important part of a CGA. Ask about:

- living situation (where, type of building, with whom, any stairs to navigate)
- birthplace, year of immigration (if applicable)
- first language or languages spoken
- highest level of education
- previous occupations, and the year and reason for retirement
- marital status and children (ask where the children live)
- substance use (smoking, alcohol, drugs)
- financial supports

Functional History

- Ask whether the patient is independent or dependent for the following tasks:
  > **ADLs:** These include dressing, eating, ambulating (ask about gait aids), toileting, and hygiene (bathing and showering).
  > **IADLs:** These include shopping, housekeeping, accounting, food preparation, and toileting.

› **Driving:** Is the patient still driving? If so, ask about recent road or written tests, recent accidents, and concerns about safety.
• Ask about vision and hearing problems and aids.
• Ask about formal supports in the patient's home.

Plans for Care

• Determine what directions the patient has in place for their care (e.g., goals of care, advance directive, power of attorney, end-of-life planning).
• If the patient has nothing in place, start a discussion about a care plan.

Physical Examination

Vital signs: orthostatic BP
Weight
Mental status:
  › **General impression:** level of alertness, orientation, appearance, speech, eye contact, cooperation, motor activity
  › **Thinking:** thought process, thought content, perceptual disturbances
  › **Emotion:** mood, affect
  › **Cognition:** orientation, attention, memory, insight, judgement
Cardiac: any abnormalities
Respiratory: any abnormalities
Abdominal: any abnormalities
Neurological:
  › A complete neurological exam is important, including cerebellar testing, and assessing for parkinsonism (tremor, rigidity, bradykinesia), and Romberg sign.
  › Conduct a gait assessment: ask the patient to stand from a sitting position (without using their arms, if possible), and to walk and turn; assess the patient's ability to do tandem gait and unipedal stance.
Skin and feet: skin breakdown, ulcerations; foot ulcers, bunions, ingrown toenails, other issues

Investigations

LABORATORY INVESTIGATIONS

Basic workup: CBC, electrolytes, renal function, liver enzymes
Workup for secondary causes of cognitive impairment: glucose, Ca, thyrotropin (TSH), vitamin B_{12}, HIV, syphilis serology, urine drug screen, serum toxicology screen
Workup for secondary causes of osteoporosis: Ca, vitamin D level, ALP, thyrotropin (TSH), serum or urine protein electrophoresis

MICROBIOLOGY

Check for results of previous urine cultures or other cultures.

CARDIAC ASSESSMENTS

ECG: arrhythmias, QT interval (these can impact medications)

Echocardiogram: EF, wall motion abnormalities

IMAGING

CT of the head: Order this depending on the clinical context to look for volume loss, infarcts, hemorrhage, and cerebrovascular disease.

COGNITIVE TESTING

General Guidelines

- Perform cognitive testing in the context of concern about cognition, and compare the results to previous tests.
- In general, avoid formal cognitive testing on delirious patients as the result may not represent their true cognitive ability.

Specific Tests

MoCA: This is best for outpatient settings; for those who speak English and have more than 12 years of education; and for suspected MCI.

MMSE: This is the most commonly used test; it is suitable for those with less than 12 years of education and is best for separating moderate dementia from normal cognitive function.

RUDAS: This is best for those whose first language is not English or who have less than 12 years of education.

Impression and Plan

ISSUES BREAKDOWN

Create a problem-based list of issues. Common issues include:

- **Cognition:** Provide:
  › a diagnosis (e.g., MCI, AD) with severity assessment
  › a workup to rule out secondary causes of cognitive impairment
  › nonpharmacological management (e.g., a referral for occupational therapy [OT] for cognitive training)
  › pharmacotherapy, as indicated
  › management of cardiovascular risk factors, as indicated
- **Falls and bone health:**
  › Provide an assessment of fall risk and send the patient for a BMD scan if indicated.
  › Describe factors that can be mitigated.
  › Refer the patient for a PT or OT assessment (specify for in-home or as an inpatient).

> Consider initiation of vitamin D and antiresorptive therapies for bone health.
- **Continence:**
  > Management is based on the etiology of incontinence.
  > Always consider nonpharmacological interventions first, then pharmacotherapy.
  > Consider referring the patient to a continence clinic.
- **Safety and functional status:**
  > Consider the patient's needs for home supports.
  > Refer the patient to a case manager if the patient is planning to move out of their home to a facility, or has complex issues requiring multiple team members.
  > Refer the patient to a community OT to evaluate equipment needs in the home.
  > Provide an assessment of the patient's competence to drive.
  > Comment on the patient's need for a power of attorney or representative if there are concerns about financial mismanagement.
  > Recommend medication management, as indicated.
- **Mood:** Refer the patient to a psychiatrist and/or prescribe pharmacotherapy, as indicated.
- **Nutrition:** Refer the patient to a dietitian, and recommend nutritional supplements (e.g., Ensure or Boost), as indicated.
- **Polypharmacy:** List medications to stop or decrease.
- **Pain:** Provide nonpharmacologic and pharmacologic options.

CARE PLANS

Clearly document discussions about care plans that have taken place with the patient or their family, including decisions made.

FOLLOW-UP

Describe plans for follow-up and consider referral to a geriatrician.

Delirium

These notes are in addition to the **general guide for all consultations** on page 1, and the **starting points for comprehensive geriatric assessments** at the beginning of this chapter.

Identification

Key information in the identification statement includes relevant comorbidities, any known cognitive impairment, and, for inpatients, the date of and reason for admission.

Reason for Referral

Common reasons for referral include altered level of consciousness (LOC), agitation, and confusion.

History of Present Illness

Collect collateral history: Delirious patients may be unreliable, so talk to caregivers, family, and other health-care providers.

Identify nursing concerns: Review the patient's chart and speak to the bedside nurse regarding their concerns about the patient's behaviour (e.g., if the patient has required security or a one-on-one sitter) and response to any medications given for delirium.

Establish the acuity of onset.

Identify key symptoms: Ask about fluctuating symptoms of disorganized thinking (incoherent speech, switching subjects, illogical conversation), changes in sensorium, and changes in the patient's sleep-wake cycle.

Clarify changes in LOC: Ask about symptoms of:
› **Hyperactive delirium:** hypervigilance, agitation, calling out, pulling at IV lines or catheters, attempting to climb out of bed
› **Hypoactive delirium:** lethargy, drowsiness, "bed seeking," minimal verbal output

Establish the patient's baseline cognition and functional status.

Clarify the course of hospitalization: Consider asking the patient to summarize this to assess for understanding and thought process.

Identify potential causes: Ask about:
› **Drugs:** new or changed medications, especially psychoactive medications (anticholinergics, opioids, benzodiazepines)
› **Infections:** focal infectious symptoms, fever, chills, sick contacts
› **Metabolic signs:** fatigue, weakness, myalgias, cold or heat intolerance, weight changes
› **Structural abnormalities:** focal neurological changes, pain, seizures
› **Retention:** last bowel movement, difficulties voiding
› **Environmental triggers:** sensory deprivation (e.g., the patient is not wearing their usual hearing aids or glasses; they are in a windowless room), lines, tubes, recent procedures

Past Medical History

Ask about:

- cognitive history:
  - › Obtain the patient's most recent MMSE, MoCA, or RUDAS score, if available.
  - › Identify specific diagnoses (e.g., MCI, AD, VD, FTD, LBD, PDD, presence of BPSD); physicians and allied health professionals following the patient in the community; and medications prescribed.
- a history of strokes

Past Surgical History

Pursue this only if the patient is postoperative.

Medications

- Identify medications the patient takes at home and whether patient is taking them as prescribed.
- For inpatients, identify hospital-administered medications and whether they differ from medications taken at home. Look for:
  - › abruptly stopped medications with potential for withdrawal (e.g., opioids, benzodiazepines)
  - › new medications (e.g., anticholinergic or psychotropic medications), their dosage, and frequency
  - › as-needed medications

Allergies

Ask about drug allergies and adverse reactions (e.g., dizziness, hypotension, nausea, confusion).

Family History

Ask about dementia and Parkinson disease.

Social History

Ask about:

- alcohol use, recreational drug use, smoking
- occupation, level of education, primary language, traumatic life events such as living through a war

Functional History

Ask about ADLs, IADLs, and, in particular, how medications are dispensed (independently or with help; from bottles, dosettes, or blister packs).

Physical Examination

Vital signs: Look specifically for trends (e.g., fever trends, trends in hyper- or hypotension, trends in oxygen saturation).

General impression: Does the patient look well or unwell? Do they appear to be their stated age? Are they well groomed or dishevelled, well nourished or cachectic, frail or robust?

Mental status: Conduct a focused exam: determine LOC (e.g., alert, agitated, somnolent), mood, affect, thought process (e.g., coherent, logical, tangential, circumferential), thought content (identify preoccupations, delusions, paranoia, and the patient's insight into their current health).

Attention:
› The Confusion Assessment Method (CAM) is a useful 4-item tool that screens for delirium.
› Other ways to assess attention at bedside include:
  » listing the days of week or the months of the year backwards
  » spelling *world* backwards
  » repeating a digit span (ask the patient to repeat a sequence of numbers after you, such as 2-4-3-5-4-8)
  » performing serial subtractions from 100 by 7
  » completing a task despite distractions (e.g., distract the patient by clapping or tapping at points during a task to see whether they can resume and complete the task)
› Note that a full cognitive exam such as an MMSE or MoCA *is not helpful in the setting of acute delirium.*

Systems: Conduct a head-to-toe exam.

Neurological: Conduct a detailed neurological exam on evidence of focal deficits.

Lines and tubes: Take note of restraints, Foley catheters, IV lines, belts, mittens, and so on.

Investigations

LABORATORY INVESTIGATIONS

Basic workup: CBC, electrolytes, urea, creatinine (eGFR), liver enzymes

Workup to rule out secondary causes of cognitive impairment: glucose, extended electrolytes (Ca level), thyrotropin (TSH), vitamin B_{12}, urine drug screen, serum toxicology if relevant

Other medical workup for etiologies of delirium: troponin, BNP, CRP, urinalysis

MICROBIOLOGY

Blood, urine, sputum cultures

CSF cultures, syphilis screening if relevant

IMAGING

Chest x-ray: Use this to assess for infection.

Abdominal x-ray: Use this to assess for fecal loading.
Postvoid residual US or scan
CT of the head: Consider this if there are focal neurological findings or concern for structural lesions.

Impression and Plan[1]
Identify the etiology of delirium: It is usually multifactorial.
Provide CAM scores.[2]
Target perpetuating factors of delirium and risk factors for delirium[1,3]:
› Cognitive: Provide frequent reorientation; use wall charts, clocks, calendars.
› Functional: Recommend early mobilization; involve PTs and OTs.
› Medications: Minimize anticholinergics, antihistamines, and benzodiazepines and "Z-drugs" (unless the patient is in withdrawal).
› Pain: Provide scheduled pain control (e.g., acetaminophen 1 g orally 3 times per day) and use opioids judiciously.
› Altered sensorium: Provide glasses, hearing aids, dentures.
› Diet: Ensure the patient has adequate nutrition and hydration.
› Bowel and bladder: Reevaluate the indication for urinary catheters and remove if appropriate; initiate a bowel regimen.
› Sleep-wake cycle derangement:
  » At minimum, establish cues to regulate the circadian rhythm: get the patient up 3 times per day with meals, and place the patient by a window in daytime.
  » Low-dose melatonin can help regulate the sleep cycle.
  » Avoid the use of antipsychotics for sleep.

MANAGING AGITATION
• If the patient poses a risk of harm to self or staff, prescribe a low-dose, nonsedating antipsychotic as a last resort: a one-to-one sitter or familiar caregiver to provide reassurance and redirection is superior to chemical restraint.
• Note that no medication is approved to treat delirium.
• When prescribing medication, always establish a maximum dose over 24 hours.
• Options include (the numbers provided in brackets are suggested 24-hour maximums):
  » Haldol: 1–2 mg every 1–2 hours IM or IV as needed (maximum 5 mg); for frail elderly, 0.5–1 mg dose range
  » Loxapine: 5–10 mg every 4 hours as needed IM or subcutaneously (maximum 20 mg); for frail elderly, 2.5–5 mg dose range
• In patients exhibiting "sundowning" behaviours, prescribe stacked loxapine or quetiapine 12.5–25 mg orally at 1600 hours and 2000 hours.

- Avoid combining antipsychotics and check the patient's QT interval; stop antipsychotics as early as possible.
- Avoid antipsychotics in patients with diagnosed or suspected Parkinson disease or Parkinson-plus syndrome.

Dementia

These notes are in addition to the **general guide for all consultations** on page 1, and the **starting points for comprehensive geriatric assessments** at the beginning of this chapter.

Identification

Key information in the identification statement includes significant comorbidities, living circumstances, and dementia symptoms with a brief timeline.

Reason for Referral

Examples of reasons for referral include impaired cognition, distinguishing dementia from dementia mimics, and/or determining the type of dementia.

History of Present Illness

A family member, friend, or caregiver is often needed for collateral information.

Characterize the memory loss:
› Establish the timeline of the memory loss.
› Ask about acuity of onset, fluctuations, progression, and rate of progression.

Ask about distinguishing symptoms:
› **Alzheimer disease (AD):** amnesia (primary feature); also aphasia (difficulty with word finding), apraxia (difficulty with simple tasks, such as pouring water or brushing teeth), agnosia (difficulty recognizing family members), and executive dysfunction (inability to organize and plan, which may present as difficulty performing higher-order tasks and IADLs)
› **Vascular dementia (VD):** executive dysfunction, apathy, depression, with a clear time course consistent with vascular insults ("stepwise" decline)
› **Lewy body dementia (LBD):** dementia and at least 2 of the following features: fluctuating cognition, recurrent visual hallucinations, parkinsonism, and REM sleep behaviour disorder

» Note the "1 year rule" for distinguishing between LBD and Parkinson disease dementia (PDD): if dementia precedes or starts within 1 year of parkinsonism, then it is LBD.

› **Frontotemporal dementia (FTD):** dementia and at least 3 of the following features: disinhibition, loss of empathy, apathy, perseveration, hyperorality, and executive dysfunction

› **Normal pressure hydrocephalus:** urinary incontinence, gait disturbance

Conduct a psychiatric review of systems: Ask about:

› depression
  » Assess with symptoms (SIGECAPS) and/or validated questionnaires (PHQ-9, Geriatric Depression Scale).
› psychosis
  » Assess for hallucinations and delusions.
› mania
› posttraumatic stress

Past Medical History

Ask about:

- results of previous MoCA or MMSE, if available
- stroke
- Parkinson disease
- cardiac disease
- type 2 diabetes
- dyslipidemia
- brain trauma
- a history of falls

Past Surgical History

Ask about cardiac and brain-related surgeries.

Medications

- Ask about medication management and compliance.
- Pay special attention to medications that can impair cognition: benzodiazepines, antidepressants, antipsychotics, opioids, antihistamines, sedatives, anticonvulsants, anticholinergics, and corticosteroids.

Allergies

Follow the **general guide for all consultations** and the **starting points for comprehensive geriatric assessments.**

Family History

Ask about dementia (clarify age of onset, and type, if known).

Social History

Ask about:

- place of birth, primary language
- level of education achieved
- occupation
- marital status, children, family
- community and social activities
- alcohol use, recreational drug use, smoking

Code Status

Determine the patient's code status and whether they have a substitute decision maker.

Functional History

Ask about:

- **The patient's level of functioning:** ability to do ADLs and IADLs; use of assistive devices, home supports, equipment, and community nursing care
  - › Apply the mnemonic DEATH for ADLs (**D**ressing, **E**ating, **A**mbulating, **T**oileting, **H**ygiene) and SHAFT for IADLs (**S**hopping, **H**ousekeeping, **A**ccounting, **F**ood preparation, **T**elephone/transportation).
- **Safety concerns:** leaving tap or stove on; getting lost; managing finances; falls; competence to drive (ask the caregiver or a family member for their assessment)
- **Caregiver burnout:** availability of respite care

Physical Examination

Vital signs

Mental status, attention: Is there evidence of active delirium?

Neurological:

- › Assess eye movements for vertical gaze palsy.
- › Assess for parkinsonian features: tremor (typically asymmetric), rigidity, bradykinesia, festinating gait, orthostasis, masked facies, and hypophonia.
- › Perform a gait assessment.
- › Assess for focal neurologic deficits.

Investigations

LABORATORY INVESTIGATIONS

Basic workup: CBC, electrolytes, renal function, liver enzymes

Workup for secondary causes of cognitive impairment: glucose, Ca, thyrotropin (TSH), vitamin B_{12}, HIV, syphilis serology, urine drug screen, serum toxicology screen

Delirium workup (if needed)
EEG:
> › Consider this in patients with a history of fluctuating mental status, risk factors such as substance use, presence of potential foci for seizures such as recent stroke, and/or recent changes to medications that can lead to lower seizure threshold.

LP:
> › Consider this in young patients, rapidly progressive impairment, or suggestive findings on CT, such as leptomeningeal enhancement.

IMAGING

Brain imaging: This is not routinely required, but indicated in patients with bleeding risk, unusual presentation (e.g., younger than 60; rapid, unexplained decline; short duration of dementia of less than 2 years; atypical cognitive presentation), suspicion of intracranial lesion (e.g., focal neurological findings), or suspicion of normal pressure hydrocephalus.
> › Findings on CT of the head include atrophy, ventriculomegaly (e.g., in normal pressure hydrocephalus), and ischemic changes.
> › MRI is more sensitive for ischemic white-matter changes.
> › Order a CT stroke protocol if the patient has focal neurologic deficits.

OTHER INVESTIGATIONS

ECG: Pursue this to rule out bradycardia and heart block, if you are considering initiating a cholinesterase inhibitor.

COGNITIVE TESTING

Test with MMSE, MoCA, or RUDAS:
• MoCA is more sensitive than MMSE, and is usually for patients with higher education and suspected minor impairment, such as MCI.
• MMSE is better for picking up more advanced impairment.
• RUDAS is better for those whose first language is not English or who have a lower education level.
• Note that these cognitive tests are more for identifying deficits across domains, not making the diagnosis of a particular type of dementia.

Testing Cognitive Domains

Attention: adding by 7s; spelling *world* backwards
Memory: repeating 3 words (e.g., *boy, ball, red*), and recalling them
Language: repeating a statement ("no ifs ands or buts"); reading a written command and then performing it
Executive function: trail-making test part B on MoCA; drawing a clock face (this is not included in the MMSE)

Visuospatial: drawing a clock face; copying intersecting pentagons; drawing a cube

Impression and Plan

Start with a summary: Include the patient's age, major comorbidities, and significant deficits in cognitive domains.

› Significant deficits in cognitive domains affect social functioning, are not associated with delirium or psychiatric illness, and are based on clinical assessment with corroboration from caregivers or family members. The domains include:
  » learning and memory
  » language
  » executive function
  » complex attention
  » perceptual motor function
  » social cognition

Indicate the etiology and severity of the dementia:
› Is this dementia?
  » The diagnostic criteria for dementia require subjective and objective cognitive deficits that interfere with independence in function.
  » Note that some patients may have "mixed dementia," which involves more than 1 type of dementia (e.g., AD and VD).
› Indicate severity as mild (few IADLs affected), moderate (needs help with ADLs), or severe (total dependence).
› Keep the differential in mind:
  » **MCI:** self-reported memory difficulty, objective cognitive deficits on testing, but no effect on daily and social functioning
  » **Delirium:** fluctuating level of consciousness, difficulty with attention and concentration, acute onset
  » **Depression, often termed "pseudodementia":** self-reported memory loss, poor effort on testing, psychomotor slowing

Describe appropriate management.

PRINCIPLES OF DEMENTIA MANAGEMENT

Provide general medical care: Screen for falls, mobility, nutrition, weight loss, incontinence, and sleep disturbance.

Evaluate and manage behavioural and psychological symptoms of dementia (BPSD).

Evaluate and manage safety risks and/or provide risk reduction: This includes:
› home OT safety assessment
› support services
› elder abuse screening
› blister packaging for medications and/or assisted or supervised administration

> driving evaluation
  » Note that you have a duty to report if the patient refuses to stop driving despite a medical recommendation to stop.

Refer caregivers for support: For example, refer them to the Alzheimer's Society or a social worker.

Encourage planning for future needs: For example, discuss putting in place goals of care and a power of attorney.

Nonpharmacologic Interventions

- **Exercise:** This has the best evidence for delaying the progression of dementia or MCI. It also improves functional ability and mitigates the risk of falls.
- **Cognitive training, social engagement:** Cognitive training in a particular domain improves performance in that domain (e.g., reasoning, processing speed, memory), but has questionable clinical relevance.
- **Other:** No evidence supports the value of certain diets or OTC supplements for treating dementia.
  > The Mediterranean diet has shown improved cognitive outcomes, but no significant impact on MCI rates; however; it has cardiovascular health benefits.

Pharmacologic Interventions

Consider:

- cholinesterase inhibitors (donepezil, galantamine, rivastigmine)
  > These provide modest improvement in cognition and functioning.
  > They are indicated for mild-moderate AD, LBD, and PDD.
- N-methyl d-aspartic acid receptor agonist (memantine)
- medications to optimize cardiovascular risk factors (e.g., hypertension, diabetes, dyslipidemia)
  > Consider acetylsalicylic acid in patients with high cardiovascular risk.
- medications to manage FTD (trazodone; SSRIs for behaviours)
  > Note that cholinesterase inhibitors have no role in FTD management.
- medications to manage BPSD
  > Provide these if nonpharmacological strategies have failed, and if symptoms are disruptive, distressing, and/or unsafe for the patient and caregivers.

Falls

These notes are in addition to the **general guide for all consultations** on page 1, and the **starting points for comprehensive geriatric assessments** at the beginning of this chapter.

Identification

Key information in the identification statement includes significant comorbidities, the timeline and circumstances of the fall, and major injuries resulting from the fall.

Reason for Referral

The referral typically seeks assessment and management of modifiable and nonmodifiable risk factors for falls.

History of Present Illness

Determine the circumstances around the fall:
› What details does the patient recollect? Did they lose consciousness?
› Were there any witnesses to the fall?
› When did the fall happen? How long was the patient down for?
› Where did the fall occur?
› Was the patient able to get up or was help needed?

Ask about prodromal symptoms: These may suggest a particular etiology.

Assess for a neurologic etiology:
› Does the patient have vision issues? Do they require visual aids?
› Did the patient have vertiginous symptoms (e.g., "room spinning")?
› Do they have decreased or changed sensation in the lower limbs? Is there new weakness?
› What is the patient's baseline level of cognition?
› Does the patient have issues with balance or gait?

Assess for a cardiovascular etiology:
› Did the patient have lightheadedness (e.g., feeling like they were "about to pass out")?
› Did they experience tunnel vision, nausea, flushing, palpitations, diaphoresis, or chest pain? Was it a sudden "drop attack"? (A fall on the face resulting in fractured facial bones or significant bruising is concerning for cardiac etiology.)
› Did they fall after changing position (e.g., from sitting to standing)?

Assess for a musculoskeletal etiology:
› Ask about prolonged malnutrition and baseline mobility (e.g., whether the patient is mostly bedbound).
› Ask about joint pain and swelling.

Ask about urinary issues.

Identify extrinsic factors: Ask about:
› environmental factors (e.g., flooring, rugs, steps)
› assistive devices, footwear

Conduct a review of systems: Exacerbation of chronic medical conditions or new diseases may contribute to falls (e.g., HF exacerbation, UTI).

Past Medical History
Ask about:
- cognitive impairment (obtain prior MoCA or MMSE scores if available)
- past falls (determine the circumstances of past falls) and frequency of falls
- osteoporosis and a history of fragility fractures
- dementia
- stroke
- chronic musculoskeletal impairment and pain (e.g., arthritis, Parkinson disease, MS)
- diabetes, in particular if it is long-standing, poorly controlled, and/or has complications such as peripheral neuropathy and chronic foot ulcers
- spinal stenosis
- visual impairment
- urinary incontinence
- cardiac disease (HF, valvulopathy, arrhythmia)

Past Surgical History
Ask about:
- fractures from falls requiring surgical fixation
- joint surgeries

Medications
- Ask about changes to medications, including new medications and changes in doses of existing medications.
- Pay special attention to culprit medications: benzodiazepines, TCAs, antihypertensives, beta-blockers, diuretics, antipsychotics, opioids, antihistamines, vasodilators, sedatives, anticonvulsants, and corticosteroids.
- Note that the patient is at risk of bleeding if taking anticoagulants.

Allergies
Follow the **general guide for all consultations** and the **starting points for comprehensive geriatric assessments**.

Family History
Ask about hip fractures and osteoporosis.

Social History

Ask about:

- alcohol and recreational drug use, including changes in level of use
- occupation, education level
- home supports, equipment, community nursing care in place

Functional History

Determine whether the patient performs ADLs and IADLs independently or with assistance.

Physical Examination

Vital signs: Pay particular attention to heart rate and orthostasis.

Mental status, attention

Visual acuity, hearing

Cognition: Perform a screening cognitive exam.

Standing and walking: Perform a timed up-and-go test:
> Ask the patient to get up from a chair, walk 3 meters, and walk back.
> A normal performance time is less than 12 seconds; times of more than 14 seconds indicate an increased risk of falls (note frail adults typically take more than 20 seconds).

Gait: Assess for:
> base (wide [greater than pelvis width] or narrow)
> symmetry
> foot clearance (look for foot drop, or high-stepping and slapping)
> arm swing
> stance phase (e.g., decreased in antalgic gait where one side is compensating for a problem on the opposite side)
> safety awareness
> righting reflex
>> Conduct a pull test: stand behind the patient and pull them gently backwards (be prepared to catch them); a normal response is a brisk step back and an abnormal response is no step back.
> gait speed in meters per second (< 0.8 m/s indicates increased fall risk)
> balance
>> Evaluate tandem gait; toe or heel walk; and unipedal stance.

Neurological:
> Assess:
>> strength (especially in the lower extremities)
>> postural stability (perform a Romberg test for visual dependence)
>> power and tone (increased tone suggests an upper motor neuron issue, or, if other suggestive features are also present [e.g., bradykinesia, cogwheeling, postural instability], parkinsonism)
>> coordination (with cerebellar testing)

» visual acuity (with Snellen chart and confrontational visual field testing)
> Assess for:
» tremors
» peripheral sensor impairment (joint position sense for proprioception; fine touch sense [posterior column]; pain and temperature sense [spinothalamic tract])
» vertigo with positional changes (perform the Dix-Hallpike manoeuvre)

Musculoskeletal: Assess:
> muscle bulk (squaring of shoulders, atrophy of quadriceps)
> deformities from arthritis
> feet (ulcers, infections, bunions, nails, neuropathy)

Cardiovascular:
> Assess for cardiac murmurs, arrhythmias, and carotid bruit.
> On high suspicion of cardiac etiology, consider carotid sinus massage if the patient is on telemetry and pacing pads are available.

Systemic disease: Perform a general examination for systemic illness.

Investigations

LABORATORY INVESTIGATIONS
CBC, glucose, creatinine, CK

OTHER INVESTIGATIONS
Holter monitor and transthoracic echocardiogram: Pursue this on suspicion of cardiac syncope.

EEG: Pursue this on suspicion of seizure.

IMAGING
CT of the head: Consider this especially in the context of focal neurological signs and/or anticoagulation.

Pelvis or other musculoskeletal imaging: Pursue this on suspicion of acute fracture.

Impression and Plan

Start with a summary: Include the patient's major comorbidities and the likely etiology of the fall (often multifactorial).

Manage urinary incontinence.

Taper or stop offending medications.

Treat underlying systemic illness: Examples include HF, COPD.

Treat osteoporosis.

Treat other contributing conditions:
> **Orthostatic hypotension:** Counsel lower-extremity muscle contractions, use of compression stockings, and better hydration; consider midodrine or fludrocortisone and salt tablets.

› **Postprandial hypotension:** Counsel frequent small meals.
› **Arrhythmias:** Prescribe antiarrhythmics and consider a pacemaker.
› **Decreased vision:** Counsel better lighting and updated glasses; refer the patient to an optometrist and/or ophthalmologist for cataracts, glaucoma, and other vision issues.
› **Vestibular dysfunction:** For benign paroxysmal positional vertigo, consider the Epley manoeuvre; for Ménière disease, consider vestibular rehabilitation.
› **Musculoskeletal pain:** Provide conservative management; prescribe oral analgesics, and steroid and/or analgesic injections.

Provide strategies for managing falls in the community setting:
Examples include:
› exercise programs with a focus on balance and strength (this provides the greatest benefit)
› a home safety assessment by an OT
› PT assessment for mobility aids and correct use
› vitamin D supplementation (this is more helpful in those who are deficient; some evidence shows vitamin D supplementation can reduce the risk of falls in ambulatory or institutionalized older adults)
› podiatry referral (foot wear, orthotics)
› thorough medication review (withdrawal of psychotropic medications reduces the rate of falls)

Consider referring the patient to a local geriatric or falls clinic.

Polypharmacy

These notes are in addition to the **general guide for all consultations** on page 1, and the **starting points for comprehensive geriatric assessments** at the beginning of this chapter.

Identification

Follow the **general guide for all consultations** and the **starting points for comprehensive geriatric assessments**.

Reason for Referral

The referral typically seeks assessment and/or management of polypharmacy, and may also include questions about specific medications or side effects.

History of Present Illness

CURRENT AND PAST MEDICATIONS

Ask about:

- what prescribed medications the patient is currently taking
- the start date for each medication, if known
- the patient's understanding of what each medication is for
- recent changes in medications (new medications; stopped medications; and changes in dose, frequency, or method of delivery)
- concerns about medications
- access to medications (delivered, picked up, brought by a family member)
- medication packaging (pill bottles, blister packs, dosettes)
- administration of medications (independent or assisted)
- missed doses (occurrence and frequency)
- compliance (whether the patient is taking medications as prescribed for dose and schedule)
  - › It is important to ask the patient about dose and schedule because it may be different than what is indicated on the patient's medication list or medical record.
- affordability of medications

ADVERSE DRUG REACTIONS THAT MAY LEAD TO A PRESCRIBING CASCADE

Screen for signs and symptoms of adverse drug reactions by system:

- **Cardiovascular:** dizziness, orthostatic symptoms, presyncope, palpitations, hypotension
- **GI:** constipation, diarrhea, reflux, abdominal pain, dehydration, dry mouth
- **Neurological:** delirium, confusion, vision changes, paresthesias, insomnia
- **Dermatological:** rashes
- **Musculoskeletal:** joint pain, fractures, falls
- **GU:** incontinence, retention

Past Medical History

Identify all conditions for which the patient is taking medications.

Past Surgical History

Follow the **general guide for all consultations** and the **starting points for comprehensive geriatric assessments.**

Medications

- Identify all medications the patient is currently taking, ensuring accuracy for dose and schedule (cross reference this information with what patient is actually taking).

- Note any recently changed medications.
- Ask about:
  › start dates of medications, if known
  › any recently discontinued medications
  › supplements, and herbal or natural medications
  › OTC medications

Allergies

- Identify drug allergies and known adverse drug reactions.
- For each, determine:
  › the medication involved
  › the reaction type
  › whether the reaction required hospitalization or medical care
  › whether the medication was continued

Family History

Ask about similar adverse reactions to particular medications in family members.

Social History

Follow the **general guide for all consultations** and the **starting points for comprehensive geriatric assessments.**

Physical Examination

Examine any systems related to potential or mentioned adverse reactions. Examples include:

- orthostatic vital signs
- neurological (EPS, parkinsonism)
- gait
- abdominal (constipation)

Investigations

LABORATORY INVESTIGATIONS

Basic investigations: Order CBC, electrolytes, and extended electrolytes.

Creatinine (eGFR): These are relevant to renal dosing.

Liver enzymes: These are relevant to hepatic dosing.

Levels of medications that can have toxicity: Examples include digoxin and lithium.

Other: Order investigations for conditions currently managed with medications to check for needed dosing corrections (e.g., order a lipid panel if the patient is on a statin).

IMAGING
Imaging is generally not required, but consider it if relevant to a medication side effect or a condition under treatment.

Impression and Plan
Review each medication:
> Is there an indication for this medication?
> Is the medication effective for the condition?
> Is the dosage correct? (For example, consider renal, liver, and age-related dosing.)
> Are the directions correct?
> Are the directions practical? (Once-a-day dosing is preferred.)
> Are there any significant drug-drug interactions?
> Are there any drug-disease interactions?
> Is there unnecessary duplication with other medications?
> Is there an alternative that is less expensive or safer?
> Pearls:
>> Always consider the patient's preferences and goals, which should direct deprescribing.
>> Consider prescribing cascades, as these can contribute to polypharmacy.

Check for potentially inappropriate medications: Consult resources such as:
> Beers Criteria[4]
> STOPP/START Criteria[5]
> FORTA List[6]

Avoid medications that are high risk for side effects: Common medications to avoid include[4]:
> anticholinergics
> anticonvulsants
> benzodiazepines
> TCAs
> NSAIDs
> digoxin (at doses > 0.125 mg)
> glyburide

GENERAL CONSIDERATIONS
- Discontinue any medications that are unsafe, not required, or causing harm that outweighs the benefits.
- Reduce the dose of medications, if possible.
- Make dosing once a day, if possible.
- Identify new medications the patient needs.
- Call the patient's pharmacy directly about changes to medications.
- Inform the patient's family physician about changes to medications.

- Provide multiple medications in blister packs.
- Apply for government programs that defray medication costs, when applicable.

References

1. Fong T, Tulebaev S, Inouye S. Delirium in elderly adults: diagnosis, prevention, and treatment. Nat Rev Neurol. 2009;5(4):210-20. doi: 10.1038/nrneurol.2009.24
2. Wong C, Holroyd-Leduc J, Simel D, et al. Does this patient have delirium?: value of bedside instruments. JAMA. 2010;304(7):779-86. doi: 10.1001/jama.2010.1182
3. Inouye S, Bogardus S, Charpentier P, et al. A multicomponent intervention to prevent delirium in hospitalized older patients. N Engl J Med. 1999;340(9):669-76. doi: 10.1056/NEJM199903043400901
4. American Geriatrics Society. 2019 updated AGS Beers Criteria for potentially inappropriate medication use in older adults. J Am Geriatr Soc. 2019;67(4):674-94. doi: 10.1111/jgs.15767
5. O'Mahony D, O'Sullivan D, Byrne S, et al. STOPP/START criteria for potentially inappropriate prescribing in older people: version 2. Age Ageing. 2014;44(2):213-8. doi: 10.1093/ageing/afu145
6. Pazan F, Weiss C, Wehling M. The EURO-FORTA (Fit fOR The Aged) list: international consensus validation of a clinical tool for improved drug treatment in older people. Drugs Aging. 2018;35(1):61-71. doi: 10.1007/s40266-017-0514-2

9

Hematology

Dr. Angelina Marinkovic
Dr. WanLi Zhou
Dr. Julia Varghese

REVIEWER
Dr. Katherine Ng

Starting Points: Hematology Consultations

These notes are in addition to the **general guide for all consultations** on page 1.

Identification

Key information in the identification statement includes relevant comorbidities and whether the patient has had any previous hematologic disorder or VTE.

Reason for Referral

The referral may seek to confirm a hematological disorder and/or clarify appropriate management.

History of Present Illness

Note that for certain hematologic issues (such as neutropenia), it may be more useful to review relevant laboratory investigations and, for inpatients, the course in hospital. The patient may not have symptoms related to the reason for referral.

Clarify why the patient has sought care: For an inpatient, clarify why the patient was admitted to hospital.

Clarify the time of onset and associated symptoms: Hematological symptoms are most important.

Clarify the chronicity and progression of symptoms.

Assess for constitutional symptoms: Ask about weight loss of more than 10% of body weight in the past 6 months; night sweats; fever; and severe pruritus.

Ask about dietary habits and/or restrictions.

Conduct a review of systems: Target the specific problem in the reason for referral.

For coagulopathy consultations, take a thorough bleeding history:
› Clarify current and prior bleeding challenges.
› Consider using a standardized tool, such as the International Society on Thrombosis and Haemostasis bleeding assessment tool (ISTH BAT).[1]

Past Medical History

Clarify the patient's hematological history: Ask about:
› hematologists involved
› hemoglobinopathies (e.g., sickle cell disease, thalassemia)
› MGUS (including results of previous serum or urine protein electrophoresis [SPEP, UPEP] and/or serum free light chains)
› previous hematological malignancies (clarify date of diagnosis and treatment)
› prior VTE

Ask about clotting and bleeding history: For example, did the patient have excessive bleeding during childbirth or wisdom teeth removal?

Review nonhematologic history: Ask about other malignancies and treatments (e.g., therapy-related myeloid neoplasm).

Ask about previous transfusions, transfusion reactions, and blood type.

Past Surgical History

Ask about valve replacement requiring anticoagulation.

Medications

• Always review the patient's medical record for start dates of new medications.
• Ask about anticoagulation.
• Take special note of chemotherapy and immunosuppression.

Allergies

• Ask about medication allergies.
• Check for documented history of heparin-induced thrombocytopenia.

Family History

Ask about hematological malignancy, VTE, sickle cell disease, thalassemia, and hemolytic disorders.

Social History
Ask about:
- health-benefit plans and/or insurance
- factors affecting the patient's ability to adhere to medication regimes or pay for medications
- alcohol use, recreational drug use, smoking
- occupation and occupational exposures
- ethnicity

Physical Examination
Vital signs: Obtain the patient's heart rate, BP, respiration rate, oxygen saturation, and temperature.

Weight: Also obtain the patient's height if BSA is required.

General exam: Perform a focused exam based on the clinical question.

Lymph nodes: Examine the lymph nodes (occipital, pre- and postauricular, submandibular, submental, cervical, supra- and infraclavicular, axillary, epitrochlear, and inguinal).

› **Tip:** Always look in the mouth for enlarged adenoids and/or tonsils (Waldeyer throat ring) as part of the lymph node exam.

Abdominal: Examine for splenomegaly and hepatomegaly.

Dermatological: Look for new rashes.

Other: Look for petechiae, purpura, and ecchymosis (look in the mouth for wet purpura).

Investigations

LABORATORY INVESTIGATIONS
CBC: Remember to assess WBC differential (e.g., neutrophils, monocytes, lymphocytes, basophils, eosinophils, blasts if present).

Peripheral blood smear

Coagulation profile

Hemolysis workup: Order reticulocyte count, LDH, bilirubin, haptoglobin, and peripheral blood film (schistocytes).

Creatinine and liver enzymes: This is important for medication dosing and assessing for contraindications to therapy.

OTHER INVESTIGATIONS
Bone marrow (BM) biopsy: Pursue this if indicated.

SPEP, UPEP, and/or serum free light chains

IMAGING
Make sure you look at images yourself: don't just read the reports. Call the radiologist directly if your specific question is not addressed in the report or if further information is required.

Impression and Plan

Start with a summary: Summarize the case, and list the presenting issues and provisional diagnoses.

Indicate the patient's stability: Discuss whether the patient is stable or unstable.

Provide the suspected etiology of the problem and differential diagnosis: Use a systematic approach (e.g., for cytopenias, generally think in terms of decreased production, increased destruction, or sequestration).

Pursue relevant laboratory investigations: Order investigations relevant to the clinical context (e.g., vitamin B_{12}, thyrotropin [TSH], liver function tests for elevated MCV).

Discuss management: Ensure you have the patient's correct weight if the therapy is weight based, and ensure there are no contraindications to the therapy proposed.

Anemia and Cytopenia

These notes are in addition to the **general guide for all consultations** on page 1, and the **starting points for hematology consultations** at the beginning of this chapter.

Identification

Key information in the identification statement includes relevant comorbidities and the patient's ethnicity.

Reason for Referral

The referral may seek to clarify the type of anemia (microcytic, normocytic, macrocytic) and whether other cell lines are affected (bicytopenia, pancytopenia).

History of Present Illness

Determine the chronicity and progression of symptoms.

Clarify symptoms:
> **Anemia:** dyspnea, chest pain, dizziness, pica symptoms, decreased exercise tolerance
> **Thrombocytopenia:** mucosal bleeding (e.g., epistaxis, GI bleeding, menorrhagia), easy bruising, other bleeding
> **Neutropenia:** recurrent infections, oral ulcers
> **Hemolysis:** jaundice, scleral icterus, tea-coloured urine

Ask about a history of bleeding: For example, ask about blood in the stools (melena) and heavy menstrual periods.

Check dietary history: Is the patient vegetarian?

Assess for possible triggers: Ask about recent viral illnesses, travel history (e.g., to areas where malaria is endemic), new medications, chemotherapy, and recent transfusions.

Conduct a rheumatologic review of systems: See the starting points for rheumatology consultations (chapter 16).

Past Medical History

Ask about:

- chronic conditions (CKD)
- inflammatory and autoimmune diseases
- conditions affecting absorption (e.g., celiac disease, prior bowel resections)
- a history of GI bleeds (e.g., ulcers, diverticular disease)
- malignancy

Medications

Ask about:

- chemotherapy and hydroxyurea
- immunosuppressants (i.e., methotrexate)
- antibiotics and antivirals

Allergies

Follow the **general guide for all consultations** and the **starting points for hematology consultations.**

Family History

Ask about:

- thalassemia and sickle cell disease
- hemolytic disorders (e.g., glucose-6-phosphate dehydrogenase deficiency, spherocytosis)
- a history of recurrent cholelithiasis or cholecystectomy

Social History

Ask about:

- alcohol use
- recreational drug use (e.g., cocaine, cutting agents such as levamisole)
- ethnicity

Physical Examination

Vital signs: tachycardia, orthostatic vitals

General nutritional status

Signs of iron-deficiency anemia: pallor of skin or conjunctiva, koilonychia

Signs of hemolysis: jaundice (check under the lingual frenulum) or scleral icterus

Signs of vitamin B$_{12}$ deficiency: "lemon-coloured skin," glossitis, cognitive impairment, loss of vibration sensitivity and/or proprioception

Dermatological: rashes (livedo reticularis suggests parvovirus, SLE)

Investigations

LABORATORY INVESTIGATIONS

CBC with differential:
› Always look at all cell lines.
› Always look at MCV as a clue to the etiology of anemia.
› Establish when the CBC was last normal and what the baseline is.

Basic workup: iron studies, reticulocytes, vitamin B$_{12}$, thyrotropin (TSH), creatinine (eGFR), liver enzymes
› Anemia is often multifactorial; thus, in clinical practice, a basic workup is often ordered as a starting point.

Microcytic anemia workup:
› **Iron studies:** Always order a ferritin test (see Table 9.1 for interpretation) and calculate the Mentzer index.
› **Hemoglobin electrophoresis:** Note that this can be falsely normal in iron deficiency, and normal in alpha thalassemia.
› **DNA testing:** Pursue this for suspected alpha thalassemia.

Normocytic anemia workup: reticulocytes; hemolytic workup (see below); SPEP and UPEP; thyrotropin (TSH)

Macrocytic anemia workup: vitamin B$_{12}$, thyrotropin (TSH), liver function tests, hemolytic workup (see below), SPEP and/or UPEP

Peripheral blood smear (PBS):
› The cellular morphology may reveal an underlying etiology such as myelodysplastic syndrome (MDS) or life-threatening causes (e.g., leukemia, microangiopathic hemolytic anemia [MAHA]).

Reticulocytes

Hemolytic workup: bilirubin, LDH, haptoglobin, PBS, reticulocytes
› Consider a direct antiglobulin test to assess for autoimmune hemolytic anemia.

Table 9.1. Iron Study Interpretation

	IRON	TIBC	FERRITIN	TSAT
IDA	↓	↑	↓	↓
ACI	↓	↓ / ↔	↑	↓

Abbreviations: ACI: anemia of chronic inflammation; IDA: iron deficiency anemia; Tsat: transferrin saturation

INR, PTT, fibrinogen, D-dimer
› Order these for suspected DIC.
Other (as indicated): viral serologies (HBV, HCV, HIV, *Parvovirus B19*), autoimmune serologies

OTHER INVESTIGATIONS
BM biopsy: Pursue this in suspected BM disorder.

IMAGING
CT with contrast: Pursue this in suspected bleeding or suspected lymphoproliferative disorder.

Impression and Plan

- Describe each cytopenia as an issue with decreased production, increased destruction, or sequestration (note that sequestration is less relevant for anemia and leukopenia).
- Describe the etiology of the anemia based on MCV (see Table 9.2).
- Always look at all cell lines.

Table 9.2. Etiology of Anemia

MICROCYTIC (MNEMONIC: TAILS)	NORMOCYTIC (LOOK AT RETICULOCYTE COUNT)	MACROCYTIC
Thalassemia (alpha or beta) ACI Iron deficiency Lead poisoning Sideroblastic	**Low/normal reticulocyte count** ACI, CKD, liver disease BM suppression BM infiltration (e.g., leukemia, myeloma, lymphoma, myelofibrosis, malignancy, granulomatous disease) BM failure or aplasia (aplastic anemia, red cell aplasia, genetic conditions) MDS Endocrine disease (e.g., hypothyroidism, hypopituitarism) Acute bleeding or hemolysis Under production anemias (early IDA/ vitamin B_{12} deficiency) **High reticulocyte count** Loss of blood from bleeding or hemolysis BM recovery (e.g., after nutrient replacement) PNH	**Megaloblastic** Vitamin B_{12} or folate deficiency (megaloblastic anemia) Medications that affect nuclear maturation (chemotherapy, MTX, HU) **Nonmegaloblastic** Hypothyroid Liver disease Excess alcohol HIV medications MDS Myeloma Hemolysis (due to reticulocytes which are larger than mature RBCs)

Abbreviations: ACI: anemia of chronic inflammation; BM: bone marrow; CKD: chronic kidney disease; HU: hydroxyurea; IDA: iron deficiency anemia; MDS: myelodysplastic syndrome; MTX: methotrexate; PNH: paroxysmal nocturnal hemoglobinuria: RBC: red blood cell

Hematologic Malignancy

These notes are in addition to the **general guide for all consultations** on page 1, and the **starting points for hematology consultations** at the beginning of this chapter.

Identification

Key information in the identification statement includes relevant comorbidities, age, and town or city of residence (to identify the nearest cancer treatment centre).

Reason for Referral

Examples of reasons for referral include the severity of the patient's symptoms, a malignancy of concern, and/or the presence of life-threatening complications (tumour lysis syndrome, DIC, leukostasis, febrile neutropenia).

History of Present Illness

Ask about symptom onset and progression (acute versus chronic).
Identify treatments tried for symptom alleviation.
Clarify symptoms:
> › **Leukemia:** bone-marrow failure symptoms, including fatigue, decreased exercise tolerance, easy bruising and bleeding, and neutropenic infections
>> » See Anemia and Cytopenia in this chapter for questions for each cytopenia.
> › **Lymphoma:** painless nodal enlargement; distribution and progression of lymphadenopathy; constitutional symptoms (fever, drenching night sweats, weight loss greater than 10% of the patient's body weight over 6 months), fatigue, anorexia
>> » **Hodgkin lymphoma:** pain at nodal sites after drinking alcohol; intense pruritus
>> » **CNS involvement of lymphoma:** neurological changes
> › **Multiple myeloma (MM):** hypercalcemia, new renal failure, symptoms of anemia, bone or back pain ("CRAB" symptoms)
> › **Hyperviscosity syndrome (a complication of Waldenström macroglobulinemia or MM):** visual disturbances, chest pain, dyspnea, oronasal bleeding, seizure
> › **Leukostasis (a complication of acute leukemia):** confusion, visual impairment, shortness of breath, stroke

Ask about rashes: These may be cutaneous manifestations of lymphoma or leukemia.
Determine the patient's performance status: For example, determine an ECOG score for the patient.

Past Medical History
Ask about:
- previous solid organ or hematopoietic cell transplantation (these increase the risk of posttransplant lymphoproliferative disorder)
- acute leukemia risk factors, including preexisting BM disease such as MDS; previous chemotherapy and/or radiation; Down syndrome or other genetic syndromes
- lymphoma risk factors, including HIV, EBV, HHV, HTLV-1, *Helicobacter pylori*, autoimmune diseases, and congenital immune deficiencies
- myeloma risk factors (i.e., previously identified monoclonal protein)

Medications
Follow the **general guide for all consultations** and the **starting points for hematology consultations.**

Allergies
Follow the **general guide for all consultations** and the **starting points for hematology consultations.**

Family History
Ask about hematological malignancies.

Social History
Ask about:
- occupational exposures, including organophosphate insecticides and benzenes
- functional baseline
- siblings (for potential stem cell donor)

Physical Examination
ECOG status
Neurological: altered mental status, focal neurological deficits (suggests CNS involvement)
Lymph nodes
Cardiovascular: volume overload
Respiratory: adventitious sounds (suggests leukostasis)
Abdominal: hepatomegaly, splenomegaly
Extremities: rashes; bruising; joint involvement; unilateral swelling (suggests thrombosis)

Investigations
Workup for all patients: CBC, liver function tests, LDH (elevation may be a clue to lymphoma), electrolytes, extended electrolytes, pregnancy testing for women of childbearing age

Additional leukemia workup: PBS to assess for blasts and Auer rods; BM biopsy (with cytogenetic and molecular analysis)

Additional lymphoma workup: CT of the chest, abdomen, and pelvis, or PET (to clarify staging and biopsy target); lymph node biopsy (excisional preferred); flow cytometry; BM biopsy (for staging in non-Hodgkin lymphoma); LP (in suspected CNS involvement)

Additional MM workup: creatinine; Ca; quantitative immunoglobulins; SPEP and immunofixation; UPEP; serum free light chain assays; BM biopsy; serum β2 microglobulin (for prognostication); skeletal survey or low dose whole body CT or MRI

EVALUATION OF COMPLICATIONS

DIC (leukemia): INR, PTT, D-dimer, fibrinogen

Tumour lysis syndrome (leukemia or aggressive lymphoma): LDH, uric acid, K, PO_4, Ca, ECG, creatinine

Hyperviscosity syndrome (Waldenström macroglobulinemia or MM): quantitative immunoglobulins, serum viscosity

Leukostasis: CBC
› Leukostasis can be seen in acute leukemia with a blast count > 50 x 10^9/L.

Impression and Plan

GENERAL APPROACH

- Describe steps or investigations needed to obtain or confirm the diagnosis and staging, and any prognostic markers needed.
- Provide scores from prognostic scoring scales for the specific malignancy.
- Indicate if the patient is willing and fit to undergo chemotherapy.
- Describe any prechemotherapy considerations: fertility counselling; echocardiogram, or pulmonary function tests (depending on the type of chemotherapy); assessment for latent or underlying diseases (HBV, HCV, HIV, TB).
- Identify life-threatening emergencies or complications that require attention.
- Provide pain and symptom management if applicable.

GUIDELINES FOR SPECIFIC ENTITIES

Lymphoma:
› Order tissue biopsy, radiologic studies for staging, BM biopsy (not required for Hodgkin lymphoma staging).
› Indicate whether the patient has indolent versus aggressive lymphoma.

> Order β2 microglobulin, SPEP, and UPEP for prognostic markers.

Leukemia: Order BM aspirate and biopsy (leukemia has more
than 20% blasts in BM or peripheral blood) for cytogenetic and
molecular analysis, and prognostication.

MM:
> Plasma cell malignancies include a spectrum of diseases ranging
from MGUS, to smoldering myeloma, to symptomatic myeloma.
> The definition of MM is[2]:
» BM with more than 10% plasma cells **plus** 1 or more CRAB symptoms
—or—
» any 1 of: BM with more than 60% plasma cells; serum free light chain assay
ratio greater than 100; or more than 1 focal lesion ≥ 5 mm in size
> Assess for CRAB features of myeloma: hypercalcemia (calcium > 0.25
mmol/L ULN); anemia (hemoglobin < 100 g/L or > 20 g/L below
normal); renal insufficiency (creatinine > 177 mol/L); bone lesions.
» Assessment requires SPEP and UPEP; serum free light chain assays; skeletal
survey; and BM biopsy.
> State immunoglobulin and/or light chain subtype.
> Order β2 microglobulin, albumin, and LDH, and assess cytogenetics
for prognostication.
> Order hepatitis serologies and an HIV test before starting chemotherapy.
> Refer the patient to a dentist before starting bisphosphonate therapy.

Thrombocytopenia

These notes are in addition to the **general guide for all
consultations** on page 1, and the **starting points for
hematology consultations** at the beginning of this chapter.

Identification
Key information in the identification statement includes age and relevant
comorbidities.

Reason for Referral
Key information in the referral includes the timeline of thrombocytopenia, the patient's baseline CBC, and assessment of key findings (e.g., concerning symptoms, bicytopenia, pancytopenia).

History of Present Illness
Ask about the onset, timing, and progression of thrombocytopenia:
> If the condition has newly developed in hospital, review the patient's
course in hospital and the overall trend of thrombocytopenia.
> Establish when the platelet count was last normal.

Clarify symptoms:
> **Bleeding symptoms:** petechiae, ecchymoses, epistaxis, gingival, conjunctival hemorrhage, other bleeding sites (e.g., intracranial hemorrhage, GI bleeding, bleeding at IV sites)
> **Thrombotic microangiopathy:** bloody diarrhea, fever, neurologic impairment
> **Heparin-induced thrombocytopenia (HIT):** recent heparin exposure, venous or arterial thromboses
  » Consider using the 4T score.[3,4]
> **Symptoms of pancytopenia:**
  » See Anemia and Cytopenia in this chapter.
> **Infectious symptoms:** fever, infectious contacts
Conduct a nutritional review: Assess for folate and/or vitamin B_{12} deficiency.
Ask about recent transfusions.
Ask about planned procedures.

Past Medical History
Ask about:
- autoimmune history
- pregnancy
- HIV, HBV, HCV
- splenomegaly (or any conditions that may lead to splenomegaly)

Medications
Conduct a careful review of medications and their relation to the timing of thrombocytopenia.

Allergies
Follow the **general guide for all consultations** and the **starting points for hematology consultations.**

Family History
Ask about:
- low platelets or platelet disorders
- congenital bone marrow failure syndromes

Social History
Follow the **general guide for all consultations** and the **starting points for hematology consultations.**

Physical Examination
Neurological:
> Assess for focal deficits that may indicate signs of intracranial hemorrhage.

Signs of DIC: bleeding in IV lines
Head and neck: mucocutaneous bleeding in nasal and oral cavity, wet
  purpura, jaundice
Dermatological: petechiae, ecchymosis, jaundice
Rheumatological: scleritis, uveitis, joint involvement, rashes
Lymph nodes
Signs of VTE

Investigations

LABORATORY INVESTIGATIONS
CBC: Always document the patient's baseline and trend, and note
  other cell lines.
PBS: Assess for schistocytes.
Hemolytic workup: Order reticulocytes, LDH, bilirubin, and
  haptoglobin.
DIC workup: Order fibrinogen, INR, PTT.
Vitamin B$_{12}$, iron studies
Serologies for HBV, HCV, HIV, *Helicobacter pylori*: Use these to assess
  for secondary ITP.

OTHER INVESTIGATIONS
Blood cultures: Order this for suspected sepsis.
HIT assay: Pursue this if clinically indicated by the patient's 4T score.
ADAMTS13 level: Pursue this in suspected TTP.
Stool culture: Assess for *Escherichia coli* 0157:H7 in suspected HUS.
Antiphospholipid antibody, ANA testing: Pursue this if applicable.
BM biopsy: Pursue this in suspected primary BM disorder.

IMAGING
Upper and/or lower extremity Doppler US: Assess for venous or
  arterial thrombosis in HIT.
Abdominal ultrasound: Assess for splenomegaly.

Impression and Plan

GENERAL APPROACH
- The approach to etiology is based on decreased production, increased
  destruction, and sequestration (see Table 9.3).
- Always first rule out life-threatening causes (HIT, MAHA, DIC).
- In the context of clinical suspicion of TTP, call the lab to review the
  slide for schistocytes.
- For patients with platelet counts < 50 x 10^9/L, hold anticoagulation.

Table 9.3. Differential Diagnosis of Thrombocytopenia

DECREASED PRODUCTION	INCREASED DESTRUCTION	OTHER
Congenital Toxins: drugs, chemotherapy, alcohol Radiation Infection Nutritional deficiency Aplastic anemia Ineffective hematopoiesis (MDS) BM infiltration (e.g., lymphoma, leukemia, MM, secondary malignancies, granulomas)	**Immune mediated** ITP (primary or secondary) HIT APS PNH Alloimmune (transplant or transfusion related) Drug induced **Nonimmune mediated** MAHA (TTP, HUS/atypical HUS, DIC, HELLP syndrome, hypertension crisis, scleroderma crisis, acute rejection) Infection, sepsis	Sequestration (splenomegaly) Pseudothrombocytopenia (repeat CBC using citrated tube) Dilutional (postresuscitation, gestational)

Abbreviations: APS: antiphospholipid syndrome; BM: bone marrow; CBC: complete blood count; DIC: disseminated intravascular coagulation; HIT: heparin-induced thrombocytopenia; HUS: hemolytic uremic syndrome; ITP: immune thrombocytopenic purpura; MAHA: microangiopathic hemolytic anemia; MDS: myelodysplastic syndrome; MM: multiple myeloma; PNH: paroxysmal nocturnal hemoglobinuria; TTP: thrombotic thrombocytopenic purpura

- Consider planned procedures, active bleeding, or ongoing fevers when considering platelet transfusion thresholds.
  › *Note:* Platelet transfusion is contraindicated in TTP and HIT.

GUIDELINES FOR SPECIFIC ENTITIES
TTP:
  › Order ADAMTS13 prior to plasmapheresis and rule out other MAHAs.
  › Order acetylsalicylic acid (ASA) and DVT prophylaxis when the platelet count is > 50 x 10^9/L.
  › TTP is a hematologic emergency: if the suspicion of TTP is high, consult a hematologist for consideration of plasmapheresis.
HIT:
  › Discontinue all heparin and heparin-containing products such as flushes.
  › Start alternate anticoagulant therapy and transition to an oral anticoagulant when the platelet count is >150 x 10^9/L.
    » The duration depends on whether thrombosis is present (obtain a Doppler US).

> List heparin as an allergy in the patient's medical record and consider a medical alert bracelet.

ITP:

> Assess for secondary causes.
> In active bleeding and a platelet count $< 50 \times 10^9$/L, provide IVIG, steroids, and platelet transfusion, and consider providing tranexamic acid.

Venous Thromboembolism

These notes are in addition to the **general guide for all consultations** on page 1, and the **starting points for hematology consultations** at the beginning of this chapter.

Identification

Key information in the identification statement includes the patient's history of malignancy, VTE, and/or thrombophilia, and obvious provoking factors (such as recent surgery or trauma).

Reason for Referral

The referral typically seeks clarification about the type of clot, such as:

- PE (lobar, segmental, or subsegmental; massive or submassive)
- DVT (proximal or distal; deep or superficial)
- superficial venous thrombophlebitis
- portal vein thrombus
- symptomatic versus incidental

History of Present Illness

Clarify the patient's presentation:

> For an inpatient, clarify why the patient was admitted to hospital.
> Ask about planned surgeries or procedures.

Ask about symptoms:

> **PE:** Ask about sudden onset shortness of breath, pleuritic chest pain, syncope or near syncope, hemoptysis, fever; assess for PE rule-out criteria (PERC) or Wells criteria.[5,6]
> **DVT:** Ask about calf pain, swelling, redness.

Identify provoking factors:

> **Major transient factors:** surgery involving more than 30 minutes of general anesthesia in the past 4 weeks; major trauma; immobilization for more than 72 hours
> **Minor transient factors:** surgery involving less than 30 minutes of general anesthetic; minor trauma (outpatient treatment); acute

medical illness; immobilization for less than 72 hours; estrogen or
OC use; pregnancy; long distance travel
› **Persistent factors:** active cancer, antiphospholipid antibody
  syndrome, hereditary thrombophilia, inflammatory bowel disease
  (IBD), inflammatory disease
› **Presence of central venous catheters in upper-extremity DVT**
Conduct a review of systems:
› **Malignancy:** Ask about change in bowel habits; lymphadenopathy;
  fevers, sweats, weight loss; and smoking history.
› **Age-appropriate malignancy screening:** For women, this
  includes mammogram, Pap smear, and colon cancer screening;
  for men, it includes PSA, testicular exams, and colon cancer
  screening.
› **Rheumatologic review of systems:** See the **starting points for
  rheumatology consultations** (chapter 16).
› **Pregnancy history:** Ask about recurrent pregnancy loss.
Ask about planned procedures: Both major and minor surgeries
require careful assessment and planning for anticoagulation.

Past Medical History
Ask about:
- VTE (identify if provoked or unprovoked)
- cancer and treatments (hormonal treatment, chemotherapy)
- inflammatory conditions (e.g., SLE, RA, IBD)
- thrombophilia (clarify if hereditary or acquired)
- factors that contribute to bleeding risk
  › Apply the mnemonic HAS-BLED[7]: uncontrolled **H**ypertension,
    Abnormal renal or liver function, **S**troke, uncontrolled **B**leeding,
    Labile INRs, **E**lderly (older than 65), and **D**rug or alcohol use.
- factors that may affect drug absorption (e.g., prior bowel surgery)

Medications
Ask about:
- anticoagulation
- OCs and hormone replacement
- chemotherapy (such as cisplatin)
- erythropoiesis stimulating agents (these may increase the risk of VTE)

Allergies
Ask about a history of HIT.

Family History
Ask about:
- VTE

- malignancy
- hematologic disorders
- thrombophilia

Social History

Ask about:

- health-benefit plans and/or insurance
- alcohol use, recreational drug use, smoking
- occupation

Physical Examination

Vitals signs: Check the patient's heart rate, BP (hemodynamic stability is important), respiration rate, and oxygen saturation.

Weight: This is important to establish for anticoagulant dosing.

Signs of RV failure: Check for distended JVP; right-sided S3; RV heave; palpable or loud P2; pulmonary regurgitation murmur; and tricuspid regurgitation murmur.

Signs of DVT: Check for:

> **Calf symptoms:** These include swelling in one calf greater than 3 cm compared to the unaffected side (10 cm below the tibial tuberosity); erythema; warmth; tenderness; palpable cord; dilated superficial veins; and edema.

> **Homan sign:** The patient has calf pain on dorsiflexion of the foot.

> **Phlegmasia cerulea dolens (rare):** This is massive proximal (iliofemoral) DVT with edema, cyanosis, pain, and compartment syndrome (venous gangrene, arterial compromise).

Signs of malignancy: Check for hepatosplenomegaly, examine the lymph nodes, and perform an age-appropriate examination (e.g., DRE, testicular exam).

Investigations

Review prior investigations for malignancy markers, such as results from fecal immunochemical testing, SPEP, and mammogram, and relevant surgical pathology (e.g., colon biopsy confirming colon cancer).

LABORATORY INVESTIGATIONS

CBC (hemoglobin, MCV, platelets): These are important to assess for the safety of starting anticoagulation, but they may also provide clues to etiology (e.g., chronic elevation in platelets may indicate a myeloproliferative neoplasm).

Creatinine (eGFR): These are important for dosing and choice of anticoagulant.

Troponin and BNP: These provide risk stratification for PE and assessment of heart strain.

Liver function tests, bilirubin: These are important to assess the safety of starting direct oral anticoagulants (DOACs).

Baseline coagulation (INR, PTT): An isolated elevated PTT may indicate the presence of a lupus anticoagulant.

Other workups:

› For patients with unusual sites of thrombosis (e.g., unexplained portal vein thrombosis), or if clinically indicated, consider a workup for antiphospholipid-antibody syndrome (APS serology, lupus anticoagulant), paroxysmal nocturnal hemoglobinuria (flow cytometry), or myeloproliferative neoplasm (e.g., JAK2).

› Consider a workup for inherited thrombophilia (e.g., factor V Leiden) only if clinically warranted.

IMAGING

Review previous imaging for malignancy (lymphadenopathy, masses, nodules) or for age-appropriate malignancy screening, and imaging demonstrating VTE or vascular abnormality (CT or MRI of the pelvis; MRI venogram).

CT pulmonary angiogram (or CT pulmonary embolism): This assesses for PE location and type (e.g., submassive PE), and may identify the presence of right heart strain.

V/Q scan:

› Pursue this when contrast is contraindicated (e.g., acute or chronic renal disease).

› Consider whether to proceed with a V/Q scan in pregnancy.

ECG: This assesses for sinus tachycardia and signs of right heart strain.

Echocardiogram: Pursue this on suspicion of heart strain.

Bilateral leg Doppler US:

› Document the baseline clot burden (note that this does not change PE management).

› If the patient has a PE and a contraindication to anticoagulation (e.g., bleeding), a Doppler ultrasound is useful to assess if a proximal DVT is present, in which case consider an inferior vena cava (IVC) filter.

Impression and Plan

Describe VTE characteristics: State the specific location of the clot (see Table 9.4); the amount of clot burden; if the clot is provoked or unprovoked; if it is cancer associated or catheter related; and if it is recurrent VTE or the patient's first VTE.

› In provoked VTE, state the kind of provoking factor (major or minor).

Table 9.4. Classification of the Venous System

		LEG VEINS	ARM VEINS
Deep	**Proximal**	Iliac; common, superficial, or deep femoral; popliteal	Radial, ulnar, brachial, axillary, subclavian
	Distal	Anterior or posterior tibial; peroneal; gastrocnemius; soleus	
Superficial		Greater saphenous and lesser saphenous	Cephalic, basilic, median

> In unprovoked VTE, screen for age-appropriate malignancies.

In PE, describe the patient's status:
> Is the patient hemodynamically stable? Do they have any RV dysfunction?
> Does the patient have an associated pulmonary infarct (which presents a risk of bleeding)?
> If US has not been done, consider bilateral Doppler US of the legs to document VTE burden.

Describe key investigations: These include investigations for malignancy and/or thrombogenic process (e.g., malignancy markers, previous imaging).

Describe anticoagulation therapy:
> The duration of anticoagulation therapy is always *at minimum 3 months* for DVT and PE.
> Consider indefinite anticoagulation therapy (with periodic reassessment) for recurrent or unprovoked VTE, or for as long as the risk factor remains (i.e., indefinite in cancer-associated VTE, with frequent reassessment).
> Consider patient factors (issues with compliance, delivery, absorption) and financial factors when choosing anticoagulation (DOACs are more expensive than warfarin).
> State if the patient has renal or liver dysfunction or failure, or any bleeding risk (this affects type of therapy used).
> Discuss the patient's bleeding risk or any potential current contraindications to anticoagulation.
>> If anticoagulants are contraindicated, consider the indications for an IVC filter.
>> If an IVC filter is being considered, arrange for a bilateral Doppler US (if not already performed) to assess for proximal DVT.

Manage anticoagulation for surgeries and procedures:
> For minor procedures, anticoagulation needs to be timed or held appropriately.

> For major surgery, consider delaying the procedure until safe, or if required urgently, consider indications for an IVC filter.
> For inpatients who have had recent surgery or severe bleeding (e.g., intracranial hemorrhage), discuss with the admitting service when anticoagulation could be safely initiated for the newly diagnosed VTE.

References

1. Gresele P, Orsini S, Noris P, et al. Validation of the ISTH/SSC bleeding assessment tool for inherited platelet disorders: a communication from the Platelet Physiology SSC. J Thromb Haemost. 2020;18(3):732-9. doi: 10.1111/jth.14683
2. Rajkumar S, Dimopoulos M, Palumbo A, et al. International Myeloma Working Group updated criteria for the diagnosis of multiple myeloma. Lancet Oncol. 2014;15(12):e538-48. doi: 10.1016/S1470-2045(14)70442-5
3. Lo G, Juhl D, Warkentin T, et al. Evaluation of pretest clinical score (4 T's) for the diagnosis of heparin-induced thrombocytopenia in two clinical settings. J Thromb Haemost. 2006;4(4):759-65. doi: 10.1111/j.1538-7836.2006.01787.x
4. Vatanparast R, Lantz S, Ward K, et al. Evaluation of a pretest scoring system (4Ts) for the diagnosis of heparin-induced thrombocytopenia in a university hospital setting. Postgrad Med. 2012;124(6):36-42. doi: 10.3810/pgm.2021.11.2611
5. Kline J, Courtney D, Kabrhel C, et al. Prospective multicenter evaluation of the pulmonary embolism rule-out criteria. J Thromb Haemost 2008 May 01;6(5):772-80. doi: 10-1111/j.1538-7836.2008.02944.x
6. Wolf S, McCubbin T, Feldhaus K, et al. Prospective validation of Wells Criteria in the evaluation of patients with suspected pulmonary embolism. Ann Emerg Med 2004 November 01;44(5):503-10. doi: 10.1016/j.annemergmed.2004.04.002
7. Lip G, Frison L, Halperin J, et al. Comparative validation of a novel risk score for predicting bleeding risk in anticoagulated patients with atrial fibrillation: the HAS-BLED (Hypertension, Abnormal Renal/Liver Function, Stroke, Bleeding History or Predisposition, Labile INR, Elderly, Drugs/AlcoholConcomitantly) score. 2011;57(2):173-80. doi: 10.1016/j.jacc.2010.09.024

10

Infectious Diseases

Dr. Rahel Zewude
Dr. Marie JeongMin Kim
Dr. Stephan Saad

REVIEWERS
Dr. Natasha Press
Dr. William J. Connors

Starting Points: Infectious Diseases Consultations

These notes are in addition to the **general guide for all consultations** on page 1.

Identification

Key information in the identification statement includes relevant known infectious disease diagnoses (e.g., HIV, prior endocarditis) and demographics (e.g., history of IV drug use).

Reason for Referral

The referral may seek to confirm an infectious disease diagnosis and/or clarify appropriate management.

History of Present Illness

Determine the chronology of illness progression, from symptom onset to present:
› Ask about prodromes.
› For inpatients, ask about the course of illness before admission to hospital, at the time of admission, and during the hospital stay.

Ask about fevers:
› Does the patient have subjective or objective fevers?
› If measured, what was the maximum temperature?
› Do the fevers follow a pattern?

Take an exposure history relevant to the specific problem: Ask about:
› sick contacts
› antibiotic use (agents, duration, compliance)
› fresh or salt-water exposure
› recent trauma, including insect bites
› HIV risk factors (vertical transmission; multiple sexual partners; unprotected anal or vaginal sex; STI; sharing contaminated needles, syringes, or other equipment; unsafe injections, transfusions; unsterile procedures such as piercing; needlestick injury in a health-care worker)
› MRSA risk factors (incarceration, hospitalization in the past year, long-term care residence, dialysis, previous MRSA screening or MRSA infection)
› TB risk factors (immigration from a country with a high rate of TB; close contacts with TB; homelessness; IV drug use; working or residing in high-risk facilities such as hospitals, shelters, military, prisons, residential homes)
› lifetime travel history (abroad and within Canada), including the purpose of travel (e.g., work, visiting friends and family, tourism), exposures, and itinerary of activities

Past Medical History

Focus mostly on the patient's history of infectious disease:
› For IV drug use, determine the patient's status for HIV, HBV, HCV, and HAV immunity or infection. Include the date of last testing in patients who are negative.
› For HIV, determine CD4 count and/or viral load, known resistance to or intolerance of antiretroviral drugs, date of diagnosis, exposure method, and history of opportunistic infections.

Ask about comorbidities: For example, does the patient have diabetes? (What type? Is it controlled? What was the latest HbA_{1c} result? Are there microvascular or macrovascular complications?)

Past Surgical History

• Ask about procedures or surgeries involving prosthetic material (vascular grafts, pacemaker insertion, prosthetic valves, prosthetic joints) including dates and material used.
• If the patient has had surgery or a drain for source control, determine if there is any remaining infection.

Medications

• Ask about currently prescribed medications and home medications.
• For recently prescribed antimicrobials, determine start and stop dates.
• For steroids, antimicrobials, and immunosuppressive agents, determine doses.

Allergies

- Determine all drug allergies and clarify the patient's reaction.
- Pay particular attention to antibiotic allergies: determine when allergic reactions occurred; reaction symptoms; the type of reaction, if diagnosed (e.g., anaphylaxis; Stevens-Johnson syndrome or toxic epidermal necrolysis); and reactions on reexposure, if applicable.
- In penicillin allergy, ask about exposure to carbapenems and cephalosporins.

Family History

Ask about conditions relevant to the presenting illness (e.g., primary immune compromise).

Social History

Ask about:

- housing status
- occupation, relationships, hobbies, social habits, and immigration status, as relevant
- recreational drug use (clarify the substance, and the frequency and route of use)

Physical Examination

Review documented fevers: Establish fever temperature, pattern, and timing.

Conduct a focused examination based on the clinical question: A complete physical examination is required when the source of infection is unknown.

Remove dressings to examine surgical sites, if relevant.

› *Note:* If the patient is less than 24 hours from surgery and the surgical team has not yet disturbed the dressing, check with the patient's nurse before removing the dressing.

Investigations

LABORATORY INVESTIGATIONS

CBC: Include differential for WBCs.

Creatinine: If abnormal, identify the patient's baseline creatinine.

Other: Order other investigations relevant to the clinical context (e.g., LP; LDH in patients with suspected *Pneumocystis jiroveci* pneumonia [PCP]; CK in patients on daptomycin; liver enzymes in patients on rifampin).

MICROBIOLOGY

Review prior microbiology results, if available.

- Identify positive cultures and serologies, and relevant negative ones.

- Determine the chronological order of positives (note the date of testing and antibiotic susceptibilities).
- For blood cultures, determine the number of sets and the sites drawn from, if known (e.g., peripheral or central line).
- Determine whether antibiotics were given before the cultures were taken, if possible.
- Assess Gram stains for polymorphonuclear neutrophils, epithelial cells, and bacteria.

IMAGING

- Make sure you look at images yourself: don't just read the reports.
- Call the radiologist directly if your specific questions are not addressed in the report or if further information is required.
- Review pertinent recent studies and relevant prior images (e.g., to look for change in the size of an abscess).

Impression and Plan

SUMMARY

State all important characteristics of the patient as host: For example, the patient may be immunocompromised or acutely ill, or have risk factors for resistant organisms.

State the leading diagnosis or give a differential diagnosis: Provide evidence that supports the leading diagnosis, or give a concise differential diagnosis with supporting or refuting findings.

Describe the "what" and the "why": Identify the infectious disease (e.g., MRSA bacteremia) and the route of infection (e.g., secondary to IV drug use), because the route of infection (the "why") affects treatment and prevention.

Consider the possibility of noninfectious causes for the patient's symptoms.

PLAN

Apply a bug-drug-host framework

Bug: What organisms may be causing the problem? Does the patient have risk factors for resistant organisms? Do they have risk factors for "unusual" organisms (e.g., because of immune compromise and/or travel history)?

Drug: Will it penetrate the affected organ? Does the patient need a bactericidal drug (e.g., for endocarditis or CNS infections)? What side effects may result? Are renal or hepatic clearance an issue?

Host: How sick is the patient? What is their hemodynamic status? Are they immunocompromised? Are allergies an issue? Is medication compliance an issue?

Arrange the plan in steps for the referring team
Treatment:
> For all antibiotics, give the dose, the route of administration, and the frequency of administration.
> When prescribing an antibiotic, consider the following factors (mnemonic: AID):
  » allergies
  » interactions with other medications
  » dosing (e.g., requirements based on renal clearance, weight, CNS penetration, organism coverage such as *Pseudomonas aeruginosa*)
> If an antibiotic requires drug-level monitoring, provide instructions.
Investigations: List these in bullet form, and provide a brief rationale if the rationale is not obvious (e.g., US to assess for liver abscess, abdominal x-ray to assess for megacolon).
Precautions: If precautions are required, explain why, and indicate when they can stop (e.g., airborne isolation for pulmonary tuberculosis until the patient has 3 negative sputum acid-fast bacilli smears).
Follow-up and/or monitoring: State key features of appropriate response to treatment (e.g., decreasing WBCs and fever) and possible complications (e.g., evidence of liver toxicity, common side effects of medications).
Infectious-disease team follow-up:
> Indicate whether the infectious-disease team will follow and when.
> If no follow-up is planned, state what should trigger further consultation with the infectious-disease team (e.g., recurrent bacteremia, echocardiogram demonstrating endocarditis, nonresponse to recommended treatment at 5 days).

Bloodstream Infections

These notes are in addition to the **general guide for all consultations** on page 1, and the **starting points for infectious diseases consultations** at the beginning of this chapter.

Identification

Key information in the identification statement includes whether the patient uses IV drugs, is immunocompromised, and/or has had recent surgery.

Reason for Referral

The referral typically seeks to clarify the infectious entity and/or appropriate management.

History of Present Illness

Clarify the patient's presenting symptoms: For inpatients, also ask about the patient's course in the ED or hospital.

Assess for specific symptoms of metastatic infection:
> **Infective endocarditis:** dyspnea, chest pain
> **Epidural abscess:** back pain, saddle anesthesia
> **Embolic infarcts:** altered mental status, focal weakness
> **Endophthalmitis:** vision changes

Conduct a review of systems: Ask about skin and soft tissue infections (SSTIs), ulcers, wounds, and any peripheral lines, central lines, dialysis lines, or urinary catheters.

Clarify antimicrobial administration: Identify specific agents, response to therapy, duration of therapy, and any adverse reactions.

Take an exposure history: Ask about:
> IV drug use
> MRSA risk factors
> travel-related exposures
> recent exposure to antimicrobials

Past Medical History

- Ask about previous bloodstream infections:
  > For each infection, clarify the source, date, treatment, and whether the patient completed the course of therapy.
  > Obtain documentation of blood culture clearances.
- If the patient has a previous history of deep-seated infections such as osteomyelitis, infective endocarditis, or septic arthritis, clarify key details (bones, valves, and joints involved; the results of tissue or bone biopsies; any surgical interventions).
- Ask about a history of immune compromise.

Past Surgical History

Follow the **general guide for all consultations** and the **starting points for infectious diseases consultations**.

Medications

Follow the **general guide for all consultations** and the **starting points for infectious diseases consultations**.

Allergies

- Ask about medication allergies and identify the specific medications.
- For allergies to antimicrobials, clarify the reaction.

Social History

Ask about:
- recreational drug use, alcohol use, smoking
- occupation (if a health-care provider, clarify role)
- housing status

Physical Examination

Vital signs:
› Obtain the patient's vital signs.
› Compare the patient's current temperature to their maximum recorded temperature, if available (note the date of the maximum temperature), and check the date of the last fever.

Signs of infective endocarditis: Look for Roth spots, Janeway lesions, Osler nodes, and splinter hemorrhages.

Signs of IV drug use: Look for track marks.

Potential sites of infection:
› Inspect any skin ulcers and wounds (obtain the diameter of wounds; clarify if purulent or nonpurulent, and whether there is bone exposure or probing to bone).
› Inspect any peripheral or central IV lines, dialysis lines, and surgical sites.
› Remove dressings to examine surgical sites, if deemed safe.

Cardiovascular: Assess JVP, auscultate for cardiac murmurs and extra heart sounds, and assess for peripheral edema (bacteremia can cause infective endocarditis which can result in heart failure).

Respiratory: Conduct a general exam, with attention to diminished breath sounds and crackles on auscultation.

Back, flanks, abdomen:
› Assess for spinal tenderness and epidural abscesses.
› If acute lower back pain, flank pain, or lower abdomen pain is present, perform a hip extension to assess for exacerbation of pain as a sign of psoas abscess.

Neurological: If altered level of consciousness is present, or on suspicion of epidural abscess or spinal osteomyelitis, conduct a neurological exam including assessment of deep tendon reflexes and muscle power.

Eyes: If altered vision is present:
› assess for conjunctival injection, extraocular movements, and associated pain
› assess visual acuity with a Snellen chart

Investigations

LABORATORY INVESTIGATIONS

CBC with differential: Assess for neutrophilia, lymphocytosis, and eosinophilia.

Creatinine: If abnormal, identify the patient's baseline creatinine.

Electrolytes

Liver enzymes

CRP and/or ESR

MICROBIOLOGY

- Determine the most recent positive cultures (i.e., within the previous 2 weeks) and the most notable positive cultures (i.e., prior resistant organisms).
- Remember to establish the timing and site from which each blood culture was obtained.
- Call the microbiology laboratory for more information as needed.
  › Laboratories can provide susceptibilities not listed in the patient's record, time to positivity, and preliminary information not yet finalized (e.g., lactose fermenter, oxidase).
  › You can provide laboratories with clinical information that may be helpful in guiding workups.

IMAGING

Chest x-ray: Assess for focal consolidations and cavitary lesions.

CT of the chest: Assess for septic pulmonary emboli.

Echocardiogram (transthoracic or transesophageal): Assess for vegetations (if present, specify the valve, size, severity of regurgitation, and EF, and whether an aortic root abscess is present).

ECG: Assess for conduction abnormalities, and assess QT and PR intervals (PR interval prolongation or heart block can indicate aortic root abscess).

Impression and Plan

Describe the source of bacteremia: Examples include SSTI, UTI, and others.

List metastases of infection: Examples include osteomyelitis, infective endocarditis, septic emboli infarcts, and others.

Discuss the patient's risk for resistant organisms: This is important when drug susceptibility is pending.

Discuss source control: In the context of local infections, abscesses, or deep-seated infections, consider the need for surgical or interventional radiology (IR) drainage.

Prescribe antibiotics:
> In deep-seated infections such as endocarditis, osteomyelitis, and CNS infections, consider organ penetration when choosing an antibiotic.
> Consider bactericidal antibiotics for endocarditis and CNS infections.
> Consider side effects, and renal and hepatic clearance.

Specify the duration of therapy:
> The duration of therapy depends on whether the bacteremia is simple or complicated (i.e., metastasis with infective endocarditis, osteomyelitis, epidural abscess).
> Include recommendations regarding a PICC line after blood culture clearance.

Discuss line removal: Consider the need to remove prosthetic devices, urinary catheters, and/or central, peripheral or dialysis lines.

Fever of Unknown Origin

These notes are in addition to the **general guide for all consultations** on page 1, and the **starting points for infectious diseases consultations** at the beginning of this chapter.

Identification

Key information in the identification statement includes:
- whether the patient is immunocompromised (e.g., infected with HIV), has a malignancy or autoimmune condition, or uses IV drugs
- ethnicity, if relevant (e.g., Mediterranean)

Reason for Referral

The referral may seek diagnosis of a fever of unknown origin and/or clarify management.

History of Present Illness

Characterize the fever:
> Ask about onset, frequency (e.g., quotidian fever in malaria), and duration.
> Ask if the fever spontaneously resolves.

Clarify associated symptoms: Ask about chills, rashes.

Conduct a review of systems: Ask about:
> **ENT:** oral sores, toothaches, change in hearing or vision, rhinorrhea, facial tenderness or swelling, nasal congestion
> **CNS:** headaches, altered level of consciousness, neck stiffness, behavioural changes, focal weakness, loss of sensation
> **Respiratory:** cough, shortness of breath, hemoptysis

> **GI:** nausea, vomiting, abdominal pain, diarrhea, constipation
> **GU:** urinary frequency or urgency, flank pain, vaginal or penile discharge, genital ulcers
> **Dermatological:** rashes, ulcers, wounds
> **Musculoskeletal:** joint pain, back pain
> **Constitutional symptoms:** weight loss, night sweats, fatigue, loss of appetite

Clarify neutropenia status: Ask if the patient is currently neutropenic or has previous history of neutropenia.

Take an exposure history: Ask about:
> international travel
> sexual history
> insect bites
> wild and domestic animals
> fresh or salt water
> sick contacts
> immunization history

Past Medical History

Ask about:

- **Immune compromise:**
  > **Malignancy:** Determine treatment administered and dates (e.g., chemotherapy).
  > **HIV:** Determine date of diagnosis, exposure method, history of opportunistic infections, most recent CD4 and viral load results, and treatment history.
- **Autoimmune conditions:** Determine date of diagnosis, recent flares, treatment course, and outpatient follow-up.
- **TB:** Determine date of diagnosis, treatment history, and subsequent exposures.
- **HBV, HCV:** Determine date of diagnosis, treatment history, and immune status.

Past Surgical History

Ask about transplantations, including solid-organ and hematopoietic stem cell transplantations (clarify transplantation anatomy, type, and source, and any history of rejection including treatment and response).

Medications

Ask about:
- **Antimicrobials:** Determine start and stop dates.
- **Immunosuppressive agents:** For chemotherapy, determine the most recent cycle date.

- **HIV therapy:** Determine all current antiretroviral therapy (ART) and doses, and ask about medication compliance.
- **All other medications:** Determine doses.

Allergies

- Ask about medication allergies.
- In allergy to antimicrobials, clarify the reaction.

Family History

Ask about:
- hereditary fever syndromes or persistent fever with no diagnosis
- autoimmune conditions
- malignancy

Social History

Ask about:
- alcohol use, recreational drug use, smoking
- occupation
- housing status
- immigration history

Physical Examination

Vital signs:
> Obtain all the patient's vital signs.
> Compare the patient's current temperature to their maximum recorded temperature, if available (note the date of the maximum temperature), and check the date of the last fever.

ENT:
> Check for oral ulcers; compromised teeth or gums; and facial tenderness.
> If the patient reports vision or hearing changes on history, assess hearing and vision with funduscopy and otoscopy.

Neurological: Perform a jolt accentuation test and nuchal rigidity assessment (this is relevant to meningitis).

Lymph nodes: Assess for lymphadenopathy (hematologic malignancy).

Cardiovascular, respiratory: Conduct a general exam.

Abdominal: Conduct a general exam with attention to hepatosplenomegaly (hematologic malignancy).

Dermatological: Look for rashes and/or purpura (connective tissue disease), and insect bites.

Musculoskeletal: Examine the joints for effusion, erythema, and tenderness.

Surgical sites, wounds: Remove dressings if deemed safe.

Investigations

LABORATORY INVESTIGATIONS

CBC: Include differential for WBCs (e.g., neutrophils, lymphocytes, eosinophils).

Peripheral smear: Assess for malaria in travellers.

Creatinine: If abnormal, identify the patient's baseline creatinine.

Liver enzymes

CRP and/or ESR

LP: Order cell count and differential, glucose, and protein.

Autoimmune investigations: Order tests for ANA, extractable nuclear antigen, rheumatoid factor, C3, C4, and antineutrophil cytoplasmic antibodies.

Other: Review previous laboratory investigations for abnormal findings.

MICROBIOLOGY

- Determine the most recent positive cultures (i.e., within the previous 2 weeks) and the most notable positive cultures (i.e., prior resistant organisms).
- Review a wide array of tissue sites including blood cultures; urine, wound, and sputum cultures, if available; and LP.

IMAGING

Chest x-ray: Assess for any focal consolidation, opacities, cavitary lesions, hilar lymphadenopathy, and other notable findings.

Abdominal imaging: Assess for hepatosplenomegaly, abdominal masses, and lymphadenopathy, and findings that suggest inflammation of the gall bladder, pancreas, or peritoneum.

Impression and Plan

Provide a summary: Apply the bug-drug-host framework.

Consider medication compliance: Consider prescribing a medication with 1 or 2 doses per day (as opposed to 3 or 4 doses per day).

Provide a differential diagnosis:

› Consider the possibility that the etiology is *not an infection.*

› The differential diagnosis for fever of unknown origin is broad and includes:

  » malignancy (hematologic and solid tumours)
  » autoimmune conditions (e.g., SLE, vasculitis, RA)
  » endocrine conditions (hyperthyroidism, pheochromocytoma)
  » drugs (cocaine, antiepileptics, antibiotics, antimalarials)

» hereditary periodic fever syndromes (e.g., familial Mediterranean fever, periodic fever with aphthous stomatitis and adenitis)
» alcoholic hepatitis

HIV

These notes are in addition to the **general guide for all consultations** on page 1, and the **starting points for infectious diseases consultations** at the beginning of this chapter.

Identification

- Key information in the identification statement includes HIV status (positive, negative, or unknown), HIV transmission risk (e.g., men who have sex with men, IV drug user, sex worker, risk of vertical transmission in women of childbearing age).
- In confirmed HIV positivity, key information includes: year of diagnosis; last CD4 results (count and fraction) and date; HIV RNA results and date; and current ART.

Reason for Referral

The referral may seek to confirm HIV infection and/or clarify appropriate management.

History of Present Illness

Clarify why the patient has sought care: In an inpatient setting, why was the patient admitted to hospital?

Clarify the context of newly diagnosed HIV infection:
› Note that, in a new diagnosis, the patient may not be aware of their HIV status.
› Determine what prompted the HIV test.

Clarify treatment and follow-up in known HIV infection:
› Determine compliance with ART and barriers to compliance (e.g., side effects, pill burden); consider objective confirmation of compliance (e.g., review pharmacy records, connect with the patient's case manager).
› Clarify the patient's primary infectious disease doctor and the date of their last appointment.

Ask about sick contacts.

Conduct a review of systems: Ask about:
› fever, night sweats, weight loss
› headache, vision changes, neck pain

> cough, rhinorrhea, sinus congestion, sore throat, anosmia
> pain with swallowing
> shortness of breath
> chest pain
> abdominal pain, nausea, vomiting, diarrhea
> dysuria, flank pain, genital discharge, genital rashes
> last menstrual period
> rash, joint pain, abscess, lymph nodes
> extremity weakness or change in sensation

Past Medical History
Ask about:
- **Other infectious diseases:**
  > Establish the dates of diagnosis and treatment history.
  > Ask about chronic active HBV, HCV (determine genotype), syphilis, endocarditis, cellulitis, osteomyelitis, pneumonia, septic arthritis, and TB.
  > Ask about past opportunistic infections such as PCP, mycobacterium avium complex (MAC), TB, CMV, toxoplasmosis, cryptococcal meningitis, esophageal candidiasis, and HIV-related cancers.
- **Comorbidities:** Check for cardiovascular disease, diabetes, osteoporosis, hypertension, end stage liver disease, cirrhosis, psychiatric diagnoses (depression, bipolar disorder, PTSD), dyslipidemia, COPD, and renal disease.
- **Obstetrical history:** Assess the patient's risk of vertical transmission.

Medications
Ask about:
- ART past and present
  > If the therapy has changed, determine why.
- pain medications
- OTC medications and herbal medications
- hormonal and dietary supplements
- immunizations
  > Determine whether the patient completed needed booster courses and the year received.
  > Ask about pneumococcal 13/23; HAV; HBV; influenza; tetanus; HPV; meningococcal meningitis; MMR; varicella; and shingles (in patients older than 50).

Allergies
Ask about hypersensitivity to antibiotics and/or ART.

Family History
Ask about HIV infection in the patient's children and mother.

Social History
Key areas of inquiry include:
- **Substance use:** Ask about:
  › a history of addiction
  › substances used (tobacco, alcohol, opioids, marijuana, stimulants)
  › route of substance use (smoking, injection, inhaling, IM, IV)
  › amounts used, duration of use, and instance of last use
  › a history of withdrawal
  › date of last IV drug use and the context of use (needle sharing, use of a safe injection site, enrollment in a harm reduction program, access to naloxone)
- **Sexual history:** Ask about:
  › the number of recent partners
  › sex and HIV status of partners
  › disclosure of HIV status to partners
  › type of sex engaged in (e.g., oral, vaginal, penile, anal)
  › use of condoms and/or contraceptives
  › previous or current role as a sex worker
- **Relationships:** Ask about marital status, number of children, family planning goals, and a history of domestic violence.
- **Housing status:** Determine where the patient lives (e.g., house or apartment, long-term care facility, shelter, treatment house).
- **Financial resources:** Ask about employment status (full-time or part-time job, retired) and other financial supports (e.g., social assistance, disability income, pension).
- **Social supports:** Ask about social networks, sense of isolation, and assistance with ADLs and IADLs.
- **Exposures:** Ask about incarceration, lifetime travel history, recent exposure to animals, and tick bites.
- **Medical care:** Determine the patient's primary care physician or clinic.

Physical Examination
Vitals signs
Weight
Head, eyes, neck: ocular disorders (funduscopy), scleral icterus, compromised dentition, mouth ulcers, candidiasis, meningeal signs
Respiratory: work of breathing, abnormal sounds (auscultation)
Cardiovascular: abnormal sounds (auscultation), peripheral edema, peripheral pulses

Abdominal: stigmata of liver disease, masses, tenderness, hepatosplenomegaly

GU: ulcers, warts, genital discharge

Anorectal: ulcers, warts, fissures, masses

Lymph nodes: generalized versus local enlargement (cervical, axillary, inguinal)

Musculoskeletal: muscle wasting, spinal tenderness, mobility

Dermatological: rashes, bruising, cutaneous lesions

Neurological: level of consciousness; focal deficits; gait; speech; signs of cognitive impairment, depression, anxiety, intoxication

Investigations

Routine investigations: CBC and differential; electrolytes; creatinine; urea; glucose; Mg; PO_4; ALT; bilirubin; INR, PTT (if the patient may have an LP); fasting lipid panel (HIV is associated with CVD); fasting glucose or HbA_{1c} (diabetes is more prevalent in HIV infection); pregnancy test; urinalysis; chest x-ray; ECG (to assess QTc)

HIV-specific investigations: lab-confirmed diagnosis; CD4 count and percentage; HIV viral load; drug-resistance testing; HLA*B5701 testing; glucose-6-phosphate dehydrogenase deficiency testing

Coinfection investigations: urine gonorrhea and chlamydia: HAV, HBV, HCV serology; syphilis

Opportunistic infection investigations:
› Patient symptoms and a past history of opportunistic infections should guide testing.
› Screen for common opportunistic infections in asymptomatic patients (see Table 10.1).

Impression and Plan

In inpatient settings, consider the reason for admission: If the patient has been admitted to hospital for a reason other than HIV infection, consider how HIV and ART might impact the clinical course.

Prescribe ART:
› Treatment guidelines recommend initiating ART within 2 weeks for most opportunistic infections (*exception*: cryptococcal and TB meningitis because of the risk of IRIS).
› When discussing ART, consider patient preference, pretreatment RNA level, pretreatment CD4 count, ability to follow-up, food requirements, renal function, osteoporosis, psychiatric illnesses, hyperlipidemia, and drug interactions.

Table 10.1. Screening Guidelines for Opportunistic Infections in Asymptomatic HIV Patients

CD4 COUNT	OPPORTUNISTIC INFECTION	INVESTIGATIONS
All levels	TB	TST, chest x-ray
	Malignancy	Age-appropriate guidelines specific to persons with HIV
	Infections (SSTI, respiratory)	No routine screening
200 (or clinical evidence of thrush)	PCP	Chest x-ray +/- CT, LDH
100	Toxoplasmosis	IgG
	Cryptococcus	Antigen (LP: include opening pressure)
50	MAC	Blood AFB x 2
	CMV	Ophthalmologic exam +/- PCR

Abbreviations: AFB: acid-fast bacilli; CD: clusters of differentiation; CMV: cytomegalovirus; CT: computed tomography; IgG: immunoglobulin G; LDH: lactate dehydrogenase; MAC: mycobacterium avium complex; PCP: *Pneumocystis jiroveci* pneumonia; PCR: polymerase chain reaction; SSTI: skin and soft tissue infection; TB: tuberculosis; TST: tuberculosis skin test

Prevent concurrent infections:
›   Consider the possibility of coinfections based on the patient's risk factors and CD4 count, and the need for testing and/or prophylaxis.
›   Recommend vaccinations, including annual influenza; DTP; pneumococcal; meningococcal; HBV; HPV (if the patient is younger than 26 years); MMR and varicella (if the patient is not already immune and has a CD4 ≥ 200 cells/µL).

Refer for psychosocial support, as indicated: This could include referral for addictions support and/or to a psychiatrist or social worker.

Skin and Soft Tissue Infections

These notes are in addition to the **general guide for all consultations** on page 1, and the **starting points for infectious diseases consultations** at the beginning of this chapter.

Identification

Key information in the identification statement includes whether the patient is immunocompromised, uses IV drugs, or has peripheral vascular disease, diabetes, or a chronic wound.

Reason for Referral

Examples of reason for referral include management of SSTI and ruling out deep tissue infection.

History of Present Illness

Ask about onset and progression of the SSTI: For inpatients, determine the patient's course in the ED, including hemodynamic status.

Clarify specific symptoms: Ask about associated drainage from wounds, severity of pain in the affected area, sensation in the affected area, fevers, chills, joint pain, back pain, ability to weight bear, and rash.

Conduct a review of systems: Ask about upper and lower respiratory symptoms, GI symptoms, urinary symptoms, and any recent hospitalizations or illnesses.

Take an exposure history: Ask about:
> IV drug use
> MRSA risk factors
> travel-related exposures
> recent exposure to antimicrobials
> animal or human bites (including fist bites)
> recent trauma

Past Medical History

Ask about:
- previous SSTIs (determine dates of diagnosis, treatment, whether the patient completed the course of therapy, and whether deep-seated infections such as osteomyelitis or septic arthritis were present)
- peripheral arterial disease
- immune compromise (in diabetes, determine the last known HbA_{1c}, and whether the patient is insulin dependent and/or has microvascular or macrovascular complications)

Past Surgical History

Follow the **general guide for all consultations** and the **starting points for infectious diseases consultations**.

Medications

Ask about:

- antimicrobials (clarify specific agents, response to therapy, duration of therapy, and any adverse reactions)
- all other prescription medications

Allergies

- Ask about medication allergies.
- In allergy to antimicrobials, clarify the reaction.

Social History

Ask about:
- recreational drug use (IV drug use; substance use with inhalation or ingestion), alcohol use, smoking
- occupation (if a health-care provider, clarify role)
- housing status
- community wound-care support for any chronic wounds (clarify frequency of visits)

Physical Examination

Vital signs:
> Obtain all the patient's vital signs.
> Compare the patient's current temperature to their maximum recorded temperature, if available (note the date of the maximum temperature), and check the date of the last fever.

Peripheral pulses

Suspected SSTI site:
> Check for erythema, swelling, and purulence (note if the border of erythema is well demarcated or irregular).
> Obtain the diameter of the wound, and determine whether there is bone exposure or probing to bone.
> Examine for crepitus, skin tenseness in the affected area, bullae, and violaceous colour (to assess for necrotizing fasciitis).
> Assess for pain with passive or active stretch, and for sensation in the area (to assess for compartment syndrome).
> Palpate for fluctuance, which suggests abscess.

Signs of IV drug use: Look for track marks.

Cardiovascular: Conduct a general exam, looking for murmurs or stigmata that suggest infective endocarditis and concomitant bacteremia.

Respiratory: Conduct a general exam.

Musculoskeletal: Examine the back for spinal tenderness.

Neurological: On suspicion of epidural abscess or spinal osteomyelitis, conduct a neurological exam including assessment of deep tendon reflexes and muscle power.

Surgical sites: Remove dressings if deemed safe.

Investigations

LABORATORY INVESTIGATIONS

CBC with differential: Assess for neutrophilia, lymphocytosis, and eosinophilia.

Creatinine: If abnormal, identify the patient's baseline creatinine.

Electrolytes: K is particularly important in possible trimethoprim-sulfamethoxazole therapy.

Liver enzymes: AST can indicate muscle damage.

CRP and/or ESR

CK: This assesses for muscle damage in compartment syndrome.

Other: Review previous laboratory investigations for abnormal findings.

MICROBIOLOGY

- Obtain previous microbiology reports with a focus on blood cultures, wound cultures, tissue biopsies, and bone biopsies.
  › In previous biopsies and wound cultures, determine the sample site.
- Determine the most recent positive cultures (i.e., within the previous 2 weeks) and the most notable positive cultures (i.e., prior resistant organisms).

IMAGING

X-ray of SSTI site: Assess for foreign bodies and bony changes.

CT of extremity:
› Review for radiologic findings that suggest necrotizing infection (e.g., gas in soft tissues).
› Assess for osteomyelitis (if the patient has a previous history of osteomyelitis, compare current and previous scans to assess for changes that indicate acute osteomyelitis).

Other: Review prior US and other imaging for evidence of abscess.

ECG: Assess QT interval.

Impression and Plan

Describe the type of SSTI: For example, indicate cellulitis or necrotizing infection.

Describe the cause of the SSTI: For example, indicate trauma such as a bite, or skin entry through IV drug use.

Discuss the patient's risk for resistant organisms:
› This is important when drug susceptibility is pending.
› MRSA is a particular concern.

Prescribe antibiotics:
> Specify IV or oral antibiotics (depending on whether the patient can take oral medications and/or is hemodynamically stable).
> Consider multiple antibiotics in polymicrobial infections.
> Include antitoxin antibiotics (i.e., clindamycin for necrotizing infection regimen).
> Consider side effects, and renal and hepatic clearance.

Provide hemodynamic support, as indicated: Septic patients may require IV fluids.

Specify the duration of therapy:
> The general rule is 5 to 7 days of therapy for mild SSTIs.
> Consider extended duration in severe infection, immunosuppression, presence of concomitant bacteremia, and/or deep tissue infection.

Discuss source control:
> Necrotizing infection requires emergent surgical exploration and intervention.
> Consider surgical or IR drainage for abscesses.

Discuss wound care: If specialized wound care and follow-up are required, consider referral to a wound care team.

11

Medical Oncology

Dr. Lidiya Luzhna
Dr. Arkhjamil Angeles
Dr. Meredith Li

REVIEWER
Dr. Howard J. Lim

Starting Points: Medical Oncology Consultations

These notes are in addition to the **general guide for all consultations** on page 1.

Identification

Follow the general guide for all consultations.

Reason for Referral

The referral may seek a workup for newly diagnosed malignancy and/or an appropriate approach to management.

History of Present Illness

Ask about events leading to diagnosis:

› What signs and symptoms did the patient have? How did these evolve between onset and diagnosis? (Ask specifically about weight loss, night sweats, unexplained pain.)

› Determine the patient's risk for malignancy (e.g., tobacco use, alcohol use, infections, chronic inflammation, environmental exposures).

› Did the diagnosis result from self-examination, screening, workup of signs and symptoms, or an incidental finding?

Determine diagnostic workup to date:

› Has a tissue biopsy been done? Determine what was biopsied and how the biopsy was performed (e.g., fine-needle aspiration, core biopsy, surgical biopsy).

› What are the pathology results? Determine important tumour-specific details such as cell type (e.g., adenocarcinoma, squamous cell carcinoma), lymphovascular or perineural invasion, nodal involvement, extranodal extension, and margins.

› If genetic testing has been done, were any targetable mutations or variants found?

› What staging investigations have been performed? When were they done? What were the results? Review pertinent laboratory and radiographic findings, including tumour markers.

› Are there any pending investigations?

Determine treatments to date:

› Has the patient undergone primary surgical resection or metastasectomy? Were there any postoperative complications?

› Has the patient had radiation therapy? Were there any complications? What was the response to treatment?

› Ask about systemic therapies (e.g., neoadjuvant, adjuvant, palliative).

› Ask for the names of other specialists involved in oncological care (e.g., radiation oncologist, surgical oncologist).

Clarify current clinical status:

› If the patient has started treatment for cancer, how is their clinical recovery?

› Clarify signs and symptoms that suggest ongoing or recurrent disease.

› Assess the patient's performance status with the Eastern Cooperative Oncology Group (ECOG) scale.

› Conduct a general review of systems (e.g., ask about pain, weight, appetite, mood, bowel and bladder symptoms).

Past Medical History

• Ask about other medical conditions.

• Ask specifically about autoimmune disease, renal and hepatic dysfunction, cardiac disease, chronic infections, and other previous cancer diagnoses.

Past Surgical History

• Ask about all surgeries.

• Ask specifically about surgeries for malignancy (primary tumour resection, metastasectomy).

Medications

Review all medications (e.g., corticosteroids, immunomodulatory agents), vitamins, herbal medications, and supplements.

Allergies

Follow the **general guide for all consultations.**

Family History

Ask about malignancy (clarify in what family member, type of cancer, and age at diagnosis, if known) and genetic disorders (e.g., BRCA mutations, Lynch syndrome, familial adenomatous polyposis).

Social History

Ask about:
- alcohol use, recreational drug use, smoking
- occupation
- supports at home

Physical Examination

Height, weight, and BSA

Tumour-specific signs: Perform a focused exam. For palpable masses and lymph nodes, note location, size, shape, borders and surface texture, mobility, and tenderness.

Investigations

LABORATORY INVESTIGATIONS

CBC with differential

Creatinine (eGFR)

Liver enzymes and liver function tests: Order INR, albumin, and bilirubin.

Electrolytes, Ca

Endocrine tests: Pursue these if considering immunotherapy (e.g., thyrotropin [TSH], morning cortisol).

Relevant tumour markers: Examples include CEA, CA-19-9 antigen, and PSA.

Genetic testing: Pursue this as indicated.

IMAGING

- Obtain relevant previous imaging and order new imaging as indicated.
- Consider what baseline investigations are needed before initiation of cancer therapy (e.g., echocardiogram, ECG, pulmonary function test).

Impression and Plan

Provide a concise diagnosis: Include the type of cancer, and clinical or pathological staging (TNM staging) based on available information.
  › Comment on features that influence the risk and aggressiveness of disease.

> Consider a pathology review of a specimen from the cancer site in the context of diagnostic uncertainty.

Summarize previous treatments and their course: Specify what treatments the patient received, response to treatment, and treatment-related complications or adverse effects.

Describe eligible treatment options: Include clinical trials and specify the intent of treatment (e.g., curative or palliative).

> Discuss the likelihood of side effects and complications associated with each treatment.
> Document patient consent or refusal of treatment.
> Indicate the dose and date of treatment, and the need for pretreatment medications.

Order pretreatment investigations:

> Order blood work, tumour markers, and imaging as needed.
> Consider genetic testing if applicable.

Order surveillance investigations, as indicated.

Discuss goals of care and code status: Provide a prognosis, if known.

Refer the patient to palliative care, if appropriate.

Febrile Neutropenia

These notes are in addition to the **general guide for all consultations** on page 1, and the **starting points for medical oncology consultations** at the beginning of this chapter.

Identification

Follow the **general guide for all consultations.**

Reason for Referral

The referral may seek to confirm febrile neutropenia (FN) and/or clarify appropriate management.

History of Present Illness

Clarify details of the cancer and systemic treatment: Determine:

> type and stage of cancer
> current ECOG performance status[1]
> current systemic therapy
> history of side effects on current therapy
> dates of the most-recent cycle of treatment (most treatments have an absolute neutrophil count [ANC] nadir at 1 to 2 weeks, and ANC recovery at 3 to 4 weeks[2])

Clarify fever and infectious symptoms: Determine:
› onset and duration of fever
› maximum recorded temperature and method of measurement (oral, tympanic)
› focal infectious symptoms (e.g., cough, dyspnea, abdominal pain, diarrhea, urinary frequency, dysuria, chills)
› risk factors for infection (e.g., central venous access, active uncontrolled cancer, mucosal disruption, hospitalization, steroid use, recent travel, sick contacts)
› history of infections, antimicrobial prophylaxis, and potential side effects to antimicrobial therapy

Past Medical History
Ask about:
- cancer diagnoses:
  › type, stage, date of diagnoses, extent of metastases
  › treatment history and dates (e.g., surgical resection, radiation, systemic therapy)
  › side effects and complications of treatment
  › name of the patient's primary medical oncologist
- medical conditions that increase risk of infection (e.g., liver disease, kidney disease, COPD, diabetes, immunosuppression)
- other medical history

Past Surgical History
Ask about:
- implantation of prosthetic material (e.g., vascular grafts, pacemakers, prosthetic valves, prosthetic joints)
- other surgical history

Medications
- Review recent antibiotic exposure.
- Review all medication administration routes. Rectal administration should be avoided in FN.

Allergies
Follow the **general guide for all consultations.**

Family History
Follow the **general guide for all consultations** and the **starting points for medical oncology consultations.**

Social History
Follow the **general guide for all consultations** and the **starting points for medical oncology consultations.**

Physical Examination

Vital signs:
> Obtain all the patient's vital signs.
> Compare the patient's current temperature to their maximum recorded temperature, if available (note the date of the maximum temperature), and check the date of the last fever.

General impression: Assess the patient's appearance, mental status, and hydration status.

Signs of infection: Perform a focused exam assessing for:
> **Head and neck:** meningismus, otitis, sinusitis, stomatitis, oral thrush, tender cervical lymph nodes, dental infection
> **Chest:** crackles, decreased air entry
> **Abdomen:** peritonitis, tenderness, hepatosplenomegaly, Murphy sign, Rovsing sign (do not perform a DRE)
> **Pelvis:** suprapubic or costovertebral angle tenderness
> **Skin:** cellulitis, HSV, perianal infections, venous access sites

Investigations

LABORATORY INVESTIGATIONS

CBC with differential: Note ANC and degree of neutropenia.

Electrolytes, urea, creatinine, glucose, Ca

Liver enzymes, bilirubin, albumin

Lactate, CRP, procalcitonin: Consider these.

MICROBIOLOGY

Review previous cultures and note prior growth of resistant organisms.

Blood cultures:
> Provide 2 sets from 2 separate peripheral IV sites.
> Draw from each venous access site (central venous catheter, PICC) plus a single peripheral IV site.[3]

Urinalysis and urine culture

Other microbiology: If clinically indicated, consider LP; sputum (Gram stain and culture, fungal culture, acid-fast bacilli), viral nasopharyngeal swab, stool culture, *Clostridium difficile* assay, and wound culture.

IMAGING

Chest x-ray

Other imaging: As clinically indicated, consider CT of the chest, abdomen, and pelvis, and abdominal US.

Impression and Plan

GENERAL APPROACH

Confirm or rule out a diagnosis of FN:
› The definition of the Infectious Disease Society of America guidelines requires: 1) a temperature of 38.0°C for 1 hour or any single temperature reading $\geq$ 38.3°C; and 2) ANC < 0.5 x 10^9/L or an expected nadir of ANC < 0.5 x 10^9/L.[4]
› Some patients may be afebrile with minimal symptoms due to chemotherapy-induced attenuation of immune response.[3]
› On evidence of infection, and if the patient is neutropenic in the context of recent systemic therapy, consider initiating treatment for FN.[5]

Decide on the appropriate treatment setting:
› Notify patient's medical oncologist.
› Stratify the patient's risk of complications using clinical judgement and validated tools such as the Multinational Association for Supportive Care in Cancer (MASCC) score[6] and Clinical Index of Stable Febrile Neutropenia (CISNE) score.[7]
  » **Low-risk FN:** This generally includes *all* of the following features: an expected duration of ANC < 0.5 x 10^9/L that is no longer than 7 days; no active comorbidities; stable hepatic and renal function; MASCC score > 21; CISNE score < 3.[3]
  » **High-risk FN:** This generally includes *any* of the following features: an expected duration of ANC < 0.5 x 10^9/L that is more than 7 days; ongoing, active comorbidities; significant hepatic dysfunction (AST or ALT > 5 times ULN) or renal dysfunction (creatinine clearance < 30 mL/min); MASCC score < 21; CISNE score $\geq$ 3; uncontrolled or progressive cancer; clinical instability.[3]
› In low-risk FN, consider outpatient treatment or short admission (4 hours or less) for observation.[3]
› In high-risk FN, admit the patient to hospital.[3]

Avoid all rectal agents in new prescriptions and reevaluate rectal administration in existing prescriptions.

INITIAL MANAGEMENT

• Provide resuscitation with IV fluids as needed.
• Start empiric antibiotics ideally *within 1 hour* of presentation to hospital and after blood cultures are drawn.[8]
• Antibiotic choice depends on allergies, presumed source of infection, recent antibiotic use, risk of nosocomial infection, and previous growth of resistant organisms or colonization with resistant organisms.

- Antibiotic coverage should include gram-positive bacteria, gram-negative bacteria, anaerobes, and *Pseudomonas*.
- Provide acetaminophen 500–1000 mg orally every 4 hours as required for fever (maximum dose: 4 g from all sources).

OUTPATIENT TREATMENT

- Provide empiric antibiotics: ciprofloxacin 750 mg orally 2 times per day, plus either amoxicillin-clavulanate 500 mg orally 2 times per day or clindamycin 600 mg orally 3 times per day.[3]
- Arrange for close follow-up.
- Reassess in 48 to 72 hours:
  › If the patient is afebrile for more than 48 hours, is clinically stable, and has an ANC $\geq$ 0.5 x 10^9/L for 2 consecutive days, take the following action: 1) consider stopping antibiotic therapy if there is no documented infection; 2) complete the antibiotic course tailored to sensitivities; or 3) hospitalize the patient if they continue to have a fever.[3]

INPATIENT TREATMENT

- Follow isolation precautions as clinically indicated: no pets, plants, or flowers nearby.
- Provide empiric antibiotics: piperacillin-tazobactam 4.5 g IV every 6 hours; imipenem plus cilastatin 500 mg IV every 6 hours; cefepime 2 g IV every 8 hours; meropenem 500 mg IV every 6 hours.[9]
- Consider adding empiric vancomycin in the context of MRSA risk factors, skin and soft tissue infection, line infection, pneumonia, mucositis, or hemodynamic instability.[9]
- Step down the antibiotics and complete the course as dictated by clinical status, source of infection, and culture sensitivities.[9]
- If no source of infection is found and the patient is clinically stable, continue empiric antibiotics until the patient is afebrile for at least 48 hours and ANC is > 0.5 x 10^9/L for 2 consecutive days.[9]
- If no source of infection is found and the patient is clinically unstable or has ongoing fevers after 4 to 7 days of antibiotics, consider broadening antibiotic coverage to include resistant organisms and fungal infections, and consult an infectious diseases specialist.[9]
- Consider removing central venous catheters in the context of tunnel infection; port pocket infection; and catheter-related bloodstream infection with *Staphylococcus aureus*, *Pseudomonas*, nontuberculous mycobacteria, or fungi.[5]
- Avoid aminoglycosides in patients on platinum chemotherapy due to increased risk of nephrotoxicity.
- G-CSF has no strong evidence for use in established FN.[10]

› Consider it in these contexts: expected prolonged neutropenia (more than 10 days) or profound neutropenia (ANC < 0.1 x 10^9/L); patients older than 65; pneumonia or other identified infections; sepsis; invasive fungal infection; history of FN; and fever that has developed in hospital.[11]

- The criteria for discharge include: afebrile for at least 48 hours, clinically stable, and ANC spontaneously recovered to > 0.5 x 10^9/L (or with G-CSF to > 1.0 x 10^9/L) for 2 consecutive days.[3]
- Consider DVT prophylaxis.

Immune-Related Adverse Event

These notes are in addition to the **general guide for all consultations** on page 1, and the **starting points for medical oncology consultations** at the beginning of this chapter.

Identification

Key information in the identification statement includes the type of cancer and current systemic therapy.

Reason for Referral

The referral may seek to confirm an immune-related adverse event and/or clarify appropriate management.

History of Present Illness

Identify the patient's cancer and systemic treatment, including checkpoint inhibitor immunotherapy:
 › Checkpoint inhibitor immunotherapy is often pursued in the setting of advanced melanoma, lung cancer, urothelial cancer, kidney cancer, and Hodgkin lymphoma.[12]
 › Clarify the dose and duration of the checkpoint inhibitor immunotherapy.
 › Ask about concurrent chemotherapy or targeted therapy.
 › Ask about the date of last treatment.

Clarify symptoms: Ask about:
 › onset and duration, whether the adverse event is infusion related, and whether there are any premedications
 › fatigue (exclude thyroid disease, adrenal insufficiency)
 › dermatologic rash, mucosal involvement
 › diarrhea or colitis (median time to onset is 6 to 8 weeks after initiation of therapy[13])

› pneumonitis with cough and/or dyspnea
› type 1 diabetes and features of diabetic ketoacidosis
› current ECOG[1] performance status

Clarify the severity of the adverse effects: Use the Common Terminology Criteria for Adverse Events from the US National Cancer Institute[14]:
› **Grade 1:** asymptomatic or mild
› **Grade 2:** moderate, limiting age-appropriate IADL
› **Grade 3:** disabling, limiting self-care ADL; severe or medically significant but not immediately life-threatening
› **Grade 4:** life-threatening consequences
› **Grade 5:** death related to adverse event

Past Medical History

Ask about:
- the patient's primary cancer, including:
  › date of diagnosis, pathology, and staging
  › treatment history (surgery, radiation, systemic therapy) and their side effects or complications
  › primary oncologist involved in the patient's care
- preexisting autoimmune disease
- other medical history

Past Surgical History

Follow the **general guide for all consultations** and the **starting points for medical oncology consultations.**

Medications

Follow the **general guide for all consultations** and the **starting points for medical oncology consultations.**

Allergies

Follow the **general guide for all consultations.**

Family History

Ask about malignancy (clarify in what family member, type of cancer, and age at diagnosis, if known) and autoimmune disorders.

Social History

Follow the **general guide for all consultations** and the **starting points for medical oncology consultations.**

Physical Examination

Vital signs: temperature for fever; BP and heart rate for hypovolemia; oxygen saturation and respiratory rate for hypoxemia

General impression
Presenting symptoms:
› Perform a focused exam based on the presenting symptoms.
Dermatologic: rash, mucous membranes
› Determine BSA involved.
› Check for blistering and other features of Stevens-Johnson syndrome.
Respiratory: decreased air entry, crackles
Abdominal: tenderness, organomegaly
Thyroid: goitre

Investigations

LABORATORY INVESTIGATIONS
CBC with differential: Eosinophilia may be a biomarker of immunotherapy toxicity.[15]
Metabolic panel
Hepatotoxicity: Order AST, ALT and other liver enzymes; bilirubin; INR, PTT; viral hepatitis serology; and serum drug levels.
Thyrotropin (TSH) and other pituitary hormones: Assess for thyroid and pituitary disease.
Random serum glucose, HbA$_{1c}$
Urine ketones: Pursue this on suspicion of diabetic ketoacidosis.
ESR/CRP: This assesses for clinical severity.

IMAGING
Chest x-ray: Pursue this to rule out pulmonary infection in patients with respiratory symptoms.
CT of the chest and/or abdomen: Assess for other pathology and metastasis.

MICROBIOLOGY
Blood cultures: Assess for systemic infection.
Others, as indicated: Examples include stool cultures, *Clostridium difficile* assay, and CMV DNA load.

Impression and Plan
Rule out other causes of presenting symptoms and rule out metastasis.
Note that immune-related adverse events are:
› more common with an anti-CTLA-4 antibody (ipilimumab) than with anti-PD-1 agents (nivolumab or pembrolizumab) or anti-PD-L1 agents (atezolizumab, durvalumab, avelumab)[16]
› most common with combined nivolumab and ipilimumab[17]
Consider premedication for infusion-related symptoms: Examples include acetaminophen or antihistamines.

Grade the severity of the observed toxicity to clarify management:
› Consider hospitalization in extreme dehydration, or in toxicity that is severe grade 2 or grade 3 and higher.[18,19]
› **Grade 1:** Monitor closely.
› **Grade 2:** Consider withholding the checkpoint inhibitor; initiate corticosteroid immunosuppression if symptoms do not resolve within a week (e.g., prednisone 0.5 mg/kg/day or its equivalent); consider resuming the checkpoint inhibitor only if toxicity is grade 1 or lower and after a risk-benefit discussion including tumour response to immunotherapy.[18,19]
› **Grade 3 or 4:** Permanently discontinue the checkpoint inhibitor, prescribe high-dose corticosteroid immunosuppression (e.g., prednisone 1–2 mg/kg/day or its equivalent) and taper when symptoms subside to grade 1 or lower.[19]

Consider prophylaxis for opportunistic infections: Prolonged immunosuppression may require this.

Consider referral for dermatological or mucosal events: Refer the patient to a dermatologist (for possible biopsy) when dermatologic or mucosal events do not promptly resolve with corticosteroid creams.

Consider referral for colitis: Refer the patient to a gastroenterologist for colitis that does not resolve after 5 days, or that recurs,[20,21] for possible treatment with infliximab.

Order routine blood work before each immunotherapy administration.

Consider alternative treatment options.

Malignant Spinal Cord Compression

These notes are in addition to the **general guide for all consultations** on page 1, and the **starting points for medical oncology consultations** at the beginning of this chapter.

Identification

Key information in the identification statement includes the type of cancer (including metastases, if known), current systemic therapy, and chief complaint (e.g., back pain).

Reason for Referral

The referral may seek to confirm malignant spinal cord compression and/or clarify appropriate management.

History of Present Illness

Clarify the patient's cancer history: Establish the type, stage of cancer, location of known metastases, current treatment, and ECOG performance status.

Clarify the presenting complaints: Establish the timeline and the character of each symptom compared to baseline function:

› **Back and neck pain:** Ask about new versus worsening pain; location along the spine; severity; band-like features; referred versus radicular pain; pain that is worse with movement, coughing, sneezing, lying down, and/or at night; pain that radiates down the arms or legs; and Lhermitte sign (sudden "electric shock" sensation down the back or extremities triggered by forward neck flexion).[22,23]

› **Weakness:** Identify muscle group affected (hips, arms), and associated gait ataxia.[22]

› **Sensory loss:** Ask about the location of the loss, ascending numbness, and saddle anesthesia (loss of feeling around the buttocks, anus, and genitals).[22,24]

› **Bowel and urinary retention or incontinence**[22]

Assess for cauda equina red flags: See sidebar.

Ask about a recent history of falls or fractures.

Ask about constitutional symptoms if the patient has no previous cancer history.

Determine ECOG performance status.

||||||||||||||||||||||||||||||||||||||||||||||||||||||||||||||||||||||||||||||||||||||||||||||||||||||||||||||||||||||||||||||||||||||||||||||||||||||||||||||||||||||||||||

RED FLAGS FOR CAUDA EQUINA[22,25]

Apply the SPINE mnemonic:

• **S**addle anesthesia
• **P**ain down 1 or both legs
• **I**ncontinence of bowel and/or bladder
• **N**umbness in legs
• **E**mergency

Past Medical History

Ask about:

• cancer-related history, including:
  › type of cancer (determine date of diagnosis, stage, and location of metastases, if known)
  › treatment history to date (determine all surgeries, radiation therapy, and all systemic therapies in chronological order; clarify side effects or complications)

› names of primary oncologist and radiation oncologist
› plan for future treatments, if known
- conditions that affect spine (e.g., spinal stenosis, degenerative spine disease, disc herniation, vertebral compression fracture)
- other medical conditions

Past Surgical History

Ask about:
- previous spinal surgeries
- presence of spinal orthopedic hardware
- all other procedures

Medications

Ask about:
- current and recent medications
- recent chemotherapy, steroids, bisphosphonates
- anticoagulants (this is important if surgery is required)

Allergies

In addition to medication allergies, ask about medication intolerances (medications that were tried but discontinued due to adverse effects), especially intolerances for steroids and bisphosphonates.

Family History

Ask about malignancy (clarify in what family member, type of cancer, and age at diagnosis, if known).

Social and Functional History

Ask about:
- alcohol use, recreational drug use, smoking
- occupation
- ADLs and IADLs (clarify baseline level of independence)
- family supports

Code Status

Clarify the patient's code status and goals of care.

Physical Examination

Vital signs: Pay attention to hypertension and tachycardia (these may be symptoms of autonomic dysfunction with progression of epidural spinal cord compression).[22,25,26]

Spine:
› Inspect for normal spine alignment during standing, walking, bending and lifting (inability to retain normal spine alignment may

be a sign of spinal instability from bony destruction or pathologic compression fractures).[23]

› Palpate and percuss the intervertebral spaces, spinal processes, and paraspinal muscles along the whole spine for localized bony tenderness.[23]

› Perform a straight leg test for sciatic pain.

Neurovital signs: Determine GCS score, and assess pupillary response, painful stimuli, and muscle strength.

Peripheral neurological signs:

› **Motor deficits:**

» Assess the tone and strength of every muscle group.

» Compression at or above the conus medullaris can cause symmetric weakness of hip and knee flexion, and ankle dorsiflexion.

» Compression above the thoracic spine can also cause symmetric weakness of upper extremity extensors (triceps, wrist).

» Cauda equina can produce more asymmetric weakness.

» Perform a DRE for rectal tone if the patient is not neutropenic.

› **Reflexes:** Examine for hyperreflexia below the level of compression and for extensor plantar response.

› **Sensory deficits:**

» These are less common than motor deficits.

» They typically occur within 1 to 5 levels below the compression level.

» Do not forget to perform a pinprick test in sacral dermatomes.

› **Gait:** New ataxia in a cancer patient should raise suspicion of spinal cord compression.

Investigations

LABORATORY INVESTIGATIONS

CBC with differential

Electrolytes, creatinine, urea, glucose, extended electrolytes, including Ca

INR, PTT

IMAGING

Plain radiographs of the spine have a very limited role in the diagnosis of malignant epidural spinal cord compression: they can show vertebral collapse but are not sensitive in detecting spinal cord compression.[24,27]

MRI of the entire spine with and without contrast:

› This is a preferred modality and should be performed within 24 hours of symptom onset.

› Assess for level of involvement (usually above the L1 level), associated vasogenic edema, grade of epidural tumour, and percent of spinal cord infarction and/or compression of lumbosacral roots.[24,25,27]

CT myelography of the spine:
> This can be used if MRI is contraindicated or not readily available.
> It may be also useful in treatment planning for radiation therapy.[24,27]

Impression and Plan

GENERAL APPROACH

Provide a definitive or provisional diagnosis:
> Base this on clinical and radiographic findings.
> Describe the spinal levels where the compression is located or suspected.

Describe key features: These include the degree of tumour bulk, spinal stability, and degree of motor impairment.

Provide rapid treatment: Malignant spinal cord compression is an oncologic emergency that requires rapid treatment for preservation of neurologic function.[25,27]

Consider the patient's life expectancy: All treatments of malignant spinal cord compression are partly palliative, and aimed to reduce pain and preserve ambulation.[28,29]

PLAN

Involve a spine surgeon for an opinion: If indicated, decompressive surgery should be performed preferably within 48 hours of symptom onset.[28-31]

Order strict bed rest on suspicion of spinal cord instability.

Administer corticosteroids:
> Do this as soon as the diagnosis is confirmed or strongly suspected to reduce spinal cord edema and back pain.[28]
> Prescribe dexamethasone 10–16 mg IV bolus, followed by 4–6 mg IV or oral every 4 hours.
> Communicate the taper plan with the primary oncologist, radiation oncologist, and spine surgeon.

Consult a radiation oncologist:
> Palliative radiation therapy is standard treatment after decompressive surgery.
> If the patient is not a candidate for surgery, radiotherapy alone is the recommended treatment.[29-31]

Consult a medical oncologist for new cancer diagnoses or notify the primary oncologist: Patients with no history or a remote history of cancer must undergo staging with CT of the chest, abdomen, and pelvis, and a bone scan followed by a diagnostic biopsy if a new likely primary tumour is identified (the biopsy may be obtained from the spinal tumour or the most readily accessible site[27]).

Consider treating the underlying cause: Patients may require, for example, resection of the primary cancer, or chemotherapy or radiotherapy.[29–31]

Discuss code status and goals of care:
> This requires careful estimation of the patient's life expectancy, the likelihood they will be ambulatory after treatment, and their overall cancer prognosis. What treatments are in line with their goals of care?
> Involve palliative care, if appropriate.

Tumour Lysis Syndrome

These notes are in addition to the **general guide for all consultations** on page 1, and the **starting points for medical oncology consultations** at the beginning of this chapter.

Identification

Key information in the identification statement includes the type of cancer, metastatic burden, current systemic therapy (and when started), whether the patient has underlying renal disease, and the presenting clinical signs of tumour lysis syndrome (TLS).

Reason for Referral

The referral may seek to confirm TLS and/or clarify appropriate management.

History of Present Illness

Clarify the patient's cancer history: Ask about:
> **Specialists:** names of the primary medical oncologist and radiation oncologist
> **Date of diagnosis**
> **Cancer characteristics:** type and stage, location of known metastases, bone marrow involvement
> **Treatment history to date in chronological order:** surgeries, bone marrow transplant, radiation therapy, systemic therapies (ask about side effects and complications, and plans for future stem cell transplantation)
> **Current treatment:** when initiated; how many days ago TLS began (TLS usually occurs within 3 days before or 7 days after chemotherapy, most often 2 to 3 days after treatment starts[32–34]); intensity of therapy, if known

› ECOG performance status
Characterize symptoms: Establish a timeline for each symptom and ask about:
  › **Variable symptoms:** nausea and vomiting, diarrhea, confusion, lethargy, muscle cramps, perioral paresthesias, decreased urine output, symptoms of fluid overload or CHF (shortness of breath, ankle swelling, syncope), flank or back pain, seizures
  › **Course in hospital to date (for inpatients):**
    » Focus on acute kidney injury (AKI), new hypertension, oliguria, electrolyte abnormalities, and delirium.
Determine TLS risk factors: Ask about acute lymphoproliferative disorders, high tumour sensitivity to chemotherapy, renal disease, and dehydration.[34,35]

Past Medical History

Ask about:
- **Preexisting renal disease:**
  › Clarify baseline creatinine (eGFR).
  › In CKD, identify the cause, especially from tumour infiltration in the kidney.
  › Ask about preexisting nephropathy from hypertension, diabetes, or gout (these patients are more predisposed to AKI from TLS[36,37]).
- **Preexisting obstructive uropathy:** Ask about BPH, ureteric stones, cancer spreads.
- **Other medical conditions:** Ask specifically about glucose-6-phosphate dehydrogenase (G6PD) deficiency. This is important to know if rasburicase treatment is being considered.[38]

Past Surgical History

- Determine all past procedures with dates.
- Ask about tumour resection, if applicable.
- Ask about renal transplantation or recent urologic procedures, if applicable.

Medications

Ask about:
- current and recent medications
- recent chemotherapy, steroids, bisphosphonates
- nephrotoxic medications (NSAIDs, ACEIs, antibiotics, diuretics)

Allergies

In addition to medication allergies, ask about medication intolerances (medications that were tried but discontinued due to adverse effects), especially intolerances for rasburicase and allopurinol.

Family History

Ask about malignancy (clarify in what family member, type of cancer, and age at diagnosis, if known).

Social and Functional History

Ask about:

- alcohol use, recreational drug use, smoking
- occupation
- ADLs and IADLs (clarify baseline level of independence)
- family supports

Code Status

Clarify the patient's code status and goals of care.

Physical Examination

Vital signs: dysrhythmia, especially bradycardia (due to hyperkalemia or hypocalcemia); hypotension (this is a risk factor for decreased urine flow and formation of crystals)

Signs of dehydration: dry mucous membranes and dry axilla, decreased skin turgor, low JVP

Cardiorespiratory: signs of HF (probably caused by hypocalcemia)

Abdominal: organomegaly (hepatomegaly, splenomegaly, or nephromegaly may indicate tumour infiltration into these organs, and increased tumour burden and risk of TLS)

Signs of hypocalcemia: Trousseau sign, Chvostek sign, tetany, muscle twitching

Investigations

LABORATORY INVESTIGATIONS

CBC with differential

Electrolytes and extended electrolytes:
> Look for low Ca, and high K, PO_4 and Mg.
> Calculate the anion gap.

Creatinine, urea

Uric acid: This causes crystal nephropathy.

LDH: This is a surrogate for tumour proliferation: the higher the level, the greater the TLS risk.

OTHER INVESTIGATIONS

Urinalysis and urine microscopy: Assess for uric acid or calcium phosphate crystals.

ECG: Look for ECG changes associated with severe electrolyte abnormalities:

> **Hyperkalemia:** peaked T waves, shortened QT, prolonged PR, wide QRS, a "sine wave"
> **Hypocalcemia:** prolonged QT without U waves

IMAGING

Renal US: Consider this to rule out postrenal AKI.

Impression and Plan

Discuss the diagnosis of TLS: The diagnosis is based on the following laboratory criteria (2 or more within 3 days[33,36,39,40]):
> serum uric acid > 475 mmol/L or 25% from baseline
> serum potassium > 6 mmol/L or 25% from baseline
> serum phosphate > 1.45 mmol/L or 25% from baseline
> serum calcium < 1.75 mmol/L or 25% from baseline

List all relevant complications of TLS[36,41]: These could include AKI, arrhythmia, and seizure.

Treat AKI and crystal nephropathy:
> Provide fluid resuscitation: initial boluses of normal saline followed by infusion of normal saline at 150–250 mL/hour.
> Consider concurrent furosemide diuresis to maintain urine output and to prevent fluid overload.
>> Do not use this in patients with hypovolemia or acute obstructive uropathy.[36]
> Insert a Foley catheter and monitor urine output; maintain output at > 100 cc/hour.
> Initiate allopurinol 300 mg orally 3 times per day for hyperuricemia (this reduces formation of uric acid); this treatment can be considered in patients at high risk of TLS even in the absence of hyperuricemia.[42,43]
> Consider rasburicase 0.05– 0.2 mg/kg IV once daily for 1 to 7 days (this degrades uric acid).
>> Consider this as a prophylactic therapy in patients at high risk of TLS.
>> Do not use in patients with a known G6PD deficiency, as it may precipitate hemolysis.[38,42,43]
> Evaluate for indications for dialysis in cases refractory to medical treatment: acidosis, electrolyte imbalance (hyperkalemia, hyperphosphatemia, hypocalcemia, hyperuricemia), overload (fluid), uremia (uremic pericarditis, encephalopathy, urea > 35–50 mM).
>> If dialysis is indicated, involve renal specialists and consider transferring the patient to ICU.
> Avoid nephrotoxic medications and review current medications for renal dose-adjustment.

Correct metabolic abnormalities:
> Treat hyperkalemia: start cardiac monitoring and calcium gluconate on findings of ECG changes; shift with 10 units of insulin regular

and 50% dextrose if symptomatic; treat with sodium polystyrene sulfonate if mild and asymptomatic.

› Treat hyperphosphatemia: remove phosphate from IV fluids and consider phosphate binders such as aluminium hydroxide for up to 2 days.

› In symptomatic hypocalcemia, consider IV calcium gluconate but monitor for acute obstructive uropathy.

› Monitor trends in electrolytes, calcium, phosphate, creatinine, uric acid, and LDH every 6 hours.

Notify the primary oncologist.

Discuss code status and goals of care:

› This requires careful estimation of the patient's life expectancy, the likelihood they will be ambulatory after treatment, and their overall cancer prognosis. What treatments are in line with their goals of care?

› Involve palliative care, if appropriate.

Consider TLS prophylaxis with IV fluids and allopurinol or rasburicase: This should be considered in all patients at high risk of clinical TLS, as in the context of a bulky tumour, high sensitivity of the tumour to chemotherapy (e.g., Burkitt lymphoma), and/or preexisting nephropathy.[34,35,38]

References

1. Oken M, Creech R, Tormey D, et al. Toxicity and response criteria of the Eastern Cooperative Oncology Group. Am J Clin Oncol. 1982;5(6):649-56. doi: 10.1097/00000421-198212000-00014

2. Moore D. Drug-induced neutropenia: a focus on rituximab-induced late-onset neutropenia. P T. 2016;41(12):765. PMID: 27990078

3. Taplitz R, Kennedy E, Bow E, et al. Outpatient management of fever and neutropenia in adults treated for malignancy: American Society of Clinical Oncology and Infectious Diseases Society of America clinical practice guideline update. J Clin Oncol. 2018;36(14):1443-53. doi: 10.1200/JCO.2017.77.6211

4. Freifeld A, Bow E, Sepkowitz K, et al. Clinical practice guideline for the use of antimicrobial agents in neutropenic patients with cancer: 2010 update by the Infectious Diseases Society of America. Clinical Infectious Diseases. 2011;52(4):e56-93. doi: 10.1093/cid/cir073

5. Klastersky J, De Naurois J, Rolston K, et al. Management of febrile neutropenia: ESMO clinical practice guidelines. Annals of Oncology. 2016;27(suppl_5):v111-18. doi: 10.1093/annonc/mdw325

6. Klastersky J, Paesmans M, Rubenstein E, et al. The Multinational Association for Supportive Care in Cancer risk index: a multinational scoring system for identifying low-risk febrile neutropenic cancer patients. J Clin Oncol. 2000;18(16):3038-51. doi: 10.1200/JCO.18.16.3038

7. Carmona-Bayonas A, Jiménez-Fonseca P, Virizuela Echaburu J, et al. Prediction of serious complications in patients with seemingly stable febrile neutropenia: validation of the Clinical Index of Stable Febrile Neutropenia in a prospective cohort of patients from the FINITE study. J Clin Oncol. 2015;33(5):465-71. doi: 10.1200/JCO.2014.57.2347

8. Rosa R, Goldani L. Cohort study of the impact of time to antibiotic administration on mortality in patients with febrile neutropenia. Antimicrob Agents Chemother. 2014;58(7):3799-803. doi: 10.1128/AAC.02561.14

9. Zimmer A, Freifeld A. Optimal management of neutropenic fever in patients with cancer. J Oncol Pract. 2019;15(1):19-24. doi: 10.1200/JOP.18.00269

10. Mhaskar R, Clark O, Lyman G, et al. Colony-stimulating factors for chemotherapy-induced febrile neutropenia. Cochrane Database Syst Rev. 2014;(10):CD003039. doi: 10.1012/14651858. CD003039.pub2

11. Smith T, Bohlke K, Lyman G, et al. Recommendations for the use of WBC growth factors: American Society of Clinical Oncology clinical practice guideline update. J Clin Oncol. 2015;33(28):3199-212. doi: 10.1200/JCO.2015.62.3488

12. Sharma P, Allison J. Immune checkpoint targeting in cancer therapy: toward combination strategies with curative potential. Cell. 2015;161(2):205-14. doi: 10.1016/j.cell.2015.03.030

13. Friedman C, Proverbs-Singh T, Postow M. Treatment of the immune-related adverse effects of immune checkpoint inhibitors; a review. JAMA Oncol. 2016;2(10):1346-53. doi: 10.1001/jamaoncol.2016.1051

14. US Department of Health and Human Services, National Institutes of Health, National Cancer Institute. Common terminology criteria for adverse events (CTCAE) [Internet]. Washington: US Department of Health and Human Services; 2017 November 27. Available from: https://ctep.cancer.gov/protocoldevelopment/ electronic_applications/docs/CTCAE_v5_Quick_Reference_8.5x11.pdf

15. Nakamura Y, Tanaka R, Maruyama H, et al. Correlation between blood cell count and outcome of melanoma patients treated with anti-PD-1 antibodies. Jpn J Clin Oncol. 2019;49(5):431-7. doi: 10.1093/jjco/hyy201

16. Horvat T, Adel N, Dang T, et al. Immune-related adverse events, need for systemic immunosuppression, and effects on survival and time to treatment failure in patients with melanoma treated with ipilimumab at Memorial Sloan Kettering Cancer Center. J Clinic Oncol. 2015;33(28):3193-98. doi: 10.1200/JCO.2015.60.8448

17. Haanen J, Carbonnel F, Robert C, et al. Management of toxicities from immunotherapy: ESMO Clinical Practice Guidelines for diagnosis, treatment and follow-up. Ann Oncol. 2018;28(suppl 4):iv119-42. doi: 10.1093/annonc/mdx225

18. Brahmer J, Lacchetti C, Schneider B, et al. Management of immune-related adverse events in patients treated with immune checkpoint inhibitor therapy: American Society of Clinical Oncology Clinical practice guideline. J Clin Oncol. 2018;36(17):1714-68. doi: 10.1200/JCO.2017.77.6385

19. Puzanov I, Diab A, Abdallah K, et al. Managing toxicities associated with immune checkpoint inhibitors: consensus recommendations from the Society for Immunotherapy of Cancer (SITC) Toxicity Management Working Group. J Immunother Cancer. 2017;5(1):95. doi:

20. Pagès C, Gornet J, Monsel G, et al. Ipilimumab-induced acute severe colitis treated by infliximab. Melanoma Res 2013; 23:227. doi: 10.1186/s40425-017-0300-z

21. Minor D, Chin K, Kashani-Sabet M. Infliximab in the treatment of anti-CTLA4 antibody (ipilimumab) induced immune-related colitis. Cancer Biother Radiopharm. 2009;24(3):321-5. doi: 10.1089/cbr.2008.0607

22. Helweg-Larsen S, Sorensen P. Symptoms and signs in metastatic spinal cord compression: a study of progression from first symptom until diagnosis in 153 patients. Eur J Cancer. 1994; 30A(3):396-8. doi: 10.1016/0959-8049(94)90263-1

23. Lawrie I. Back pain in malignant disease - metastatic spinal cord compression? Rev Pain. 2010; 4(2):14-17. doi: 10.1177/204946371000400204

24. Perrin R, Laxton A. Metastatic spine disease: epidemiology, pathophysiology, and evaluation of patients. Neurosurg Clin N Am. 2004; 15(4):365-73. doi: 10.1016/j. ned.2004.04.018

25. Macdonald A, Lynch D, Garbett I, et al. Malignant spinal cord compression. J R Coll Physicians Edinb. 2019;49(2):151-6. doi: 10.4997/JRCPE.2019.217

26. Cole J, Patchell R. Metastatic epidural spinal cord compression. Lancet Neurol. 2008;7(5):459-66. doi: 10.1016/S1474-4422(08)70089-9

27. Boussios S, Cooke D, Hayward C, et al. Metastatic spinal cord compression: unraveling the diagnostic and therapeutic challenges. Anticancer Res. 2018;38(9):4987-97. doi: 10.21873/anticanres.12817

28. Kumar A, Weber M, Gokaslan Z, et al. Metastatic spinal cord compression and steroid treatment: a systematic review. Clin Spine Surg. 2017;30(4):156-63. doi: 10.1097/BSD.0000000000000528

29. Laufer I, Rubin D, Lis E, et al. The NOMS framework: approach to the treatment of spinal metastatic tumors. Oncologist. 2013;18(6):744-51. doi: 10.1634/theoncologist.2012-0293

30. Abrahm J. Assessment and treatment of patients with malignant spinal cord compression. J Support Oncol. 2004;2(5):377-88. PMID: 15524067

31. Ribas E, Schiff D. Spinal cord compression. Curr Treat Options Neurol. 2012;14(4):391-401. doi: 10.1007/s11940-012-0176-7

32. Gupta A, Moore J. Tumor lysis syndrome. JAMA Oncol. 2018;4(6):895. doi: 10.1001/jamaoncol.2018.0613

33. Findakly D, Luther R, Wang J. Tumor lysis syndrome in solid tumors: a comprehensive literature review, new insights, and novel strategies to improve outcomes. Cureus. 2020;12(5):e8355. PMID: 32494548

34. Cairo M, Coiffier B, Reiter A, et al; TLS Expert Panel. Recommendations for the evaluation of risk and prophylaxis of tumor lysis syndrome (TLS) in adults and children with malignant disease: an expert TLS panel consensus. Br J Haematol. 2010;149(4):578-86. doi: 10.1111/j.1365-2141.2010.08143.x

35. Belay Y, Yirdaw K, Enawgaw B. Tumor lysis syndrome in patients with hematological malignancies. J Oncol. 2017;2017:9684909. doi: 10.1155/2017/9684909

36. Perry Wilson F, Berns J. Onco-nephrology: tumor lysis syndrome. Clin j Am Soc Nephrol. 2012;7(10):1730-9. doi: 10.2215/CJN.03150312

37. Mirrakhimov A, Prakruthi V, Khan M, et al. Tumor lysis syndrome: a clinical review. World J Crit Care Med. 2015; May;4(2):130-8. doi: 10.5492/wjccm.v4.i2.130

38. Bessmertny O, Robitaille L, Cairo M. Rasburicase: a new approach for preventing and/or treating tumor lysis syndrome. Curr Pharm Des. 2005;11(32):4177-85. doi: 10.2174/1381612057749413291

39. Mughal T, Ejaz A, Foringer J, et al. An integrated clinical approach for the identification, prevention, and treatment of tumor lysis syndrome. Cancer Treat Rev. 2010;36(2):164-76. doi: 10.1016/j.ctrv.2009.11.001

40. Mirrakhimov A, Ali A, Khan M, et al. Tumor lysis syndrome in solid tumors: an up to date review of the literature. Rare Tumors. 2014;6(2):5389. doi: 10.4081/rt.2014.5389

41. Thandra K, Salah Z, Chawla S. Oncologic emergencies-the old, the new, and the deadly. J Intensive Care Med. 2020;35(1):3-13. doi: 10.1177/0885066618803863

42. Alakel N, Middeke JM, Schetelig J, et al. Prevention and treatment of tumor lysis syndrome, and the efficacy and role of rasburicase. Onco Targets Ther. 2017;10:597-605. doi: 10.2147/OTT.S103864

43. Coiffier B, Altman A, Pui CH, et al. Guidelines for the management of pediatric and adult tumor lysis syndrome: an evidence-based review. J Clin Oncol. 2008;26(16):2767-78. doi: 10.1200/JCO.2007.15.0177

12

Nephrology

Dr. Jordan Friedmann
Dr. Julia Zazoulina
Dr. Teresa Tai
Dr. Alastair K. Williams
Dr. Sabina Freiman
Dr. Wayne Hung

REVIEWER
Dr. Nadia Zalunardo

Starting Points: Nephrology Consultations

These notes are in addition to the **general guide for all consultations** on page 1.

Identification

Key information in the identification statement includes baseline creatinine (GFR) and relevant comorbidities.

Reason for Referral

The referral may seek to confirm kidney disease and/or clarify appropriate management.

History of Present Illness[1-3]

Focus this history on assessing for a potential cause of the issue and the presence of its consequences.

Clarify the patient's renal history:
> Determine the patient's baseline kidney function, latest creatinine result (including the date), and the trend in creatinine, if applicable.
> In known CKD, clarify the cause (and whether it is presumed or proven on biopsy), and determine the most recent GFR and the degree of albuminuria.

› Clarify the patient's dialysis history (hemodialysis versus peritoneal dialysis; access site; schedule; target weight).

Assess for temporal relationships with precipitants: For example, in acute kidney injury (AKI), apply the prerenal-renal-postrenal approach.

Assess for uremic symptoms: Ask about altered mental status, seizures, nausea, vomiting, chest pain, pruritus, altered taste, and anorexia.

Assess for volume overload: Ask about shortness of breath on exertion, orthopnea, paroxysmal nocturnal dyspnea, and swelling of the extremities.

Assess for urinary abnormalities: Ask about colour, frothiness, amount, obstructive symptoms, and UTI symptoms.

Determine trends in urine output and weights.

Ask about therapies trialed and response so far.

Past Medical History[3,4]
Ask about:
- urologic history (previous ureteric stones, infections)
- consideration or workup for renal transplantation
- hypertension (including average BP, if known)
- diabetes mellitus and associated complications
- autoimmune disorders
- cardiac history (including EF, if available)

Past Surgical History
Ask about:
- urologic surgeries and procedures
- renal transplantation (including the date of surgery, and whether the donor was alive or deceased)

Medications[3,4]
- Ask about recent use of relevant medications (e.g., NSAIDs, IV contrast, antibiotics, loop and thiazide diuretics, lithium).
- Ask about herbal supplements.
- Assess for medications that require dosing adjustment for renal impairment (antibiotics, DVT prophylaxis).
- In known CKD, check for erythropoietin and phosphate binders.

Allergies
Follow the **general guide for all consultations.**

Family History
Ask about:
- renal disease
- malignancy
- autoimmune disorders

Social History
Ask about:
- alcohol use, recreational drug use, smoking
- occupation
- ability to perform ADLs and IADLs
- current supports (e.g., family, personal support workers)
- factors limiting the patient's ability to adhere to, or pay for, medications

Code Status
Clarify the patient's code status and goals of care.

Physical Examination
Weight: Compare the patient's current weight to previous recorded weights; identify trends.

Volume status:
> Check for dry mucous membranes; assess JVP level and BP; and assess for bibasilar lung crackles (on auscultation) and peripheral edema.
> Consider a point-of-care US.[1]

Signs of uremia: Signs of uremia may indicate a need to start dialysis; assess for decreased level of consciousness, asterixis, and pericardial rub.[1]

Cardiorespiratory: Conduct a general exam.

Abdominal: Conduct a general exam.

Urine output: Review available documentation about the patient's 24-hour urine output.

Investigations
LABORATORY INVESTIGATIONS
Obtain results from relevant past workups.

Creatinine, urea:
> Pay attention to trends.
> In ESRD, expect elevated urea.

Electrolytes and extended electrolytes (Mg, PO_4, Ca): In ESRD, expect elevated K and PO_4, and decreased Ca and HCO_3.[1,4]

CBC:
> Assess for anemia related to CKD, the chronicity of anemia, and the presence of other hematologic derangements (e.g., thrombocytopenia, eosinophilia).
> In new or worsening anemia, consider iron studies, vitamin B_{12}, and serum or urine protein electrophoresis (SPEP, UPEP) to rule out other causes.[5]

Urine studies[3]**:** These include:
> urinalysis with or without culture and sensitivity
> microscopy
> electrolytes (if relevant)
> albumin-to-creatinine ratio
> 24-hour output

OTHER INVESTIGATIONS

ECG: This is especially important in patients with K or Ca abnormalities.

IMAGING

Renal ultrasound: Pursue this to rule out a postrenal cause for AKI and look for evidence of CKD (e.g., atrophic kidneys).[3]

Impression and Plan

Describe the patient's baseline condition (creatinine, weight) compared to the present.

Order monitoring: This includes:
> fluid intake and urine output
> weight (taken daily)

Consider specifying a diet: Appropriate diets could restrict sodium, potassium, and/or fluids.

Consider changes to medications: Suggest holding potentially nephrotoxic medications (e.g., ACEIs or ARBs, NSAIDs, diuretics, sodium-glucose cotransporter-2 inhibitors), and those that may need dosing adjustment for renal impairment (e.g., antibiotics, anticoagulation, metformin).

Discuss volume status: Indicate if volume repletion or diuresis is needed.

Discuss renal replacement therapy: Mention why the patient is or is not meeting indications for dialysis at present.
> Apply the mnemonic AEIOU to assess indications for dialysis (in inadequate response to medical therapy): **A**cidosis, **E**lectrolyte imbalance (potassium), **I**ntoxication, **O**verload (fluid), and **U**remia (encephalopathy, uremic pericarditis).[3]

Acute Kidney Injury and Hemodialysis Start

These notes are in addition to the **general guide for all consultations** on page 1, and the **starting points for nephrology consultations** at the beginning of this chapter.

Identification

Key information in the identification statement includes the patient's preexisting medical conditions that could affect renal function, such as vascular disease, BPH, known baseline CKD, diabetes, and conditions associated with glomerulonephritis (GN).

Reason for Referral

The referral may seek to identify the cause of AKI and/or clarify appropriate management, including the need for dialysis.

History of Present Illness

A goal of this history is to understand the chronology of issues leading to the present illness, especially if it involves a long or complex course.

Clarify the patient's renal history:
› Establish the patient's baseline creatinine (eGFR) and proteinuria measurements (including the date last checked and recent trends).
› Has CKD been proven on biopsy?
› Ask for the name of the patient's nephrologist and the date of their last appointment.

Clarify why the patient has sought care: For inpatients, clarify the course in hospital.

Clarify the patient's current clinical status:
› This is especially relevant in critical care settings.
› Clarify the patient's hemodynamic status, use of vasopressors, and fluid intake versus urine output.
› Is there access for hemodialysis?
› Determine the details of continuous renal replacement therapy (CRRT) if applicable, (indication, duration, volume off, when stopped).[6-9]

Identify causes and contributing factors: These include:
› **Past events:** serious AKI, stones, prior dialysis, pyelonephritis, recurrent UTIs
› **Recent events:** nephrotoxic exposures (medications, contrast agents) and how they correlate to creatinine changes; new cardiac or hepatic

dysfunction (these increase the risk of hepatorenal syndrome and cardiorenal syndrome)
> **Risk of prerenal insult:** known or suspected poor oral intake; increase in losses (diarrhea, vomiting, high volume urine output, bleeding); risk factors for renal hypoperfusion (surgery, hypotension, sepsis)
> **Risk of postrenal obstruction:** BPH, prostate cancer, intraabdominal malignancy[6-9]

Identify consequences: Determine:
> symptoms of volume overload (e.g., shortness of breath, oxygen requirements, edema) or volume depletion
> recent voiding history (hematuria, polyuria, oliguria, dysuria, change in urine colour, foamy urine, change in frequency)
> 24-hour urine output and weight trend, if available
> electrolyte disturbances, acid-base disturbances
> uremia (altered level of consciousness, features of pericarditis, nausea and vomiting, itchiness)
> treatments attempted (fluids, diuretics, monoamine oxidase)[5-8]

Past Medical History
Ask about renal-related history:
> What caused the patient's CKD? If it is biopsy proven, what was found on the biopsy and when?
> What plans for dialysis are in place (fistula creation, peritoneal dialysis catheter insertion)?
> What is the patient's history with acid-base disturbances, electrolyte derangements, and albumin-to-creatinine ratios?

Identify conditions that could affect renal health: These include:
> nephrolithiasis, BPH
> CAD, peripheral vascular disease, hypertension, diabetes, HF (check for transthoracic echocardiogram results)
> autoimmune disorders (e.g., SLE, vasculitis)
> liver disease (this increases the risk of hepatorenal syndrome)
> cardiac dysfunction (this increases the risk of cardiorenal syndrome)[6-9]

Past Surgical and Procedural History
Ask about:
• procedures affecting the renal system (lithotripsy for stones, cystoscopy, nephrectomy, stents inserted, transplant surgeries)
• surgery requiring cardiopulmonary bypass[8]

Medications
Ask about:
• current medications, with special attention to newly started, modified, or stopped medications

- immunosuppressive medications (e.g., for organ transplantation)
- herbal and OTC supplements

Allergies

- In addition to medication allergies, ask about medication intolerances (medications that were tried but discontinued due to adverse effects), which is especially relevant in immunosuppression for transplantation.
- Ask about past AKI due to medications.

Family History

Ask about kidney disease (including polycystic kidney disease), malignancies, and autoimmune disorders.[8]

Social and Functional History

Ask about:

- alcohol use, recreational drug use, smoking
- occupation
- baseline independence with ADLs and IADLs
- cognitive status (this affects dialysis modality options)
- geographic location (this affects access to hemodialysis)
- current supports (e.g., family, personal support workers)
- factors limiting the patient's ability to adhere to, or pay for, medications
- vaccinations

Code Status

Follow the **general guide for all consultations** and the **starting points for nephrology consultations**.

Physical Examination

Vital signs: Assess for hypotension, tachycardia, fever, oxygenation, and elevated respiration rate (this is a sign of pulmonary edema).

Volume status: Assess JVP, and assess for peripheral edema and lung crackles. Consider a point-of-care US.

Dialysis access: Assess fistulas (thrills, bruits, and skin integrity), and lines (signs of infection).

Cardiovascular: Assess for CAD, HF, edema, and irregular heart rate.

Abdominal: Assess for ascites, stigmata of chronic liver disease, and suprapubic tenderness.

Uremic signs: Assess for pericardial rub, signs of excoriation, asterixis, and mental status and orientation.

Dermatological, musculoskeletal: Assess for allergic or vasculitic rash; SLE rash; lower limb ischemia ("trash foot") in the context of recent catheterization; and painful and/or swollen joints.

Monitoring data: Check the patient's recent fluid intake versus urine output and daily weight measurements.[6-9]

Investigations

LABORATORY INVESTIGATIONS

Obtain results from relevant past workups.

CBC with differential, liver panel, INR, albumin, CK, lactate

Creatinine, urea: Assess current results against baseline, and determine trends and maximums.

Electrolytes: Assess for disturbances (e.g., acid-base disturbances, hyponatremia, hyperkalemia, hyperphosphatemia, calcium disorders).[6-9]

Urine studies: These include:
> dipstick (assess for proteinuria, hematuria, elevated WBCs)
> microscopy (use this to better quantify RBCs, including dysmorphic RBCs, and WBCs, and assess for the presence of casts)
> culture and sensitivity (for possible infection)
> tests for suspected prerenal state or hepatorenal syndrome (albumin-to-creatinine ratio, urine osmolality, urine electrolytes)[5-8]

OTHER INVESTIGATIONS

ECG: Assess for signs of electrolyte abnormalities, pericarditis, LVH, ischemia, and arrhythmia.[6,8]

IMAGING

Renal US: Assess for postrenal obstruction and kidney size.

CT-KUB: Pursue this on suspicion of stones.

Angiogram or CTA: Check for recent imaging because these pose a risk for contrast-induced nephropathy.[5-8]

||||||||||||||||||||||||||||||||||||||||||||||||||||||||||||||||||||||||||||||||||||||||||||||||||||||||||||||||

BRIEF NOTE ON UNDERSTANDING DIALYSIS ORDERS

Orders are usually written by a nephrology fellow or by staff.

Standard information: This includes:
- electrolyte bath concentrations (e.g., potassium at 2–3 mmol/L)
- ultrafiltration volume (this depends on how overloaded the patient is)

- dialyzer size (higher surface area delivers more efficiency)
- heparin contraindications (e.g., avoid heparin in patients with bleeding risk)
- access site (e.g., fistula, permanent catheter, temporary line)

Uremic patients:

- Uremia typically occurs in the context of CKD.
- Begin dialysis with short runs, and no or low ultrafiltration (this is intentionally "inefficient" to avoid complications such as dialysis disequilibrium syndrome and hypotension).[6,8,9]

Acute toxic ingestion: The goal is high-efficiency hemodialysis (e.g., longer duration, dialyzer with a higher surface area).

CRRT: CRRT can be used in critical care settings to provide "gentle" 24-hour-per-day dialysis (this is better tolerated in hemodynamically unstable patients); however, it is much less efficient than conventional HD, thus not first-line therapy for toxic ingestions.[6,8]

Impression and Plan

Begin your plan with a summary that includes the patient's baseline creatinine (eGFR) and your impression of the cause of AKI based on pertinent positive and negatives.

AKI MANAGEMENT[6-8,10]

Prerenal AKI:

> **True volume depletion:** Hold diuretics and give IV fluids.
> **Cardiorenal syndrome suspected:** Provide diuresis.
>> If the gut is edematous, oral furosemide may be poorly absorbed: use IV furosemide.
>> Patients with low GFR require a higher dose of furosemide.

Renal AKI: Consider acute tubular necrosis, contrast-induced nephropathy, GN, vascular causes, and acute interstitial nephritis.

Postrenal AKI: Order tests for BPH, malignancy, and stones; and a renal US with or without a Foley catheter.

Additional considerations in transplantation patients: These include surgical complications, acute or chronic rejection, and failing grafts.

Additional investigations and orders: These include:

> fluid intake and urine output monitoring
> Foley catheter insertion (only if needed)
> daily weight measurement

› urine studies as indicated (urinalysis and microscopy; albumin-to-creatinine ratio; culture and sensitivity; urine osmolality; and electrolytes)

Medication review: Consider renal dosing adjustments and hold nephrotoxic medications.

Code status: If the patient may require dialysis, does dialysis align with their goals of care?

AEIOU MANAGEMENT[6-8,10]

Acidosis: Treat the cause (bicarbonate is the treatment in some cases).

Electrolyte derangements:
› Shift potassium (dextrose, insulin, salbutamol) or eliminate potassium (furosemide or polystyrene sulfonate, when appropriate).
› Monitor the patient with ECG and provide calcium for membrane stabilization.
› Cardiac monitoring is recommended in severe hyperkalemia.

Ingestion: Monitor substance levels, provide supportive care, and consult a poison control centre.

Overload: Provide diuresis and ensure the patient has no urinary obstruction.

Uremia: Assess for clinical findings.

INDICATIONS FOR DIALYSIS

Assess for indications:
› Apply the mnemonic AEIOU.
› Consider the patient's response to medical therapy.
› Ensure the nephrology fellow and staff are aware of the patient's condition.

If the patient requires dialysis:
› Describe how urgently and the patient's hemodynamic status.
› Consider the setting: in acutely unwell patients, or toxicity requiring close monitoring, involve ICU or the high acuity unit.
› Discuss access for hemodialysis, including plans to put in a line.
› Discuss whether the patient is a good candidate for dialysis: consider the patient's frailty, quality of life, and likelihood of renal recovery. Also consider whether dialysis is appropriate in the long term.

Glomerular Disease

These notes are in addition to the **general guide for all consultations** on page 1, and the **starting points for nephrology consultations** at the beginning of this chapter.

Identification

Key information in the identification statement includes pertinent comorbidities and baseline creatinine (GFR).

Reason for Referral

The referral may seek to confirm a nephritic or nephrotic syndrome and/or clarify appropriate management.

History of Present Illness

Glomerular disease occurs on a spectrum from nephrotic to nephritic syndromes; cases may occur with features of both. Focus the history on the causes and consequences of glomerular disease, and characterize the pertinent findings (e.g., the severity of the patient's edema).

Causes of disease[11–13]:

> **Drugs:** Ask about NSAIDs, cocaine, heroin, hydralazine, gold, penicillamine, bisphosphonates, and immunomodulators (e.g., anti-vascular endothelial growth factors, TNF inhibitors, checkpoint inhibitors).

> **Autoimmune:** Conduct a rheumatological review of systems, with a specific focus on SLE and vasculitis.

> **Infectious:** Ask about HIV, HCV, endocarditis, cellulitis, pharyngitis, and other streptococcal or staphylococcal infections.

> **Malignancy:** Ask about solid organ tumours (GI, lung, breast), lymphoma, leukemia, and monoclonal gammopathy.

> **Other:** Ask about known glomerular disease (which is often relapsing-remitting), diabetes, and hypertension (hypertension is a common cause of nephrotic-range proteinuria, but not full nephrotic syndrome).

Consequences of disease: Ask about:

> **General:** constitutional symptoms[11,12]

> **Urinary symptoms:** tea- or cola-coloured urine, frothy urine, oliguria (100–500 mL/day), anuria (< 100 mL/day)[11,12]

> **Elevated creatinine:** a rise in creatinine over time (clarify timeline)

> **Uremia:** anorexia, nausea, vomiting, confusion, pruritus, pleuritis, pericarditis[12]

> **Volume overload:** anasarca, dyspnea, abdominal distention, orthopnea[12]

> **Pulmonary-renal syndrome:** hemoptysis, dyspnea[11,12]

> **Vasculitis-specific complications:** epistaxis, sinusitis, neuropathy (mononeuritis multiplex), palpable purpuric rash, arthritis, myalgias, visual changes[11,12]

> **Protein loss complications:** venous thromboembolism, infections[11,12]

Past Medical History

Ask about:

- nephrology-related history, including:
  - › known glomerular disorder
  - › underlying CKD (obtain the baseline GFR and a detailed account of previous renal function)
  - › albuminuria
- known hypertension or diabetes (characterize the severity)
- malignancy, including the status of disease and treatments
- autoimmune disorders
- HIV, HBV, HCV
- asthma, atopy, sinusitis
- other medical history

Past Surgical History

Ask about:

- past biopsies (obtain results, if relevant)
- urological surgery

Medications

- Ask about all current medications:
  - › Note those that could cause glomerular disease.
  - › Note nephrotoxic drugs and anticipate dosing adjustments.
- Ask about anticoagulation and antiplatelet agents (this is important if biopsy is required).

Allergies

Follow the **general guide for all consultations.**

Family History

Follow the **general guide for all consultations** and the **starting points for nephrology consultations.**

Social History

Ask about:

- ethnicity
- functional capacity
- drug use, especially IV drug use

Code Status

Follow the **general guide for all consultations** and the **starting points for nephrology consultations.**

Physical Examination

Vital signs: clinical stability; signs of volume overload or pulmonary hemorrhage (respiratory rate, hypoxemia); hypertension[12,13]

General impression: body habitus, work of breathing, anasarca[12,13]

Signs of uremia: altered level of consciousness; asterixis; pleural and/or pericardial rubs[12,13]

Volume status: JVP, edema, chest sounds[11-13]

Systemic manifestations of disease: saddle nose deformity; nasal septal defect; sinusitis; scleritis; respiratory wheeze; rash; arthritis; stigmata of endocarditis; mononeuritis[11-13]

Monitoring data:
> Check the patient's recent fluid intake versus urine output.

Other:
> Consider bedside US to look for pericardial effusion, pleural effusions, and new ascites, and to assess inferior vena cava calibre and jugular veins (for possible dialysis line placement).

Investigations

LABORATORY INVESTIGATIONS

CBC with differential: Assess for anemia, eosinophilia, and platelets.[11,14]

Creatinine, urea: Look up baseline creatinine and determine the trend.[11,14]

Electrolytes: Order K, HCO_3, PO_4, and Ca.[11,14]

Urinalysis and microscopy: Look for casts, dysmorphic RBCs, and oval fat bodies.[11,12,14]

Coagulation panel: This anticipates possible line insertion or biopsy.

CRP[11,14]

Albumin-to-creatinine ratio: Look up the baseline, if available.[11,14]

Nephritic investigations:
> Consider these as indicated; the decision for each test depends on clinical context.
> Consider antineutrophil cytoplasmic antibody (ANCA), anti-glomerular basement membrane (anti-GBM), ANA, anti-double stranded DNA (anti-dsDNA), C3, C4, cryoglobulins (or rheumatoid factor), HIV, HBV, HCV, antistreptolysin O titre, SPEP, UPEP, and serum free light chains.[11,12,14]

Nephrotic investigations: Consider these as indicated, including lipid panel, albumin level, SPEP, UPEP, serum free light chains, HbA_{1c}, HIV, HBV, HCV, ANA, anti-dsDNA, C3, C4, and 24-hour urine protein collection.[11,12,14]

MICROBIOLOGY

Blood cultures: Pursue these on suspicion of endocarditis.[11,12,14]

Swabs: If relevant, obtain the results of recent wound or throat swabs to assess for streptococcus or staphylococcus-associated GN.

IMAGING

Chest x-ray

CT of the chest: Consider this on concern for pulmonary-renal syndrome.

Renal US: Pursue this if the patient may need a biopsy.

OTHER

Renal biopsy: This is urgent in the setting of rapidly progressive GN.

Impression and Plan

Start with a summary:
> Describe the patient's presentation and highlight the acuity, severity, and dominant syndrome (nephritic versus nephrotic versus mixed).
> Use the clinical presentation and urine sediment to identify the glomerular syndrome.
> If you suspect an inpatient has acute GN, inform the nephrology fellow and staff early.

Provide a differential diagnosis: Develop a differential diagnosis based on the syndrome (initiate a preliminary workup):
> **Nephritic syndromes:** anti-GBM, ANCA-associated vasculitis, immune complex mediated GN (e.g., lupus nephritis, postinfectious GN)
>> In general, nephritic syndromes are more likely to be associated with acute renal dysfunction, so early identification is crucial.
> **Nephrotic syndromes:** minimal change disease, membranous GN, focal segmental glomerulosclerosis, renal amyloid, and diabetic nephropathy
> **Overlap syndromes:** IgA nephropathy, membranoproliferative GN

Describe initial management:
> For inpatients, discuss initial management with the nephrology fellow or staff.
> Indications for acute hemodialysis include uremia, refractory hyperkalemia, acidosis, and volume overload.
> Consider early intervention in anuric patients.
> The regimen for immunosuppression or plasma exchange depends on the etiology and severity.

Provide a plan for renal biopsy, if indicated:
> Hold anticoagulation and/or antiplatelets.
> Try to arrange for an urgent renal US prior to the biopsy.

› Order a CBC and coagulation panel.
› Note that the target for systolic BP is < 140/90 mmHg to reduce the risk of bleeding.

Review medications:
› Hold nephrotoxic medications.
› Adjust the dose of medications as needed.

Discuss goals of care: Is the patient a candidate for dialysis? Would they want it if needed?

Hyponatremia

These notes are in addition to the **general guide for all consultations** on page 1, and the **starting points for nephrology consultations** at the beginning of this chapter.

Identification

Follow the **general guide for all consultations** and the **starting points for nephrology consultations.**

Reason for Referral

- The referral may seek to confirm the cause of hyponatremia and/or clarify appropriate management.
- It may specify the acuity of hyponatremia:
  › **Mild:** serum sodium 130–134 mmol/L
  › **Moderate:** serum sodium 125–129 mmol/L
  › **Severe:** serum sodium < 125 mmol/L

History of Present Illness[15]

Characterize the hyponatremia:
› When was the hyponatremia first identified? What has been the trend in serum sodium?
› Are there other electrolyte disturbances (acute or chronic)?

Clarify causes:
› Determine sources of free water, including diet, IV fluids, medications (oral or IV), and recent surgery (e.g., involving irrigation or instillation of hypotonic fluids).
› Determine fluid losses leading to absolute or relative hypovolemia, including GI (vomiting, diarrhea), skin (burns), and third spacing (pancreatitis, sepsis).
› Ask about symptoms of poor forward flow or volume overload: swelling, weight gain, bloating, and orthopnea and/or paroxysmal nocturnal dyspnea.

› Ask about physiologic triggers for antidiuretic hormone: nausea, pain, and malignancy (which can manifest as constitutional symptoms).

› Review the patient's diet for solute intake (e.g., "tea and toast" diet) and alcohol consumption (beer potomania).

Clarify consequences:
› Severe symptoms include seizure and coma, and require immediate treatment.
› Moderate symptoms include nausea and vomiting, and confusion or drowsiness.
› Mild symptoms include headache and decreased attention span.
› Ask about treatments that have been attempted (e.g., IV fluids, desmopressin, diuretics, salt tablets) and their effect.

Past Medical History

Clarify nephrology-related history: Ask about:
› **CKD:** Determine etiology, and most recent tests for creatinine (eGFR) and other markers of renal function (e.g., albumin-to-creatinine ratio).
› **Nephrotic syndrome**
› **Known history of syndrome of inappropriate antidiuretic hormone secretion (SIADH):** Clarify etiology (if known) and any treatments.

Determine nonnephrology-related history: Ask about:
› **Volume-overload states that can cause hyponatremia:** These include HF and liver failure (cirrhosis).
› **Endocrine disease:** These include diabetes; adrenal insufficiency (primary or secondary); and thyroid disease.
› **Psychiatric disease:** This can lead to primary polydipsia.
› **Possible causes for SIADH:** These include malignancy, and pulmonary or CNS disease.

Medications

Ask about:
• recent medication changes
• diuretics (thiazides and thiazide-like diuretics are most likely to cause hyponatremia)
  › Determine start date, dose, compliance, and route of administration.
• desmopressin
  › Determine start date and time of administration, dose, and whether it involves chronic use.
• medications associated with acute hyponatremia (e.g., desmopressin, vasopressin, oxytocin, bowel prep, 3,4-methylenedioxymethamphetamine, cyclophosphamide)

- possible medications associated with SIADH (e.g., antidepressants, anticonvulsants, antipsychotics)
- other medications as relevant

Allergies

Follow the **general guide for all consultations.**

Physical Examination[16]

Vital signs: Pay particular attention to heart rate, BP, and trends.

Fluid balance: Consult the nursing chart and/or medication administration record for:

> **Fluid input:** fluid in diet, current IV fluids (determine composition and rate), IV medications

> **Fluid output:** urine output (insert a Foley catheter if the patient cannot reliably collect urine for quantification), stool output (e.g., diarrhea)

Neurological: Assess for impaired mental status (level of consciousness, orientation, language, attention); impaired cranial nerves; and jerking or seizure-like movements.

Volume status:

> Note that clinical assessment is imperfect and rarely leads to diagnosis.

> Assess for symptoms of hypovolemia: orthostatic vital signs, capillary refill, extremity temperature, mucous membrane moisture (eyes, mouth, and tongue), and skin turgor.

> Assess for symptoms of hypervolemia: elevated JVP, peripheral edema, ascites, and pulmonary edema.

Investigations[17,18]

BLOOD

Serial sodium with serum osmolality: This distinguishes between types of hyponatremia, which determines a workup to pursue:

> **Hyperosmolar (> 295 mmol/kg):** Order tests for severe hyperglycemia with dehydration and mannitol.

> **Iso-osmolar (280–295 mmol/kg):** Order tests for pseudohyponatremia (hyperlipidemia, hyperproteinemia) and hyperglycemia.

> **Hypo-osmolar (< 280 mmol/kg):** This is the most common type.

Other electrolytes: K, Cl, HCO_3

Creatinine (eGFR), urea, glucose

URINE

Dipstick: Specific gravity provides clues to osmolality (for an approximation, multiply the last two digits by 30).

Urine osmolality: See Table 12.1.
Urine Na: See Table 12.1.

INVESTIGATIONS FOR SUSPECTED ETIOLOGY
Order further tests depending on the suspected etiology.
Adrenal insufficiency: morning cortisol, low-dose ACTH stimulation test
Hypothyroidism (severe): thyrotropin (TSH), free T_4, T_3
SIADH: pulmonary or CNS imaging; infectious disease workup
HF: BNP, echocardiogram
Liver failure: liver enzymes and metabolic function; abdominal ultrasound
Kidney disease: standard workup (note that kidney disease is not a cause or consequence of hyponatremia per se, but determines whether urine studies are interpretable and how the hyponatremia should be managed)

Table 12.1. Urine Osmolality, Serum Osmolality, and Urine Sodium in Hyponatremia

FINDING	INTERPRETATION
$U_{Osm} < S_{Osm}$ $U_{Osm} < 100$ mmol/L	Suspect a non-ADH-mediated cause: primary polydipsia, "tea and toast" diet, excessive alcohol.
$U_{Osm} < S_{Osm}$ $U_{Osm} > 100$ mmol/L	This is a "grey zone" where ADH may be playing a role.
$U_{Osm} > S_{Osm}$ $U_{Osm} > 100$ mmol/L	Suspect an ADH-mediated cause and/or low rate of delivery of filtrate to the distal nephron: check urine sodium and/or chlorine.
Urine sodium < 30 mmol/day	This indicates low EABV (either hypo- or hypervolemia).
Urine sodium > 30 mmol/day	This points to diuretics, adrenal insufficiency, severe hypothyroidism, SIADH, or renal or cerebral salt wasting.

Abbreviations: ADH: antidiuretic hormone; EABV: effective arterial blood volume; S_{Osm}: serum osmolality; SIADH: syndrome of inappropriate antidiuretic hormone secretion; U_{Osm}: urine osmolality

Impression and Plan
Start with a summary: Include the temporal pattern of the hyponatremia (length and tempo), and the clinical syndrome (detail symptoms, signs, and investigations, both positive and negative).

Engage general principles[16]:
› Determine the tempo of the hyponatremia (acute versus chronic), its severity, and whether the patient is symptomatic (do not assume hyponatremia is solely responsible for symptoms).
› Does the patient have severe symptoms necessitating immediate treatment? If so, use hypertonic 3% saline (100 mL aliquots over 10 minutes, repeated 2 to 3 times as needed) to raise serum sodium by about 5 mmol/L.
› Patient-specific tolerances should guide the rate of raising serum sodium levels, and not (solely) equations.
› If giving IV fluids, use small aliquots with frequent checking of patient status, urine output, and electrolytes (e.g., every 2 hours).
› In stable patients where there is uncertainty about tempo, restrict all fluid intake, stop IV fluids, and closely monitor urine output.

Describe immediate management decisions[17,18]:
› Symptomatic patients who are definitely acute require rapid initial correction (as described above): there is no upper limit to the correction rate in acute hyponatremia.
› Patients with possible or definite chronic hyponatremia are at risk of osmotic demyelination syndrome (ODS) during correction: the rise in serum sodium should not exceed 8 mmol/L in any 24-hour period (target a rise of 4–6 mmol/L).
› Indicate the frequency of blood work for serum sodium, rate and composition of IV fluids (if any), and when to be concerned for overcorrection (e.g., specify a urine output).
› Identify patients at high risk for ODS (serum sodium ≤ 105 mmol/L, hypokalemia, alcohol use disorder, malnutrition, liver disease) and monitor them more closely.
› If overcorrection occurs, lower serum sodium with IV dextrose 5% in water (maximum 250 mL/hour) and desmopressin (2–4 mcg IV once, then reassess).

Specify management depending on etiology:
› Stop thiazide diuretics.
› In extracellular fluid volume contraction, cautiously restore extracellular volume with small IV aliquots of normal saline or balanced crystalloid, and check the patient frequently.
› A sudden increase in urine output to > 100 mL/hour signals increased risk of overly rapid rise in serum sodium concentration.
› In extracellular fluid volume expansion, restrict salt and free water intake, and administer loop diuretics.
› In primary polydipsia, restrict free water intake.
› In SIADH, restrict free water intake, and consider increasing solute intake with sodium chloride tablets (use caution with normal saline as it may worsen hyponatremia due to desalination).

› Treat relevant underlying conditions (e.g., adrenal insufficiency, hypothyroidism, diabetes).

› Correct other electrolyte abnormalities (remember that use of potassium chloride to correct coexisting hypokalemia will cause a rise in serum sodium similar to what occurs with the administration of an equivalent amount of sodium chloride).

Peritoneal Dialysis–Associated Peritonitis

These notes are in addition to the **general guide for all consultations** on page 1, and the **starting points for nephrology consultations** at the beginning of this chapter.

Identification

Follow the **general guide for all consultations** and the **starting points for nephrology consultations.**

Reason for Referral

The referral may seek to confirm peritoneal dialysis–associated peritonitis (PD peritonitis) and/or clarify appropriate management.

History of Present Illness

Clarify the presenting complaint: For inpatients, what has been the course in hospital to date?

Characterize the problem: Are there symptoms of peritoneal inflammation (e.g., abdominal pain, cloudy peritoneal effluent, nausea, vomiting, diarrhea, fever)?[19]

Assess for causes of peritonitis:

› **Primary peritonitis:** Ask about breaks in PD technique and contamination.

› **Secondary peritonitis:** Ask about underlying GI or GU pathology, ischemic bowel, and recent endoscopy or other procedures.[19]

Determine the consequences of the problem: Is the patient systemically unwell?

Clarify the patient's renal history: Ask about:

› **Primary nephrologist:** Who is following the patient?

› **End stage kidney disease (ESKD) history:** What is the etiology of ESKD? Has it been proven on biopsy? If so, what was the date and diagnosis on pathology?

› **Dialysis history:** Determine how long the patient has been on dialysis, and the date of PD catheter insertion; ask about a previous history of hemodialysis, alternative hemodialysis access, and plans to transition to hemodialysis.

› **PD prescription:**
  » For continuous ambulatory PD (CAPD), determine the number of exchanges per day, fill volume, and solution strengths and types.
  » For continuous cycling PD (CCPD), determine the duration on cycler, solution strengths and type, and daytime exchanges.
  » Has the patient had any recent changes in PD prescription?
  » What is the patient's goal weight and net fluid removal? Is there any residual urine output?
› **PD administration:** How has the PD been going? Are there issues with compliance or hygiene? Who does the PD (patient, family, or caregiver)?
› **Symptoms of hypotension, and volume overload or depletion**
› **History of PD complications:** These include:
  » PD peritonitis (determine date, organism grown, antibiotic type, and duration of treatment)
  » exit site infections (determine date, organism grown, antibiotic type, and duration of treatment)
  » mechanical blockage, leaks
› **CKD complications:** Assess for acid-base disturbances, anemia, electrolyte derangements, and mineral bone disease.

Past Medical History

Ask about nonrenal-related history, including:

- CAD, hypertension, HF, peripheral vascular disease
- diabetes mellitus
- GI diseases
- malignancy
- immune compromise

Past Surgical History

- Ask about all procedures.
- Abdominopelvic surgery is particularly important.

Medications

- Determine start and stop dates of current and recent antimicrobials.
- Pay particular attention to renal medications (e.g., erythropoiesis stimulating agents, iron, diuretics, antihypertensives, phosphate binders, vitamin D analogues).

Allergies

Follow the **general guide for all consultations.**

Family History
Ask about:
- kidney disease
- malignancy
- autoimmune disease

Social History
Ask about:
- alcohol use, recreational drug use, smoking
- occupation
- factors limiting PD compliance (e.g., financial burdens; independence with ADLs and IADLs; cognitive status; social supports)

Physical Examination
Vital signs: BP (hypotension), heart rate (tachycardia), temperature (fever), respiratory rate, oxygen requirements
General impression: respiratory distress, GCS score
Weight
Drained dialysate: cloudiness, fecal material (secondary peritonitis)
Alternate HD access: fistula, lines
Volume status: JVP, respiratory crackles, mucous membranes, peripheral edema, ascites
Abdominal: tenderness, rebound
PD catheter: exit site erythema and/or discharge; tunnel tenderness
Uremic symptoms: pericardial rub, asterixis

Investigations

LABORATORY INVESTIGATIONS
CBC with differential
Glucose, liver enzymes, lipase, lactate
Creatinine, urea
Investigations for ESKD complications: acid-base balance, Na, K, HCO_3, PO_4, Mg, Ca, parathyroid hormone, albumin, ferritin, transferrin saturation

PERITONEAL FLUID ANALYSIS
Cell count and differential: WBCs, percentage of polymorphonuclear leukocytes (PMNs)
Gram stain
Culture and sensitivity

MICROBIOLOGY

Check for previous PD peritonitis organisms cultured (determine date, species, sensitivities) and previous blood cultures (determine date, species, sensitivities).

Exit site culture: Pursue this if the exit site appears purulent.

Blood cultures: Pursue these if the patient appears septic.

IMAGING

Abdominal x-ray: Assess the position of the PD catheter.

CT of the abdomen and/or pelvis: Pursue this as clinically indicated to rule out secondary causes of peritonitis.

Impression and Plan

Start with a summary: Include the type of PD, the presenting complaint, results of significant investigations (PD analysis, exit site culture, blood cultures), and observations about possible etiology (primary PD peritonitis versus secondary PD peritonitis versus other causes).

Discuss PD peritonitis as a diagnosis: The diagnosis requires at least 2 of[20]:

> › signs and symptoms of peritoneal inflammation (e.g., abdominal pain, cloudy effluent)
> › positive dialysate culture
> › PD fluid with a WBC count > 100 x 10^9/L and more than 50% PMNs

Start empiric intraperitoneal (IP) antibiotics for gram-positive and gram-negative bacteria: Don't wait for a positive culture if you are clinically suspicious of PD peritonitis.[20]

> › For inpatients, consult with the nephrology fellow or attending physician on call before prescribing IP antibiotics.
> › Refer to the local PD peritonitis order set.
> › Substitute IV antibiotics if the patient is septic or systemically unwell, or on suspicion of secondary peritonitis.
> › Adjust antibiotics based on the culture and sensitivity results.[19]

Start antifungal prophylaxis on starting antibiotics: This is due to the risk of fungal infections (e.g., order oral fluconazole 100 mg daily, and nystatin swish and swallow 4 times per day).[20]

Monitor response with repeat peritoneal fluid analysis daily for 3 days.

Correct any metabolic and electrolyte derangements.

Do *not* stop PD.

Consider whether to remove the PD catheter: The PD catheter may require removal in the following circumstances: infection refractory to an appropriate course of antibiotics; recurrent peritonitis;

fungal or mycobacterial infection; tunnel infection; and peritonitis secondary to intraabdominal pathology.[20]
› Continue antibiotics for at least 2 weeks after removal.
› Switch to hemodialysis: consider the patient's code status, wishes, and vascular access.

‖‖‖

UNDERSTANDING PERITONEAL DIALYSIS ORDERS

Refer to the local PD prescription order set.

Breakdown of PD Order Components

PD type (this is usually CAPD in hospital)	Solution type and strength for overnight dwell
Number of exchanges per day	Fill volume
Solution type and strength during the day	Target weight
	Heparin (this is added on findings of fibrin strands)

Types of PD

CAPD (3 to 4 exchanges in the day; 1 overnight dwell)	CCPD (continuous exchange via cycler overnight; 1 to 2 dwells in the day)

PD Solutions

Dianeal (0.5%, 1.5% (fluid neutral), 2.5%, 4.25% dextrose)	Physioneal (1.36%, 2.27%, 3.86% glucose)
Extraneal (7.5% icodextrin)	Nutrineal (1.1% amino acid)

Adjusting Solution Strength Based on Volume Status

In volume-overloaded patients, increase the solution strength.	In volume-depleted patients, decrease the solution strength.

References

1. Waikar S, Bonventre J. Acute kidney injury. In: Kasper D, Fauci A, Hauser S, et al, editors. Harrison's principles of internal medicine. 19th ed. New York: McGraw-Hill Education; 2015. p. 1800-10.
2. Bargman J, Skoreki K. Chronic kidney disease. In: Kasper D, Fauci A, Hauser S, et al, editors. Harrison's principles of internal medicine. 19th ed. New York: McGraw-Hill Education; 2015. p. 1811-21.
3. Kidney International. KDIGO clinical practice guideline for acute kidney injury [Internet]. Kidney International Supplements. 2012;2(1) [cited 2022 Jan 11]. Chapter 2.3, Evaluation and general management of patients with or at risk for AKI, p. 25-7; Chapter 2.4, Clinical applications, p. 28-32; Chapter 2.5, Diagnostic approach to alterations in kidney function and structure, p. 33-6; Chapter 5.1, Timing of renal replacement therapy in AKI, p. 89-92. Available from: https://kdigo.org/wp-content/uploads/2016/10/KDIGO-2012-AKI-Guideline-English.pdf

4. Rosenberg M. Overview of the management of chronic kidney disease in adults. Curhan G, ed. UpToDate [Internet]. Waltham (MA); UpToDate Inc; 2020 Jul [cited 2020 Aug 11]. Available from: https://www.uptodate.com/ contents/overview-of-the-management-of-chronic-kidney-disease-in-adults?search=chronic%20 kidney%20disease&source=search_result&selectedTitle=1~150&usage_ type=default&display_rank=1#H7

5. Kidney International. KDIGO clinical practice guideline for anemia in chronic kidney disease [Internet]. 2012; 2(4): [cited 2022 Jan 11]. Chapter 1, Diagnostics and evaluation of anemia in CKD, p. 288-91; Chapter 2, Use of iron to treat anemia in CKD, p. 292-8; Chapter 3, Use of ESAs and other agents to treat anemia in CKD, p. 299-310. Available from: https://kdigo.org/guidelines/anemia-in-ckd/

6. Waikar S, Murray P, Singh A, editors. Core concepts in acute kidney injury. New York: Springer (ebook); 2018.

7. Levey A, James M. Acute kidney injury. Ann Intern Med [Internet]. 2017 Nov 7 [cited 2020 Aug 23]. Available from: https://www.acpjournals.org/doi/abs/10.7326/ AITC201711070

8. Khwaja A. KDIGO clinical practice guidelines for acute kidney injury. Nephron Clin Pract. 2012;120(4):c179-84. doi: 10.1159/000339789

9. Fatehi P, Hsu C-y. Evaluation of acute kidney injury among hospitalized adult patients. Palevsky P, ed. UpToDate [Internet]. Waltham (MA); UpToDate Inc; 2019 Dec 12 [cited 2020 Aug 24]. Available from: https://www.uptodate.com/contents/ evaluation-of-acute-kidney-injury-among-hospitalized-adult-patients?search=aki&s ource=search_result&selectedTitle=3~150&usage_type=default&display_rank=2

10. Okusa M, Rosner M. Overview of the management of acute kidney injury (AKI) in adults. Palevsky P, ed. UpToDate [Internet]. Waltham (MA); UpToDate Inc; 2021 Dec 10 [cited 2022 Jan 12]. Available from: https://www.uptodate. com/contents/overview-of-the-management-of-acute-kidney-injury-aki-in-adults?search=aki&source=search_result&selectedTitle=1~150&usage_ type=default&display_rank=1

11. Lin J, Denker B. Azotemia and urinary abnormalities. In: Longo D, Fauci A, Kasper D, et al, editors. Harrison's principles of internal medicine. 18th ed. New York: McGraw-Hill Education; 2012. p. 334-60.

12. Jennette J, Falk R. Glomerular diseases. In: Gilbert S, Weiner D, Bomback A, et al, editors. National Kidney Foundation's primer on kidney diseases. 7th ed. Amsterdam (Netherlands): Elsevier; 2018. p. 161-290.

13. Radhakrishnan J. Glomerular disease: evaluation and differential diagnosis in adults. Glassock R, Rovin B, eds. UpToDate [Internet]. Waltham (MA); UpToDate Inc; 2020 Jul [cited 2020 Aug 1] Available from: https://www.uptodate.com/contents/glomerular-disease-evaluation-and-differential-diagnosis-in-adults?search=glomerular%20 disease&source=search_result&selectedTitle=1~150&usage_type=default&display_ rank=1

14. Madaio M, Harrington J. The diagnosis of glomerular diseases: acute glomerulonephritis and the nephrotic syndrome. Arch Inter Med. 2001;161(1):25-34. doi: 10.1001/archinte.16.1.25

15. Seay N, Lehrich R, Greenberg A. Diagnosis and management if disorders of body tonicity – hyponatremia and hypernatremia: core curriculum 2020. Am J Kidney Dis. 2020; 75(2):272-86. doi: 10.1053/j.ajkd.2019.07.014

16. Kamel K, Halperin M. Fluid, electrolyte and acid-base physiology. 5th ed. Philadelphia: Elsevier; 2016. Chapter 10, Hyponatremia; p. 265-308.

17. Verbalis J, Goldsmith S, Greenberg A, et al. Diagnosis, evaluation, and treatment of hyponatremia: expert panel recommendations. Am J Med. 2013;126(10 suppl 1):S1-42. doi: 10.1016/j.amjmed.2013.07.006

18. Spasovski G, Vanholder R, Allolio B, et al. Clinical practice guideline on diagnosis and treatment of hypnatremia. Eur J Endocrinol. 2014;170(3):G1-47. doi: 10.1530/ EJE-13-1020

19. Burkart J. Clinical manifestations and diagnosis of peritonitis in peritoneal dialysis. UpToDate [Internet]. Waltham (MA); UpToDate Inc; 2020 May [cited 2020 May 1]. Available from: https://www.uptodate.com/contents/clinical-manifestations-and-diagnosis-of-peritonitis-in-peritoneal-dialysis

20. Li P, Szeto C, Piraino B, et al. ISPD peritonitis recommendations: 2016 update on prevention and treatment. Perit Dial Int. 2016;36(5):481-508. doi:10.3747/pdi.2016.00078

13

Neurology

Dr. Sina Marzoughi*
Dr. Olivia Marais*
Dr. Meshari Alsaeed
Dr. Jason Jeet Randhawa
*These authors contributed equally to this chapter.

REVIEWER
Dr. Tychicus Chen

Starting Points: Neurology Consultations

These notes are in addition to the **general guide for all consultations** on page 1.

Identification

Key information in the identification statement includes handedness, vascular risk factors, previous neurologic diagnoses, presenting complaint, the patient's first language, and the source of information about the patient.

Reason for Referral

The referral may seek to confirm a neurologic disorder and/or clarify appropriate management.

History of Present Illness

Clarify individual symptoms: For each symptom, determine:
> **Onset:** Was it sudden or gradual? What was the patient doing when they first noticed the symptom?
> **Progression:** Is the symptom stable, fluctuating, or gradually worsening?
> **Triggering factors:** Examples of inciting incidents include head injury, prodromal illness, and preceding infection.
> **Quality:** Note the patient's own words.

> **Location and radiation:** Ask about this if relevant (e.g., pain).
> **Severity:** Attempt to quantify this (e.g., 50% decrease in sensation).
> **Timing:** Clarify duration and frequency.
> **Aggravating and alleviating factors:** Examples include position, standing, lying down, the Valsalva maneuver, and medications.
> **Associated symptoms**

Conduct a **neurologic review of systems:** Ask about headache, diplopia, visual disturbances, hearing loss, tinnitus, vertigo, dysarthria, dysphagia, weakness, sensory changes, and gait disturbance.

Ask about previous similar episodes.

Assess for constitutional symptoms: Ask about fevers, chills, night sweats, and unexplained weight loss.

Ask about recent sick contacts.

Past Medical History

Ask about:

- previous neurologic diagnoses
- psychiatric diagnoses
- vascular risk factors, including type 2 diabetes, hypertension, dyslipidemia, smoking
- immunodeficiency
- malignancy, including treatments received and current status

Past Surgical History

- Ask about all surgeries.
- Neurosurgical procedures are especially important.

Medications

Identify all current medications, including OTC medications such as acetylsalicylic acid (ASA), vitamins, supplements, and herbal medications.

Allergies

Follow the **general guide for all consultations.**

Family History

Ask about:

- neurologic conditions, such as epilepsy and developmental disorders
- early onset cardiac disease

Social History

Ask about:

- occupation and living situation

- functional baseline (ADLs and IADLs)
- name of a substitute decision maker
- ethnicity and languages spoken
- substance use (alcohol, tobacco, recreational drugs)
- diet
- sexual activity, travel history
- infectious exposures (e.g., cat litter, tics) and toxin exposures (e.g., paralytic shellfish, poison, botulinum toxin)

Physical Examination

Vital signs: Pay particular attention to temperature and BP.

General impression: Does the patient look well or unwell?

CONSCIOUS PATIENTS

This exam is divided into components. Some components, however, provide information relevant to multiple systems.

Mental status: Consider a screening test such as the Montreal Cognitive Assessment (MoCA) or MMSE. Assess:

> **Alertness:** Is the patient alert, drowsy, stuporous, or comatose?

> **Attention:** Ask the patient to spell *world* backwards and to perform serial 7 subtractions.

> **Orientation to person, place, and time:** Note details of the patient's response.

> **Memory:** Assess delayed recall of 3 to 5 words.

> **Language:**
>> At minimum, assess fluency, naming (high and low frequency words), and repetition.
>> Other assessments include: comprehension (3-step command), reading, and writing.

> **Neglect:** For example, does the patient recognize only one side of their body as their own?

> **Ideomotor apraxia:** Ask the patient to act out common daily tasks such as brushing their teeth.

Cranial nerves (CNs):

> **Funduscopy (CN II):** Look for abnormalities such as blurred optic disc margins, abnormal cup-to-disc ratio, optic disc pallor, flame-shaped hemorrhages, cherry red spot, drusen, and retinitis pigmentosa.

> **Pupils (CN II, III):** Assess size, shape, and symmetry.
>> Check pupil size in the dark and light if anisocoria is present (i.e., sympathetic or parasympathetic failure).
>> Check direct and indirect response to light (i.e., integrity of optic and tectotegmental tracts) and response to accommodation.
>> Check for relative afferent pupillary defect with a swinging light test.

> **Visual acuity (CN II):** Assess best-corrected response in *each eye* (i.e., with glasses or a pinhole to exclude refractive error).
  » **Preferred method:** wall eye chart
  » **Alternatives:** finger counting, hand movement, or light perception
> **Visual fields (CN II):** Assess via finger counting or movement in each quadrant; test each eye separately.
> **Colour vision (CN II):** Look for red desaturation or formally assess with pseudoisochromatic plates.
> **Extraocular movements (CN III, IV, VI):** Ask the patient to follow an object or light in an H pattern.
> **Facial sensation (CN V):** Assess light touch, pinprick, and temperature (if applicable) to the forehead, cheeks, and mandible.
> **Facial muscles (CN VII):** Ask the patient to raise their eyebrows, close their eyes tightly, smile, and show their teeth.
> **Hearing (CN VIII):** Assess for gross symmetry; perform a Rinne test and a Weber test, if applicable, to determine conductive or sensorineural hearing loss.
> **Dysarthria (third trigeminal nerve [V3]; CN VII, IX, X, XII):** Assess labial articulation (ask the patient to say "pa, pa, pa"); labial-lingual articulation ("ta ta ta"); and lingual-guttural articulation ("ka ka ka").
> **Palate elevation (CN IX, X):** Look for symmetry and any deviation of uvula.
> **Gag reflex (CN IX, X):** This is useful in select cases (test each side separately).
> **Head and shoulder movement (CN XI):** Ask the patient to turn their head each way and shrug each shoulder.
> **Tongue movement (CN XII):** Assess for deviation on protrusion, or asymmetry in bulk or speed of side-to-side movements; assess strength of lateral tongue protrusion in the cheek against your finger.

Motor system: Compare findings on each side for:
> **Muscle bulk:** Assess atrophy, fasciculations, hypertrophy, and symmetry.
> **Abnormal movements:** Examples include tremor, chorea, and myoclonus.
> **Tone in all 4 extremities:** Assess for normal tone versus flaccidity, rigidity, or spasticity.
> **Power:** Grade each of the following on a scale of 0 to 5:
  » shoulder abduction (fifth cervical nerve root [C5]; axillary nerve)
  » elbow flexion (C5, C6; musculocutaneous nerve)
  » elbow extension (C7; radial nerve)
  » wrist extension (C6; radial nerve)
  » finger extension (C7; radial nerve)
  » finger abduction (C8, first thoracic nerve root [T1]; ulnar nerve)
  » hip flexion (second lumbar nerve root [L2], L3; femoral nerve)

» knee flexion (first sacral nerve root [S1]; sciatic nerve)
» knee extension (L3, L4; femoral nerve)
» ankle dorsiflexion (L4, L5; deep peroneal nerve)
» plantarflexion (S1; tibial nerve)
» big toe extension (L5; deep peroneal nerve)
› **Deep tendon reflexes:** Grade each reflex on a scale of 0 to 4+, including biceps, triceps, brachioradialis, patellar, and ankle.
› **Other upper motor neuron signs:** These include pronator drift, Hoffmann sign, plantar response (Babinski sign), and asymmetric crossed adductor reflex.

Sensation:
› Assess sensation in all 4 extremities: first with either pinprick or temperature (spinothalamic tract); then with either vibration or proprioception (dorsal column medial lemniscus).
  » Test all modalities if any abnormality is found.
› If there is a sensory symptom, perform more detailed testing across the nerve distribution and dermatomes (or along the trunk to test for a sensory level).

Coordination: Assess:
› speech rhythm and eye movements (e.g., saccadic intrusions, hypermetric or hypometric saccades)
› finger-to-nose manoeuvres
› heel-to-shin manoeuvres
› rapid alternating movements
› fine finger movements
› speech rhythm
› eye movements (saccadic intrusions, hypo- or hypermetric scaccades)
› Romberg sign (note: this is mainly a test of proprioception)

Gait: Assess:
› normal gait (base, stride length, heel strike, time spent on each leg, posture of trunk, arm swing)
› tandem gait (walking heel-to-toe in a straight line)
› heel walk and toe walk

UNCONSCIOUS PATIENTS
Examination of a comatose patient may provide clues about their neurological status. However, this does not apply to patients on sedation (e.g., propofol): in this context, a neurological examination for prognostication should be delayed until sedation has been stopped for at least 24 hours.
Vitals signs:
› Obtain all vital signs.

› Determine ventilator settings.

› Assess respiratory pattern.

Mental status: The examination of the unconscious patient can be summarized briefly using the GCS notation $E_xV_xM_x$ (to record eye, verbal, and motor scores); note, however, that the GCS was designed to assess consciousness after head injury (but its use is typically extrapolated to unconscious patients) and the FOUR score[1] is emerging as a better tool for examining comatose patients.

› Does the patient arouse to voice?

› Does the patient arouse to painful stimulus (e.g., sternal rub)?

› Can they follow commands?

› Can they verbalize (if not intubated)?

› Is there spontaneous movement or eye opening?

Cranial nerves:

› **Funduscopy:** This exam may be limited by positioning.

› **Pupils:** Assess as for conscious patients, and assess for hippus.

› **Eye movements:** Assess for roving or spontaneous movements.

› **Horizontal and vertical tracking with eyes open:** Consider using a mirror (selfie mode on cell phone).

› **Vestibuloocular reflex:** Omit in patients on C-spine precautions (caloric testing can be performed); ensure endotracheal tube remains in place.

› **Corneal reflexes:** Use gauze or saline drop.

› **Gag or cough reflex:** Consider asking the bedside nurse to elicit this by suctioning the endotracheal tube.

Motor system: For each limb, assess:

› **Muscle bulk, abnormal movements, and tone:** Assess as for conscious patients.

› **Spontaneous movements**

› **Movement to commands:** Ask the patient to give a thumbs up, make a peace sign, and make a fist; do not apply painful stimulus if the patient is obeying commands.

› **Localization to pain:** Squeeze the trapezius or apply pressure to the supraorbital notch; the limb being tested must cross the midline and act against gravity to show localization to pain.

› **Withdrawal to pain:** Apply pressure on a nail bed; be wary of triple flexion response in the legs, which is a reflex and not true withdrawal.

› **Reflexes**

› **Plantar response**

Investigations

LABORATORY INVESTIGATIONS

CBC, electrolytes, extended electrolytes, urea, creatinine

Other: Order other investigations depending on the clinical presentation (e.g., liver panel; ammonia; HbA_{1c}; thyrotropin [TSH]; vitamin B_{12}; serum protein electrophoresis; peripheral smear; syphilis serology; HIV; hepatitis serology screen; CRP; ANA and/or extractable nuclear antigen; double-stranded DNA; C3, C4; ACE; vitamin E; serum copper; serum zinc; ceruloplasmin; paraneoplastic panel; autoimmune encephalitis panel).

IMAGING[2]
Structural: CT or MRI of the brain, spine, and/or plexus
Vascular: CT angiogram of the cerebral arteries (arch to vertex or circle of Willis)

OTHER INVESTIGATIONS
Urinalysis: UTI can cause pseudorelapse in MS.
EEG: Pursue this in suspected seizure or encephalopathy.
LP: Have a low threshold of suspicion to perform LP for CSF collection (remember to check opening pressure).

Impression and Plan
Start with a summary: Include:
› relevant previous diagnoses
› time course of the illness (acute, subacute, or chronic)
› pattern of the illness (episodic, gradual worsening, stepwise progression)
› presenting symptoms
› pertinent positive findings on neurological exam
Describe possible localizations (e.g., for weakness): These include:
› muscle
› neuromuscular junction
› peripheral nerve
› plexus
› nerve root
› anterior horn cell
› spinal cord
› brainstem (medulla, pons, midbrain)
› thalamus
› internal capsule
› corona radiata
› cortex
Provide a differential diagnosis for suspected lesions:
› Discuss the *localization of the lesion* in detail before discussing differential diagnoses.

› Differential diagnoses include the following disorders: vascular; autoimmune; neoplastic or paraneoplastic; infectious; traumatic; metabolic; hereditary; degenerative; and functional.

Headache

These notes are in addition to the **general guide for all consultations** on page 1, and the **starting points for neurology consultations** at the beginning of this chapter.

Identification

Follow the **general guide for all consultations** and the **starting points for neurology consultations**.

Reason for Referral

The referral may seek to clarify the etiology or type of headache and/or appropriate management.

History of Present Illness

Characterize the onset of the headache: Was it gradual or sudden?
› If severity reaches 10 out of 10 within 60 seconds of onset, this is a **thunderclap headache** and requires an urgent noncontrast CT of the head to assess for subarachnoid hemorrhage.

Ask about Valsalva-maneuver-related triggers[3]: Examples include coughing, sneezing, defecating, and lifting weights.

Characterize the quality of the headache:
› dull/aching or throbbing/pulsatile (migraine)
› pressure or tight band-like sensation (tension type)
› knife-like stabbing (trigeminal autonomic cephalalgia [TAC])

Characterize other key features:
› **Location:** For example, is the headache unilateral, temporal, occipital, retroorbital, or side locked?
› **Severity:** Grade severity on a scale out of 1 to 10.
› **Duration:** Do the headaches last seconds, minutes, hours, days, or months?
› **Frequency:** How many headaches does the patient have per day? How many headache days does the patient have per month?
› **Radiation of pain**
› **Alleviating and aggravating factors**[3-5]: Ask about:
» medications
» change in position (lying down or standing up)
» time of day (headache that is worse in the morning suggests increased intracranial pressure)

» activity (headache that is worse with activity suggests migraine)

Clarify associated symptoms[3–5]: Ask about:
> › focal neurologic symptoms
> › fever, meningismus, neck stiffness, altered level of consciousness (LOC)
> › nausea, vomiting
> › preceding visual aura (scotomas, scintillating lines)
> › photo- or phonophobia
> › transient visual obscurations
> › diplopia
> › temporal or scalp tenderness
> › jaw claudication
> › unilateral autonomic symptoms (conjunctival injection, lacrimation, ptosis, miosis, eyelid edema, nasal congestion, rhinorrhea, forehead or facial sweating)
> › pulsatile tinnitus
> › recent neck manipulation or head trauma
> › constitutional symptoms
> › CSF rhinorrhea or otorrhea (spontaneous intracranial hypotension)

‖‖‖

RED FLAGS IN HEADACHE

Focal neurologic findings

Thunderclap headache

Fever, neck stiffness, or altered LOC (this may indicate meningitis or encephalitis)

Transient monocular vision loss (giant cell arteritis or TIA from internal carotid artery stenosis)

Acute or subacute neck pain with Horner syndrome (cervical artery dissection)

Constitutional symptoms, particularly if the patient is older than 50 (malignancy)

Triggered by Valsalva maneuver (mass lesion or vascular malformation)

Headache worse in the morning (this suggests a component of edema, which could indicate a brain mass[5])

Prominent positional component (worse on standing suggests intracranial hypotension; worse on lying flat suggests intracranial hypertension)

New headache or a new headache pattern[5]

Past Medical History

Ask about:
- headache history (determine the types of headache, treatment received, and efficacy of treatment)

- stroke or TIA
- head trauma associated with loss of consciousness or amnesia
- neurologic conditions
- malignancy
- immunodeficiency (e.g., HIV, organ transplantation, autoimmune disease)

Past Surgical History
Ask about:
- neurosurgery
- ventriculoperitoneal shunt

Medications
Ask about:
- medications to treat headache, and how many days per month the patient uses them (this is relevant to medication-overuse headache)
- immunosuppressive agents (posterior reversible encephalopathy syndrome [PRES])
- SSRIs and OTC nasal decongestants (reversible cerebral vasoconstriction syndrome [RCVS])
- isotretinoin and tetracyclines (idiopathic intracranial hypertension)

Allergies
Follow the **general guide for all consultations.**

Family History
Ask about:
- migraine and other headache types
- neurologic conditions

Social History
In addition to a standard social history, pay particular attention to:
- substance use, particularly cocaine and marijuana (this is relevant to RCVS)
- recent sick contacts, travel

Physical Examination
Perform a complete neurological exam, with particular attention to:
- **Vital signs:** If the patient is febrile, consider infectious causes of headache; if BP is high relative to the patient's normal, with altered LOC and seizure, consider PRES.
- **Meningismus:** Check for neck rigidity, Kernig sign, and Brudzinski sign; perform a jolt accentuation test.

- Mental status
- **Funduscopy:** Check for papilledema and spontaneous venous pulsations.
- Visual acuity
- Visual fields
- Ocular or cranial bruit
- Extraocular movements

Investigations

LABORATORY INVESTIGATIONS

CBC and differential

Electrolytes, creatinine

INR, PTT

CRP/ESR

β-HCG: Pursue this in females of reproductive age.

LP:

> › If the patient has signs of increased intracranial pressure, perform a CT of the head before performing LP to rule out an intracranial mass (which would be a contraindication to proceeding).
> › Check opening pressure during the procedure.
> › Check CSF appearance (e.g., if xanthochromia: subarachnoid hemorrhage; if straw-coloured fluid: infection or inflammation).
> › Send CSF for cell count and differential; protein, glucose, and lactate; cytology; Gram stain and culture; and PCR for HSV, VZV, and enterovirus.
> » Add acid-fast bacilli testing and/or TB culture, and cryptococcal antigen and fungal culture, if the patient is immunocompromised and/or has chronic headache.
> » Add CSF VDRL on clinical suspicion of STI (for neurosyphilis).
> › On suspicion of TB meningitis, perform multiple LPs because CSF acid-fast bacilli cultures have low sensitivity.
> › Consider involving infectious disease specialists, if indicated.
> › Consider assessing for oligoclonal bands.

IMAGING

Make sure you look at images yourself: don't just read the reports. Call the radiologist directly if your specific question is not addressed in the report or if further information is required.

Noncontrast CT of the head:

> › Pursue this on suspicion of hemorrhage or stroke.
> › Special considerations for subarachnoid hemorrhage (SAH):
> » Noncontrast CT of the head is sensitive for SAH if done within 6 hours of onset; sensitivity diminishes after that.

» If noncontrast CT of the head is done after 6 hours of symptom onset, an LP is required 12 hours after symptom onset; xanthochromia in the CSF typically appears 12 hours after onset of SAH, and can persist for up to 2 weeks.

» CT arch-to-vertex angiogram must be done with presentation of SAH to assess for ruptured aneurysm as the cause.

CT arch-to-vertex angiogram with contrast: Assess for large vessel occlusion, aneurysm, cervical artery dissection, or vasculitic changes to vessels.

CT of the head postcontrast: Pursue this on suspicion of malignancy or abscess.

MRI of the brain without contrast: Note that this is often sufficient (MRI with contrast is often not needed).

MRI of the brain with contrast (gadolinium): Discuss this with a radiologist if needed.

Impression and Plan

DIFFERENTIAL DIAGNOSIS
See Table 13.1.

MANAGEMENT
Primary Causes of Headache[3]
Abortive therapies: If no contraindications, consider:
› IV fluids
› acetaminophen
› NSAIDs, such as ketorolac
  » indomethacin if features of TAC are present
› antiemetics, such as metoclopramide
› IV dexamethasone
› triptans, such as sumatriptan
› dihydroergotamine (cannot be given within 24 hours of triptan use)
› supraorbital or occipital nerve block in select cases
Prophylactic therapies (in patients with multiple headaches per week)[3]: Consider:
› riboflavin, magnesium, and coenzyme Q10
› TCAs (amitriptyline), beta-blockers (propranolol), or antiseizure medications (topiramate)
› botulinum toxin or calcitonin gene-related peptide inhibitors in refractory headache (these are not available on most hospital formulary and generally need special approval)
Secondary Causes of Headache
• Treat the underlying cause.

Table 13.1. Differential Diagnosis of Headache

PRIMARY HEADACHE			
Tension-type headache Migraine headache Trigeminal autonomic cephalalgia Other (e.g., primary stabbing headache, primary exertional headache)			

SECONDARY HEADACHE			
STRUCTURAL	**INFECTIOUS/ INFLAMMATORY**		**VASCULAR**
SAH or SDH Stroke Neoplasm Abscess CSF leak Trauma Idiopathic intracranial hypertension CVST Hydrocephalus Colloid cyst Pituitary apoplexy	Meningitis • bacterial • viral • fungal (subacute or insidious presentation possible) • aseptic	Encephalitis • HSV (this is the most common form and is highly treatable; high morbidity and mortality if not treated) • autoimmune	Giant cell arteritis (in patients over 50) RCVS CNS vasculitis PRES Arterial dissection Genetic conditions such as CADASIL

Abbreviations: CADASIL: cerebral autosomal dominant arteriopathy with subcortical infarcts and leukoencephalopathy; CNS: central nervous system; CSF: cerebrospinal fluid; CVST: cerebral venous sinus thrombosis; HSV: herpes simplex virus; PRES: posterior reversible encephalopathy syndrome; RCVS: reversible cerebral vasoconstriction syndrome; SAH: subarachnoid hemorrhage; SDH: subdural hematoma

- Treat symptoms as for primary headache, but also consider acetazolamide for idiopathic intracranial hypertension (consider shunting if refractory) and hydration, caffeine, and abdominal binder for CSF leaks (consider epidural blood patch if refractory).
- Be cautious about using triptans in the setting of vasospasm and/or RCVS due to vasoconstriction.
- In patients with RCVS, avoid using glucocorticoids because these can worsen outcomes.[6]
- Consider CCBs and magnesium in the setting of vasospasm and/or RCVS (however, evidence is limited).
- Subarachnoid hemorrhage and obstructive hydrocephalus are **medical emergencies** and require prompt neurosurgical consultation.

Seizure

These notes are in addition to the **general guide for all consultations** on page 1, and the **starting points for neurology consultations** at the beginning of this chapter.

Identification

Follow the **general guide for all consultations** and the **starting points for neurology consultations**.

Reason for Referral

The referral may seek to confirm a diagnosis of seizure and/or clarify appropriate management.

History of Present Illness[7]

Identify provoking factors for seizure: Ask about:
› sleep deprivation
› starvation
› menstruation
› stress
› substance use
› alcohol withdrawal
› missed antiseizure medications
› infection
› new medications (e.g., bupropion)
› electrolyte disturbances (e.g., hyponatremia)
› metabolic disturbance (e.g., hepatic, renal)
› structural brain lesion (e.g., malignancy, stroke, head injury)

Clarify preictal phase:
› What was the patient doing prior to the event?
› Ask about prodromal or warning symptoms (aura):
» olfactory, gustatory, or other sensory hallucinations
» déja vu or jamais vu
» sense of impending doom
» rising epigastric sensation
» presyncope
» nausea

Clarify ictal phase: Ask about:
› duration of the event
› whether it was witnessed or unwitnessed (determine what the patient remembers and what witnesses saw)
› loss of consciousness versus retained awareness

> abnormal movements (generalized or focal; rhythmic or nonrhythmic; symmetric or asymmetric)
> course of movement progression (where the abnormal movement started and where it spread to next)
> early head turn
> gaze deviation, eyes open or closed
> tongue biting (lateral or central)
> urinary incontinence
> ictal cry
> spontaneous resolution versus resolution through medication

Clarify postictal phase: Ask about:
> weakness or other focal neurological symptoms (e.g., Todd paralysis, postictal aphasia)
> drowsiness, lethargy, and/or confusion
> agitation or psychosis
> how long until the patient was back to baseline

Conduct a seizure-related review of systems: Ask about:
> myoclonic jerks (e.g., dropping objects)
> staring spells
> unexplained tongue biting
> nocturnal incontinence
> automatisms (e.g., lip smacking, purposeless hand movements)
> memory gaps
> anxiety, panic attacks, or other paroxysmal psychiatric symptoms

Past Medical History

SEIZURES

- Ask specifically about febrile seizures as a child and diagnosis of epilepsy.
  > In a history of status epilepticus, ask about interventions required (e.g., intubation).
- Clarify the types of seizure (patients may have multiple types) and details for each type, including[7]:
  > aura
  > seizure semiology
  > frequency and last occurrence
  > typical duration of postictal state
  > time of day for occurrence (nocturnal events are more likely to be epileptic)
  > self-injury (e.g., falls, shoulder dislocations, tongue bites)
- Ask for the name of the patient's neurologist, the date of their last appointment, and any recent changes to antiseizure medications.

- Ask about adherence to antiseizure medications.
- Determine the last serum level of antiseizure medication.

OTHER KEY ENTITIES
Ask about:
- meningitis or encephalitis
- significant head trauma (leading to loss of consciousness, prolonged amnesia, or structural abnormalities in the brain)
- stroke
- malignancy
- renal or hepatic failure
- complications in pregnancy or birth
- neonatal asphyxia
- developmental delay
- psychiatric history

Past Surgical History
Clarify the details of any neurological surgery.

Medications
- Ask about all medications.
- Ask specifically about recent medication changes (e.g., recently starting certain seizure-threshold lowering antibiotics or abruptly stopping long-term benzodiazepines).

Allergies
Follow the **general guide for all consultations**.

Family History
Ask about:
- epilepsy or seizures
- neurocognitive or developmental disorders, and neurocutaneous syndromes

Social History
In addition to a standard social history, pay particular attention to:
- alcohol use, including: drinks per day; date or time of last drink; history of delirium tremens; and history of alcohol withdrawal seizures
- substance use, including: name of substance; route of consumption (e.g., inhalation, injection); amount used per day; date or time of last use
- recent stressors
- driving status, occupational hazards (e.g., ladders, power tools)

Physical Examination

Airway, breathing, circulation (ABCs): Call ICU early about patients who are or may become unstable.

Investigations

LABORATORY INVESTIGATIONS[7,8]

CBC and differential

Electrolytes: Look for hyponatremia.

Glucose

Creatinine, urea, liver enzymes, ammonia level: Look for metabolic disturbances.

CK, lactate: These are often elevated following a generalized tonic-clonic seizure.

Extended electrolytes: Order Mg, PO_4, and Ca.

CSF

Pursue CSF investigations if indicated.

Cell count and differential

Cytology

Glucose and protein

Gram stain and culture

PCR for HSV, VZV

Opening pressure

ADDITIONAL TESTS

Pursue these depending on the clinical picture (e.g., VDRL, cryptococcal antigen, fungal culture, oligoclonal bands, autoimmune antibodies).

IMAGING

- If the patient has known epilepsy and they are presenting with their known seizure type(s), imaging is not indicated.
- For first presentation of seizure, if there is a high suspicion of intracranial lesion, order an urgent CT of the head to assess for structural abnormalities (e.g., stroke, hemorrhage, mass).
- For first presentation of seizure in which the patient has returned to baseline and there is low suspicion of an intracranial lesion, arrange for an outpatient MRI brain seizure protocol.

EEG

- On concern for nonconvulsive status epilepticus, obtain an urgent EEG.
- EEG is not necessary in patients with known epilepsy presenting with their usual seizure type.

- In patients presenting with their first seizure, obtain an EEG as soon as possible (ideally within the 24 hours) to maximize yield.
- Depending on the degree of clinical suspicion, and what the first EEG reveals, a prolonged or sleep-deprived EEG may be indicated.

Impression and Plan

Consider the differential diagnosis: Was this a seizure?
> The differential diagnosis includes TIA, syncope, migraine, and psychogenic nonepileptic spell.

Treat the patient if they are still seizing:
> Stabilize the patient and follow institutional protocols for status epilepticus (SE).
> Consider convulsive SE in patients with generalized seizure activity lasting more than 5 minutes, or 2 or more seizures without return to baseline in between.
> Consider nonconvulsive SE in patients with persistent altered LOC not explained by other obvious causes.
> Call ICU if you suspect the patient may need intubation and sedation.
> Arrange for an urgent EEG.

Consider whether the seizure was provoked or unprovoked:
> If provoked, treat the underlying causes.
> If unprovoked, consider the diagnosis of epilepsy.

For epileptic seizure, describe the seizure and epilepsy type:
> Was it focal or generalized?
> Where is the seizure focus (e.g., left or right hemisphere, temporal lobe)?
> Consult the current International League Against Epilepsy (ILAE) classification for further details.[9,10]

Consider starting antiseizure medications:
> Determine if the patient meets diagnostic criteria for epilepsy (i.e., more than 1 unprovoked seizure 24 hours apart, or high chance of recurrent seizures based on risk factors or interictal epileptiform discharges on EEG).
> Determine which medication and why (see Table 13.2).
> Consider rational polypharmacy and patient comorbidities; refer the patient to a tertiary epilepsy centre if seizures are refractory to 2 or more appropriately dosed and tolerated antiseizure medications.

Provide counselling, as needed: Make sure the patient knows seizure precautions and local driving restrictions.

Table 13.2. Antiepileptic Medications Classified by Seizure Type

PRIMARY GENERALIZED	ABSENCE
Levetiracetam, valproic acid, lamotrigine, topiramate	Valproic acid, ethosuximide, lamotrigine, topiramate, benzodiazepines
MYOCLONIC	**FOCAL EPILEPSY**
Valproic acid, levetiracetam, clonazepam, topiramate (**avoid** phenytoin, carbamazepine)	Carbamazepine, oxcarbazepine, levetiracetam, lamotrigine, phenytoin, lacosamide

Stroke

These notes are in addition to the **general guide for all consultations** on page 1, and the **starting points for neurology consultations** at the beginning of this chapter.

Identification

Follow the **general guide for all consultations** and the **starting points for neurology consultations**.

Reason for Referral

The referral may seek to confirm a diagnosis (e.g., hemorrhagic stroke, ischemic stroke, subacute stroke, TIA) and/or clarify appropriate management (e.g., revascularization therapies).

History of Present Illness

Clarify the symptoms: Ask about weakness, numbness, vision loss, diplopia, dysarthria, vertigo, and other symptoms.

Determine when the patient was last seen normal:
› If the patient is within the window for acute intervention, determine the exact time (as close as possible) because this affects their eligibility for treatment.
› If the patient cannot provide a reliable history, obtain a collateral history from paramedics or family.
› If the patient woke up with deficits (e.g., in the morning after a night's sleep), ask about possible events during the night when they were last seen well (e.g., their partner noticed them getting up to use the bathroom).
› If they returned to baseline, determine how long their symptoms lasted (this is relevant to TIA).

Determine if patient takes anticoagulants or antiplatelets:
› Note that ASA is usually not listed on the pharmacy profiles because it is an OTC medication.

> What time was their last dose?
> What was their last INR/PTT?
> Have they received heparin recently?

Ask about recent head or neck trauma, including chiropractic neck manipulation.

Determine the patient's functional baseline: Are they living independently at home or do they require assistance with ADLs?

Past Medical History
Ask about:
- previous stroke or TIAs (determine stroke type, date of occurrence, stroke mechanism, residual deficits, and treatment received)
- previous head trauma
- previous MI or known CAD
- AF (clarify anticoagulation)
- hypertension
- type 1 or 2 diabetes mellitus
- dyslipidemia
- coagulopathy, or history of PE and/or DVT

Past Surgical History
Ask about:
- recent surgery or cardiac catheterization (determine if stents were placed)
- recent arterial puncture at a noncompressible site
- neurosurgical procedures

Medications
Ask about:
- anticoagulants (determine the time of last dose, and most recent INR/PTT)
- antiplatelets (ASA, clopidogrel)

Allergies
Follow the **general guide for all consultations.**

Family History
Ask about:
- stroke or MI at a young age
- thrombophilia or autoimmune disorders

Social History
Ask about:
- occupation

- living situation
- functional baseline (ADLs and IADLs)
- ethnicity and languages spoken
- substance use (alcohol, smoking, recreational drugs)
  - › For smoking, quantify packs per day.
  - › Ask specifically about IV use (this increases the risk for infective endocarditis causing embolic infarcts and/or mycotic aneurysms).

Code Status
Identify advanced directives, code status, and substitute decision makers, if applicable.

Physical Examination
Vital signs: Assess:
  - › **Temperature**
  - › **BP:** Patients are usually hypertensive in stroke; if hypotensive, look for an atypical cause (e.g., infective endocarditis) and check BP in both arms (aortic dissection).
  - › **Heart rate:** Look for irregular rhythm.
  - › **Respiration rate and oxygen saturation:** Ensure the patient is protecting their airway.
  - › **Glucose:** Don't forget to check this.

Signs of stroke: Conduct an exam based on the National Institutes of Health stroke score.[11]

Investigations

LABORATORY INVESTIGATIONS
CBC, differential, electrolytes, with special attention to glucose
Creatinine: Note that chronic or acute kidney disease is not an absolute contraindication to CT angiogram with contrast, which should still be considered in acute stroke as it may dictate life-altering management.
INR, PTT
Blood cultures: Pursue this on concern for infective endocarditis.
HbA$_{1c}$
Lipid panel
Thrombophilia testing: Pursue this (e.g., antiphospholipid antibodies) in stroke in patients younger than 50.

IMAGING
Noncontrast[2] CT of the head: Pursue this to rule out intracranial hemorrhage and to assess for early infarct changes (use the Alberta Stroke Program Early CT Score [ASPECTS]) and hyperdense vessel signs.

CT arch-to-vertex angiography:
› Assess for large-vessel occlusion or significant carotid stenosis.
› Hold metformin for 48 hours after use of contrast.
› Order a carotid Doppler ultrasound if a CT angiogram is not possible.

CT perfusion of the head: Pursue this if available, at the discretion of the stroke neurologist, to determine the size of tissue at risk (ischemic penumbra).

MRI stroke protocol: Pursue this in certain circumstances, such as concern for posterior circulation stroke not visualized on CT.

Transthoracic echocardiogram: Assess for the source of the embolus; consider a transesophageal echocardiogram if the finding is negative and clinical suspicion is high.

OTHER INVESTIGATIONS

24-hour Holter monitor: Assess for AF; consider prolonged cardiac monitoring if the finding is negative and clinical suspicion is high.

Impression and Plan

Start with a summary: Include patient demographics, chief complaint, neurologic deficits, and findings from imaging. *For example:* "78-year-old, right-hand-dominant male presenting with sudden onset right-sided weakness and aphasia at approximately 22:00. NIH score is 15. Imaging reveals early infarct changes in the left middle cerebral artery and a hyperdense vessel sign."

Localize the lesion: Does it best fit with a cortical, subcortical, brainstem, cerebellum, spinal, or peripheral nervous system localization?

Consider the differential diagnosis: In stroke not confirmed on imaging, consider stroke mimic (e.g., seizure, migraine, amyloid spell); in confirmed stroke, consider the most likely etiology of the stroke (e.g., cardioembolic, large-vessel atherosclerosis, small-vessel disease).

Provide treatment: See the sidebar on stroke management.

|||||||||||||||||||||||||||||||||||||||||||||||||||||||||||||||||||||||||||||||||||||||||||||||||||||||||||||||||||||||||||||||||||||||||||||||

STROKE MANAGEMENT

Management decisions are guided by time of onset, evidence of established infarct, collateral circulation, and CT perfusion if available.

Code stroke protocols: Follow institutional code stroke protocols[2,12,13] and don't hesitate to ask for help: time is brain!

Key initial information: When was the patient last seen well? Are they taking anticoagulants or antiplatelets? Review tPA contraindications.

CT scan: Obtain an urgent CT of the head noncontrast and a CT arch-to-vertex angiogram. Accompany the patient to the scanner. Let radiology know you would like interpretation of the images ASAP (also look at them yourself).

Acute ischemic stroke: Follow the "flat and fluids" protocol (put the head of the bed at 0 degrees if the patient can tolerate it, start IV fluids, and allow permissive hypertension).

Administration of tPA: Administer tPA within 4.5 hours of onset in disabling stroke with no hemorrhage found on noncontrast CT of the head. BP must be < 185/110 mmHg prior to tPA, and < 180/105 mmHg after tPA. Do not administer tPA in patients with active hemorrhage or high risk of major hemorrhage.

In large-vessel occlusion: Arrange for an endovascular thrombectomy within 6 hours of stroke (within 24 hours on a case-by-case basis: discuss with the interventionist on call).

In hemorrhagic stroke: BP control is key. Target BP is typically < 140/90 mmHg; use IV antihypertensives. Elevate the head of the bed above 30 degrees. Consult a neurosurgeon in patients with significant mass effect or midline shift (especially in the posterior fossa). Reverse anticoagulation with FFP or prothrombin complex concentrate.

In TIA or minor ischemic stroke: Provide dual-antiplatelet therapy for 21 days. Provide oral ASA 325 mg once and clopidogrel 300 mg once; next morning, start ASA 81 mg once daily and clopidogrel 75 mg once daily for 21 days followed by ASA monotherapy. Imaging carotid arteries is essential as the patient may be a candidate for revascularization and this is most beneficial when performed within 48 hours to 2 weeks.

Weakness

These notes are in addition to the **general guide for all consultations** on page 1, and the **starting points for neurology consultations** at the beginning of this chapter.

Identification

Follow the **general guide for all consultations** and the **starting points for neurology consultations**.

Reason for Referral

The referral may seek to clarify the etiology of weakness and/or appropriate management.

History of Present Illness

Clarify the onset and course of symptoms[14]:
› Was the onset sudden, stepwise, or insidious?
› Have the symptoms been continuous, progressive, episodic (characterize duration and frequency of episodes), or with diurnal variation?

Clarify precipitating factors: Ask about:
› trauma, immobility (e.g., compression, traction)
› surgery
› prolonged ICU or hospital stay
› preceding illness
› metabolic derangements
› specific activities

Determine the pattern of weakness: Ask about:
› focal versus multifocal symptoms
› catching toes when walking, difficulty turning a key
› symmetric versus asymmetric symptoms
› unilateral findings with or without facial involvement
› ascending weakness (acute inflammatory demyelinating polyneuropathy [AIDP])
› where symptoms began and spread (in progressive symptoms)

Identify associated symptoms[14]: Ask about:
› higher cortical functions (e.g., aphasia, neglect, anosognosia, eye deviation)
› visual symptoms (diplopia)
› bulbar symptoms (dysarthria, dysphagia, speech changes)
› sensory symptoms (clarify the pattern of sensory abnormality)
  » presence or absence of pain
  » numbness

» burning, tingling, or electric shock–like pain
» allodynia and/or hyperalgesia
› cerebellar symptoms (vertigo, ataxia, vomiting)
› neck pain
› radicular-type pain
› Lhermitte phenomenon (electric shock–like sensation down the back with flexion of neck)
› dyspnea or anxiety
› squeezing or band-like sensation around the torso
› lower back pain
› urinary or fecal incontinence
› myalgias
› autonomic symptoms
› rashes (e.g., shawl sign, V-sign, holster sign, heliotrope rash)
› arthralgias
› constitutional symptoms
› GI symptoms

Identify alleviating or aggravating factors: Ask about the effect of:
› rest
› activity, particularly repeated use of the same muscle
› particular positions or postures
› extremes of temperature (e.g., warm bath or shower, cold weather)
› medications

||||||||||||||||||||||||||||||||||||||||||||||||||||||||||||||||||||||||||||||||||||||||||||||||||||||

RED FLAGS IN WEAKNESS

Fever, chills, night sweats, weight loss (these suggest infection such as spinal epidural abscess, or malignancy)

Sudden onset unilateral weakness (stroke or TIA)

Rapidly ascending weakness (AIDP, botulism)

Dyspnea (diaphragmatic weakness)

Inability to hold the head up or speak in full sentences (this may signal impending respiratory compromise)

Bulbar symptoms (myasthenia gravis, Miller Fisher variant of AIDP, and other neuromuscular conditions)

Acute or subacute loss of ambulation

Leg weakness with associated saddle anesthesia, urinary retention or incontinence, fecal incontinence (cauda equina syndrome)

Past Medical History
Ask about:
- prior neurologic diagnoses
- vascular risk factors
- immune compromise
- malignancy and details of treatment
- endocrine disorders (e.g., diabetes, hypothyroidism)

Past Surgical History
Ask about:
- neurosurgical procedures
- other surgeries, including gastric procedures that may lead to vitamin deficiencies

Medications
Ask about:
- current medications
- vitamins and supplements
- statin or steroid exposure

Allergies
Follow the **general guide for all consultations.**

Family History
Ask about:
- neurologic or autoimmune conditions
- neurodevelopmental disorders

Social History
In addition to a standard social history, pay particular attention to:
- diet
- alcohol use
- sick contacts
- toxin exposure
- tick bites

Physical Examination
Vital signs
General appearance: Look for foot deformities, surgical scars, and rashes.
Mental status
Cranial nerves

Motor system: Compare one side to the other for each of the
following:
> **Muscle bulk:** Assess for atrophy, hypertrophy, and fasciculations.
> **Abnormal movements:** Examples include tremor and myoclonus.
> **Tone in all 4 extremities:** Assess for normal tone versus flaccidity,
rigidity, or spasticity.
> **Power in all 4 extremities**
> **Power to perform neck flexion and extension:** This is a proxy for
diaphragmatic weakness.
> **Deep tendon reflexes**
> **Upper motor neuron signs**
Sensation:
> In addition to a routine sensory examination, assess for a sensory
level bilaterally.
> Assess perianal sensation if there is concern for myelopathy.
Coordination
Other: See Table 13.3.

Investigations

SERUM
CBC and differential
Electrolytes, creatinine: This is helpful in rhabdomyolysis.
CRP
CK, LDH: This is helpful in myopathy and rhabdomyolysis.
Thyrotropin (TSH), vitamin B_{12}, HbA_{1c}
Serum protein electrophoresis, urine protein electrophoresis
HIV, HBV, HCV
ANA, rheumatoid factor: This is helpful in myopathy.
Antibody testing for specific syndromes: For example, test for
acetylcholine receptor antibody on suspicion of myasthenia gravis.
HTLV 1 and 2, vitamin E: Pursue these in the setting of ataxia.

CSF
LP is indicated if the suspected etiology is infectious or inflammatory.
Cell count and differential
Cytology
Protein and glucose
Culture and Gram stain
Viral PCR
VDRL
Oligoclonal bands (on suspicion of inflammatory cause)

Table 13.3. Special Tests for Motor Impairment

TEST	DESCRIPTION
Ice pack test	In a patient with ptosis, place an ice pack (covered in cloth to avoid discomfort) over the patient's closed eyes for 5 minutes and observe for any improvement in ptosis (myasthenia gravis).
Sustained upgaze	Ask the patient to focus on an object with a sustained upgaze for 60 to 180 seconds. Observe for ptosis of the eyelids (myasthenia gravis).
Single-breath counting	Ask the patient to take a deep breath and count as far as they can without taking another breath. A normal count is more than 20. This test is a proxy for forced vital capacity testing in myasthenia gravis and AIDP.
Jaw jerk reflex	Ask the patient to open their jaw slightly, then place your fingers on the patient's chin and tap with your reflex hammer. Brisk reflexes in the extremities with a normal jaw jerk suggests a cervical spine lesion
Neck flexion/ extension	Assess the strength of neck flexion and extension while the patient is lying down. This is used as a proxy for diaphragmatic weakness: these muscles are innervated by the same cervical nerve roots.
Spurling test	Passively extend the patient's neck and rotate the head to the affected side, then apply an axial load to the spine. The test is positive when the patient experiences radicular pain down the arm ipsilateral to the rotation of the head (suggests cervical radiculopathy).
Fatigability, facilitation	Perform repeated shoulder abductions and check for reduced or increased power or emergence of previously absent reflexes. You can test other muscles the same way (myasthenia gravis, LEMS).
Give-way weakness	Assess for a pattern of weakness in which the patient has normal power transiently, which then gives way.
Tinel sign	Lightly percuss over the course of a nerve. The test is positive if this elicits a sensation of tingling or burning in the nerve distribution. This is a useful test where nerves are superficial, such as the carpal tunnel (median nerve), medial aspect of the elbow (ulnar nerve), or lateral aspect of the knee (fibular nerve).
Phalen maneuver	Ask the patient to fully flex their wrists and place the dorsum of the hands together for 60 seconds. The test is positive if it produces paresthesias in the median nerve distribution (suggests carpal tunnel syndrome).
Abdominal reflexes	Assess abdominal muscle contraction in response to cutaneous stimulation in each of the 4 abdominal quadrants. These are absent below the level of a spinal cord injury, but may be physiologically absent.
Bulbocavernosus reflex	Look for contraction of the internal and/or external anal sphincter while pulling on an in situ Foley catheter.

Continued on p. 328

Table 13.3. *Continued from p. 327*

TEST	DESCRIPTION
Straight leg raise	With the patient in a supine position, passively flex the hip with the knee in extension (i.e., raise the patient's leg while straight). The test is positive if the patient has pain along the distribution of the lower radicular nerve roots (suggests lumbar or lumbosacral disc herniation).

Abbreviations: AIDP: acute inflammatory demyelinating polyneuropathy; LEMS: Lambert-Eaton myasthenic syndrome

EMG OR NERVE CONDUCTION STUDY
- Pursue this to characterize a nerve injury (e.g., axonal versus demyelinating; sensory versus motor versus mixed) or myopathy.
- It is most useful 10 to 14 days after the onset of symptoms.
- It may help in selecting a target for muscle or nerve biopsy in selected cases.

IMAGING
MRI: This can help assess muscles, plexus, spinal nerve roots, and the spinal cord.

US: Ultrasound of the extremities may be helpful in cases of peripheral nerve compression.

CT of chest, abdomen, and pelvis: These may be needed to assess for malignancy (e.g., thymoma or thymic hyperplasia in myasthenia gravis) or related complications (e.g., inflammatory myopathies are associated with interstitial lung disease).

OTHER
FVC: Obtain this for patients who may have respiratory muscle compromise.

Impression and Plan
Describe the pattern of weakness:
> › Is it acute, subacute, or chronic?
> › Clarify whether the pattern is consistent with an upper motor neuron lesion or lower motor neuron lesion (see Table 13.4).

Localize the lesion along the motor tract:
> › CNS (upper motor neuron):
>> » **Primary motor cortex:** impaired higher cortical functions (typically)
>> » **Centrum semiovale/corona radiata:** unilateral motor and/or sensory findings typically affecting the face, arm, and leg, with unequal distribution of weakness and often without cortical findings
>> » **Internal capsule:** unilateral motor and/or sensory findings often affecting the face, arm, and leg equally
>> » **Brainstem:** long tract signs with or without cranial nerve deficits

» **Spinal cord**[15]: possible sensory level findings, bowel or bladder dysfunction, mixed upper and lower motor neuron findings
› **Peripheral nervous system (lower motor neuron):**
  » **Anterior horn cell:** no sensory symptoms (the anterior horn is technically part of the peripheral nervous system, but it is located in the spinal cord)
  » **Spinal nerve root** (radiculopathy)
  » **Plexus** (brachial or lumbosacral)
  » **Peripheral nerves:** mononeuropathy (single nerve); mononeuritis multiplex (this involves multiple distinct nerves in a random pattern, usually in multiple limbs, and is typically painful); polyneuropathy (this is usually length dependent; affects distal areas first, beginning in the legs; and often starts involving the hands when it reaches the knees)
  » **Neuromuscular junction:** fatigability or facilitation; no sensory symptoms (myasthenia gravis, Lambert-Eaton myasthenic syndrome [LEMS], botulism)
  » **Muscle:** possible findings in the proximal shoulder or hip girdle, typically without sensory symptoms (this suggests inflammatory myopathies; toxic or viral myopathies; critical illness myopathy; toxic or viral myopathies)

Discuss the differential diagnosis: Examples include (note that the differential diagnosis depends on the specific or suspected localization):
› **Vascular:** stroke, TIA, vasculitis
› **Trauma:** compression or traction
› **Inflammatory or autoimmune:** MS; AIDP or chronic inflammatory demyelinating polyneuropathy; myasthenia gravis; necrotizing myopathy; dermatomyositis
› **Infectious:** brain abscess, epidural abscess, leprosy, Lyme disease

Table 13.4. Clinical Features of Upper and Lower Motor Neuron Lesions

FEATURE	UPPER MOTOR NEURON LESION	LOWER MOTOR NEURON LESION
Muscle bulk	Normal (atrophic after months)	Atrophic
Tone	Increased (spastic)	Decreased
Distribution of weakness	Pyramidal pattern (extensors weaker in upper extremities, flexors weaker in lower extremities)	**Distal:** polyneuropathy **Segmental:** radiculopathy **Proximal:** myopathy
Reflexes	Increased	Decreased or Absent
Plantar response	Extensor response	Mute or plantar response

> **Infiltrative:** lymphoma, tuberculosis, sarcoidosis
> **Malignancy:** primary CNS malignancy, lymphoma, metastatic disease
> **Metabolic or toxic:** rhabdomyolysis, organophosphate poisoning, botulism, heavy metal toxicity, chemotherapy, radiation
> **Hereditary:** Charcot-Marie-Tooth disease, muscular dystrophies, mitochondrial disorders, hereditary spastic paresis, myopathies
> **Functional:** conversion disorder, malingering, depression

References

1. Wijdicks E, Bamlet W, Maramattom B, et al. Validation of a new coma scale: the FOUR score. Ann. Neurol. 2005;58(4):585-93. doi: 10.1002/ana.20611
2. Menon B. Neuroimaging in acute stroke. Continuum (Mineap Minn). 2020:26(2):287-309. doi: 10.1212/CON.0000000000000839
3. Vargas B. Acute treatment of migraine. Continuum (Mineap Minn). 2018;24(4, Headache):1032-51. doi: 10.1212/CON.0000000000000639
4. Karsan N, Bose P, Goadsby PJ. The migraine premonitory phase. Continuum (Mineap Minn). 2018;24(4, Headache):996-1008. doi: 10.1212/CON.0000000000000624
5. Chou D. Secondary headache syndromes. Continuum (Mineap Minn). 2018;24(4, Headache):1079-91. doi: 10.1212/CON.0000000000000640
6. Singhal A, Topcuoglu M. Glucocorticoid-associated worsening in reversible cerebral vasoconstriction syndrome. Neurology. 2017;88(3):228-36. doi:10.1212/WNL.0000000000003510
7. Schuele S. Evaluation of seizure etiology from routine testing to genetic evaluation. Continuum (Mineap Minn). 2019;25(2):322-42. doi: 10.1212/CON.0000000000000723
8. Pack A. Epilepsy overview and revised classification of seizures and epilepsies. Continuum (Mineap Minn). 2019;25(2):306-21. doi: 10.1212/CON.0000000000000707
9. Fisher R, Cross J, French J, et al. Operational classification of seizure types by the international league against epilepsy: position paper of the ILAE Commission for Classification and Terminology. Epilepsia. 2017;58(4):522-30. doi: 10.1111/epi.13670
10. Scheffer I, Berkovic S, Capovilla G, et al. ILAE classification of the epilepsies: position paper of the ILAE Commission for Classification and Terminology. Epilepsia. 2017;58(4);512-21. doi: 10.1111/epi.13709
11. National Institutes of Neurological Disorders and Stroke. NIH stroke scale [Internet]. Bestheda (MD): US Department of Health and Human Services; 2003 [cited 2020 Oct 10]. Available from: https://www.stroke.nih.gov/documents/NIH_Stroke_Scale_508C.pdf
12. Rabinstein A. Update on treatment of acute ischemic stroke. Continuum (Mineap Minn). 2020;26(2):268-86. doi: 10.1212/CON.0000000000000840
13. Kim A. Medical management for secondary stroke prevention. Continuum (Mineap Minn). 2020:26(2):435-56. doi: 10.1212/CON.0000000000000849
14. London Z. A structured approach to the diagnosis of peripheral nervous system disorders. Continuum (Mineap Minn). 2020;26(5):1130-60. doi: 10.1212/CON.0000000000000922
15. Kirschblum S, Burns S, Biering-Sorensen F, et al. International standards for neurological classification of spinal cord injury (revised 2011). J Spinal Cord Med. 2011:34(6):535-46. doi: 10.1179/204577211X13207446293695

14

Palliative Medicine

Dr. Arunima Soma Dalai
Dr. Adrianna Gunton
Dr. Jowon L. Kim
Dr. Natanya S. Russek
Dr. Hayden Rubensohn

REVIEWER
Dr. Rose Hatala

Starting Points: Palliative Consultations

These notes are in addition to the **general guide for all consultations** on page 1.

Identification

Follow the **general guide for all consultations.**

Reason for Referral

Examples of reason for referral include assistance in symptom management at the end of life and management of dyspnea in class IV heart failure.

History of Present Illness

Clarify the course in hospital (for inpatients): This includes clarifying the patient's initial presentation.

Clarify details of the leading palliative care diagnosis: Determine the date of diagnosis, dates of recurrence (if oncologic), disease progression, medications, treatments received (chemotherapy, radiation, surgery), and secondary complications.

Conduct a review of systems:
› Ask about pain, dyspnea, nausea and vomiting, bowel function, bladder function, appetite, sleep, confusion, energy, mood, anxiety, pruritus, xerostomia, and hiccups.
› Apply the OPQRST AAA mnemonic.

Past Medical History

Ask about significant medical diagnoses.

Past Surgical History

Pursue this as relevant to the patient's symptoms and major illnesses.

Medications

Ask about:

- all current medications, including nonprescription and herbal medicines
- side effects of medications
- the efficacy of medications for symptom control

Allergies

Follow the **general guide for all consultations**.

Family History

Pursue this if it is relevant to the patient's underlying conditions (family history is often omitted from palliative consultations).

Social History

Ask about:

- the patient's birthplace, hometown, and occupation
- significant family and friends (including names, relationships, and physical proximity), hobbies, clubs
- the role of religion and spirituality in the patient's life, including: how it manifests; how it should be addressed in care; specific beliefs that impact care; spiritual leaders who should be involved in goals of care
  - » Consider using the FICA tool for spiritual history.[1]
- financial stability
- current living situation, current community and home supports in place, safety at home
- substance use
- whether the patient has completed an advanced directive

Functional History

Ask about:

- ADLs (eating, dressing, grooming, bathing, toileting)
- IADLs (cooking, cleaning, laundry, appointments, driving, groceries, finances)
- mobility aids
- equipment at home

- time course of functional decline
- anticipated future needs

Code Status

Ask about:
> the patient's understanding of their diagnosis, disease progression, prognosis, and treatment
> the patient's perception of their quality of life
> the patient's goals for their care in the future (e.g., curative, pain and symptom management, quality of life)
> presence of a power of attorney, surrogate decision maker, advanced directive
> code status

Physical Examination

Vitals signs: This is often omitted for patients at the end of life.

General impression: Assess appearance, cognition, functional status, and mobility.

Relevant signs: Perform a focused exam tailored to the patient's medical history and symptoms.

Neurological: Pursue this if indicated by clinical features or the location of pain; assess cognition, motor functioning, sensation, reflexes, gait, and coordination.

Pain: Consider using tools such as a body map to illustrate sites of pain, or clinical questionnaires such as the Brief Pain Inventory.

Investigations

Pursue relevant blood work and imaging, and determine trends in relevant tumour markers.

Impression and Plan

Provide the leading palliative care diagnosis: Include:
> staging, prognosis
> current treatment plan
> the names of consulting and following physicians
> palliative indicators (use the Palliative Performance Scale [PPS][2] and/or ECOG scale [for oncology patients] [3]).

Describe goals of care:
> List the patient's goals regarding focus of care.
> Indicate the patient's code status.
> Involve the most-responsible physician in significant conversations around code status (they can include a recommendation, if needed).

Break down each symptom: Outline:
> **Etiology:** Provide the most likely cause and a differential for alternative etiologies.
> **Recommended investigations**
> **Management plan:**
>> Organize the plan by priority issue.
>> Include recommendations for titration of therapy.
>> Comment on who will initiate and manage therapy (e.g., palliative care or most-responsible physician).
> **Recommended supports:** These could include allied health involvement and community supports.

Provide care coordination:
> Describe follow-up plans, both in hospital and in the community.
> State whether a palliative care team will continue to follow the patient.

Dyspnea

These notes are in addition to the **general guide for all consultations** on page 1, and the **starting points for palliative consultations** at the beginning of this chapter.

Identification

Key information in the identification statement includes the patient's leading palliative care diagnosis, major comorbidities, and code status.

Reason for Referral

The referral may seek to clarify the etiology of dyspnea and/or appropriate management.

History of Present Illness

Clarify the leading palliative care diagnosis: In addition to standard questions, ask about relevant medical therapy (i.e., LV enhancement therapy, puffers for COPD).

Ask the patient to describe the dyspnea in their own words.

Characterize the dyspnea:
> Apply the OPQRST AAA mnemonic.
> What emotions are associated with the dyspnea?
> Identify associated symptoms (e.g., cough, fever, sputum production, pleuritic chest pain, chest pain, presyncope, weakness, fatigue).

Grade the dyspnea: Consider using a validated tool such as the Edmonton Symptom Assessment System.[4]

Identify risk factors for thromboembolism: Examples include travel, immobilization, hormone use, and active cancer.

Clarify the impact of the dyspnea on functional status.

Past Medical History
- Ask about all medical diagnoses.
- Ask specifically about previous respiratory, cardiac, neurologic, psychiatric, hematologic, and endocrine conditions.

Past Surgical History
Follow the **general guide for all consultations** and the **starting points for palliative consultations.**

Medications
Follow the **general guide for all consultations** and the **starting points for palliative consultations.**

Allergies
Follow the **general guide for all consultations.**

Family History
Consider asking about respiratory and cardiac disorders (family history is often omitted).

Social History
In addition to standard questions, ask about smoking and new environmental exposures (e.g., dust, mould, pets).

Code Status
Follow the **general guide for all consultations** and the **starting points for palliative consultations.**

Physical Examination
Vital signs

General impression:
> › Assess the level of respiratory distress.
> › Look for evidence of anemia.

Signs of respiratory failure: Look stridor, cyanosis, marked tachypnea, tachycardia, and altered level of consciousness.

Cardiovascular (focused exam): Assess for HF, ACS, and valvular disease.

Respiratory (focused exam): Assess muscle use and breathing pattern; assess for posturing, signs of airway obstruction, signs of chronic lung disease, abnormal breath sounds, and presence of effusion.

Abdominal (focused exam): Assess for tense ascites and large masses.

Investigations

- If consistent with the patient's goals and wishes, it is important to do a full workup for other medical causes, even if the cause of dyspnea seems obvious (e.g., metastatic lung cancer).
- Generally, avoid investigations when the patient is at the end of life.

LABORATORY INVESTIGATIONS

CBC

Hemoglobin

Electrolytes

Creatinine

Liver function tests

Blood gas: Try to order venous blood gas instead of ABG since the latter can be quite painful, unless clinically indicated.

Peak flow, maximum inhalation pressure, maximum exhalation pressure: Consider these if there is concern for obstructive disease or neuromuscular weakness.

MICROBIOLOGY

Blood, sputum, urine cultures: Pursue these as indicated on suspicion for infection.

IMAGING

Chest x-ray: Assess for pneumonia, CHF exacerbation, mass, and effusion.

ECG: Pursue this to rule out a cardiac cause.

CT of the chest: Consider on suspicion of a mass lesion or metastases.

CT for PE or V/Q scan: Consider this if clinically indicated.

Echocardiogram: Consider this as clinically indicated in patients with a significant cardiac history or underlying malignancy (patients with malignancy are at risk of pericardial effusion and/or tamponade, which can contribute to dyspnea).

Impression and Plan

GENERAL APPROACH

Focus on reversible causes of dyspnea: Balance judicious use of investigations with appropriate workup so as not to miss reversible causes.

Confirm symptoms with the patient: Dyspnea is a subjective symptom that the patient needs to confirm.

Clinical signs may not correlate with dyspnea: Pulmonary function tests and oxygen saturation, in particular, may not correlate with dyspnea.

Consider whether to check oxygen saturation: Generally avoid checking oxygen saturation if the patient is at the end of life.

Include the patient's goals of care.

LEADING PALLIATIVE CARE DIAGNOSIS

Outline a plan for the leading palliative care diagnosis: Include relevant investigations and treatments.

Consult specialists as indicated: On suspicion of the leading palliative care diagnosis as the cause of dyspnea, consult relevant specialists for the management plan.

DYSPNEA

Keep the differential diagnosis broad: The etiology of dyspnea is often multifactorial; consider respiratory, cardiac, neurologic, hematologic, endocrine, and psychiatric causes.

Optimize medical therapy as a priority: Consider whether the patient's medical therapy for the most likely etiology is optimal; if not, optimize the medical therapy.

Include pharmacologic and nonpharmacologic treatment in the management plan:
› **Pharmacologic treatment:** opioids, benzodiazepines
› **Nonpharmacologic treatment:** mobility aids, exercise, breathing techniques (this has the most supportive evidence), use of a fan, controlled air humidity and flow, head-of-bed angle, relaxation techniques

Use opioids judiciously: Typically, dyspnea requires lower doses of opioids than pain.
› For opioid-naive patients, consider starting with hydromorphone 0.25 mg orally every hour as needed.
› If the patient reports activities that provoke dyspnea, consider dosing 15 minutes before those activities; monitor the patient's opioid use to determine the benefit of regular dosing.

Constant dyspnea requires constant opioids: It may require immediate regular dosing; if the dyspnea doesn't disturb the patient at night, a reasonable starting frequency is 4 times per day.

Use oxygen therapy appropriately:
› Oxygen therapy is generally only beneficial for hypoxemic patients (some exceptions apply, such as COPD patients).
› For nonhypoxemic patients, any air flow may help (e.g., via a fan) for relieving symptoms of dyspnea.

Nausea and Vomiting

These notes are in addition to the **general guide for all consultations** on page 1, and the **starting points for palliative consultations** at the beginning of this chapter.

Identification

Follow the **general guide for all consultations.**

Reason for Referral

The referral may seek to clarify the etiology of nausea and vomiting, and/or clarify appropriate management.

History of Present Illness

Clarify why the patient has sought care: For inpatients, clarify the course in hospital.

Clarify nausea history: Ask about:

› triggers, onset
› associated symptoms
  » rumination about eating (check whether the patient has had a psychiatric screen)
  » dizziness, motion sickness
  » anxiety
  » medications (especially opioids, chemotherapy)
› frequency
› intensity and fluctuation

Clarify vomiting history: Ask about:

› frequency
› inciting and relieving factors
› associated symptoms
  » abdominal pain (apply the OPQRST AAA mnemonic)
  » reflux or GERD (distinguish emesis from passive regurgitation)
  » difficulty swallowing
  » early satiety, flatulence
  » symptoms of increased intracranial pressure (morning headache, altered level of consciousness, cranial neuropathies, headaches worse with coughing or Valsalva maneuver)
› blood or bright green emesis
› appetite (ability to keep food down, hydration status, typical intake)
› bowel movements (constipation, bloating)
  » symptoms of gastric stasis, ileus, or obstruction
  » diarrhea (assess for infectious causes)
› prior treatments

Conduct a review of systems: Follow the starting points for palliative consultations.

Past Medical History
Follow the **general guide for all consultations** and the **starting points for palliative consultations.**

Surgical History
Follow the **general guide for all consultations** and the **starting points for palliative consultations.**

Medications
Ask about medications that cause constipation or have known side effects of nausea and vomiting.

Allergies
Follow the **general guide for all consultations.**

Family history
Follow the **general guide for all consultations** and the **starting points for palliative consultations.**

Social History
Ask about cannabis use.

Physical Examination
Vital signs
General impression: pallor, jaundice, alertness, fatigue
Head and neck: tumours, dentition
> **Oral lesions:** *Candida*, CMV (AIDS), HSV in immunocompromised patients
> **Meningeal irritation:** intracerebral tumours and bony metastases to base of skull

Abdominal: ascites, hepatosplenomegaly, abdominal distension, signs of obstruction (e.g., high-pitched bowel sounds)
Lines and tubes: nasogastric tube

Investigations
LABORATORY INVESTIGATIONS
CBC with differential
Ca (preferably ionized)
Electrolytes
Creatinine, urea

Liver enzymes
Thyrotropin (TSH)
Stool investigations: Pursue this on suspicion of infectious etiology.

IMAGING

Abdominal x-ray: Pursue this to rule out fecal loading and constipation.

CT of the head: Assess for intracranial metastases and increased intracranial pressure.

Impression and Plan

DIFFERENTIAL DIAGNOSIS

The differential for nausea and vomiting is broad and often classified according to mechanism[5]:

- **Drugs:** Opioids and metabolic waste accumulation (hypercalcemia) can trigger a variety of receptors, typically the chemotherapy-trigger zone in the CNS.
- **Gastric stasis:** Ascites, hepatomegaly, PUD, gastritis, anticholinergics, and opioids can trigger acetylcholine (ACh) and dopamine-2 (D2) receptors in the GI tract.
- **GI stretch:** Intestinal obstruction via metastases or constipation can trigger ACh, D2, and 5-HT3 receptors in the GI tract, triggering nausea and vomiting.
- **Infectious cause:** Consider GI tract infections including colitis and gastroenteritis, and extraintestinal sources such as meningitis; immunocompromised patients and those with frequent health-care exposures may be at increased risk for opportunistic or hospital-acquired pathogens, respectively.
- **Raised intracranial pressure:** Causes include meningeal irritation, skull metastases, cerebral infection, and intracranial tumour, edema, or bleeding, which can stimulate D2, ACh, and histamine$_1$ (H1) receptors in the CNS.
- **Motion sickness:** This is more common in ambulatory patients on opioids, which affect H1 and mu receptors in the CNS.
- **Anxiety:** This can centre on the patient's illness or arise in anticipation of treatment.

PLAN

Consider the patient's goals of care: Make sure any proposed treatment aligns with their goals.

Consider nonpharmacologic measures: Reduce nauseating environmental stimuli

› Minimize unpleasant odours from infected and/or necrotic tumours.

› Provide small meals, cool fizzy drinks, and ginger.

Consider pharmacologic management: Identify 1 or several etiologies, determine the neurotransmitters involved, and provide antagonist therapy (see Table 14.1).

› Choose 1 antiemetic at a time when possible.[5]

Consider surgical management: This could include venting a gastrostomy tube or nasogastric tube.

Table 14.1. Common Pharmacologic Treatments for Nausea and Vomiting[6]

DRUG AND CLASS	RECEPTORS	INDICATIONS
Butyrophenones Haloperidol	D2 (CNS)	Opioid-induced Chemical, metabolic-induced
Prokinetics Metoclopramide Domperidone	Mainly D2 (CNS + GI)	Gastric stasis, ileus
Phenothiazines Prochlorperazine	D2 (CNS + GI), H1, ACh	GI obstruction, peritoneal irritation, raised ICP, vestibular causes, N/V NYD
Antihistamines Diphenhydramine	mACh, H1	
Anticholinergics Scopolamine	mACh	GI obstruction, peritoneal irritation, raised ICP, excess secretions
5-HT3 antagonists Ondansetron	5-HT3 (CNS + GI)	Chemotherapy, abdominal radiotherapy, postoperative
NK1 antagonists Aprepitant	NK1	Late-onset chemotherapy related
Steroids Dexamethasone	CNS receptors	Brain metastases, chemotherapy, malignant bowel obstruction
Cannabinoids Nabilone	Cannabinoid receptors	Chemotherapy, radiotherapy

Abbreviations: ACh: acetylcholine; mACh: muscarinic acetylcholine; CNS: central nervous system; D2: dopamine-2; GI: gastrointestinal; H1: histamine$_1$; ICP: intracranial pressure; N/V NYD: nausea and vomiting, not yet determined

Pain Management

These notes are in addition to the **general guide for all consultations** on page 1, and the **starting points for palliative consultations** at the beginning of this chapter.

Identification

Follow the general guide for all consultations.

Reason for Referral

The referral may seek to clarify the cause of pain and/or appropriate management.

History of Present Illness

Clarify the patient's pain history: Use the OPQRST AAA mnemonic with special attention to:

› **Characterization of pain:** Ask about nociceptive pain (aching, throbbing, gnawing, cramping) versus neuropathic pain (numbness, burning, shooting, tingling, and sensations of hot or cold).

› **Impacts on the patient:** Ask about how it affects quality of life, ADLs, and functioning.

› **Total pain:** Ask about social, existential, and psychological contributors to pain.

Determine pharmacologic and nonpharmacologic treatment strategies to date.

Past Medical History

Follow the general guide for all consultations and the starting points for palliative consultations.

Past Surgical History

Follow the general guide for all consultations and the starting points for palliative consultations.

Medications

- Obtain a detailed account of the patient's current pain control regimen, including doses, intervals, routes, and duration of pain control.
  › Ask about opioid and nonopioid analgesics, and adjuvant medications.
  › Ask about as-needed medications: determine usage per day, triggers for using, and efficacy.
- Ask about previous pain medications tried (determine doses if possible) and the reasons for discontinuing these medications.

Allergies
In addition to standard questions, ask about opioid side effects to distinguish allergy from side effects.

Family History
Follow the **general guide for all consultations** and the **starting points for palliative consultations.**

Social History
In addition to standard questions, ask specifically about:
- social, spiritual, and financial aspects of the patient's life, and their potential contribution to total pain
- risk factors for opioid abuse or diversion
  - › Consider assessing with a standardized tool such as the Opioid Risk Tool.[7]
  - › Risk factors are not a contraindication to the use of opioids for pain management in a palliative setting, but the patient plan must address them.

Code Status
Follow the **general guide for all consultations** and the **starting points for palliative consultations.**

Physical Examination
Vital signs
Relevant signs: Perform a focused exam tailored to the patient's medical history and symptoms.

Investigations
LABORATORY INVESTIGATIONS
CBC
Electrolytes and extended electrolytes
Creatinine, urea
Liver enzymes

IMAGING
Pursue imaging as indicated on suspicion of a mass or metastases contributing to the pain.

Impression and Plan
GENERAL APPROACH
- Consult the World Health Organization's analgesic ladder for pain management.[8]

- Morphine is a good first-line opioid analgesic: whenever possible, provide it orally.
  › Be cautious with morphine dosing in patients with renal failure.
- Continuous pain requires continuous analgesia.
  › Start with a short-acting formulation every 4 hours to achieve good control; when the pain is stable, switch to a long-acting formulation every 12 hours.
  › **Do not** use transdermal fentanyl for uncontrolled pain or opioid-naive patients.
- Adjust the plan to reflect the patient's goals of care.

BREAKTHROUGH PAIN

- The starting dose is 10% of the total daily dose and given every hour as needed (usually, the as-needed medication is the same opioid as for baseline treatment).
- Reassess pain control if the patient is using 3 to 4 as-needed doses in 24 hours.
- Distinguish breakthrough pain from end-of-dose failure (end-of dose failure requires an increase in the baseline opioid dose, rather than an increase in as-needed doses or a decrease in the baseline dosing interval).
- When increasing the baseline dose, also increase the as-needed dose.

SWITCHING TO TRANSDERMAL FENTANYL

- Calculate the 24-hour morphine milligram equivalents (MME) and refer to Table 14.2 for conversion.
- Overlap the transdermal fentanyl and current opioid by 8 to 16 hours.
- Do not titrate the dose for at least 3 days.
- Use morphine or hydromorphone for breakthrough pain: convert the fentanyl dose to a 24-hour MME and then calculate the breakthrough dose.

ADJUVANT MEDICATIONS

Add adjuvant medications in patients who have a suboptimal response to the main analgesic or neuropathic pain.

- **Neuropathic pain:** TCAs (nortriptyline, amitriptyline), gabapentin, pregabalin, duloxetine
- **Pain due to swelling or compression with inflammation:** dexamethasone
- **Malignant bowel obstruction:** octreotide, dexamethasone
- **Bone pain:** bisphosphonates, calcitonin, dexamethasone, NSAIDs, gabapentin, radiation

Table 14.2. Calculating Morphine Milligram Equivalents (MME)[9]

OPIOID (IN MG/DAY EXCEPT WHEN NOTED)	CONVERSION FACTOR*
Codeine	0.15
Fentanyl transdermal (mcg/hr)**	2.4
Hydrocodone	1
Hydromorphone	4
Methadone	
1–20 mg/day	4
21–40 mg/day	8
41–60 mg/day	10
≥ 61–80 mg/day	12
Morphine	1
Oxycodone	1.5
Oxymorphone	3

*Use caution when prescribing ≥ 50 MME per day.

**Note that transdermal fentanyl is dosed in mcg/hr, and absorption can be affected by heat and other factors.

NONPHARMACOLOGICAL APPROACHES

- Consider radiation therapy, palliative surgery, transcutaneous nerve stimulation, cryoablation, radiofrequency ablation, embolization, nerve blocks, and PT and occupational therapy.
- Consider how social, existential, and psychological factors contribute to the patient's total pain, and address these through appropriate supports (e.g., psychological support, spiritual counselling, community supports, social-worker assessment).

OPIOID SIDE EFFECTS

- Prevention of common side effects includes:
  › **Constipation:** Provide regular senna with or without polyethylene glycol.
  › **Nausea:** This usually resolves after 3 to 5 days; consider short-term metoclopramide, haloperidol, or olanzapine.
  › **Somnolence:** This usually resolves after 3 to 5 days.
    » If persistent, reevaluate the dose or consider switching to another opioid.
    » For effective pain control with excess sedation, consider the addition of a psychostimulant (methylphenidate is usually preferred).

- Consider opioid rotation:
  › Reasons to rotate opioids include dose-limiting side effects and signs of opioid neurotoxicity.
  › Calculate the equianalgesic dose MME (see Table 14.2) and reduce the new dose by 20% to 30%.

ACUTE PAIN CRISES

- Provide parenteral opioids (subcutaneous administration is preferred because IV administration has a quick onset and quick decline).
- High-dose corticosteroids may be appropriate in specific scenarios.

Wish for Hastened Death

These notes are in addition to the **general guide for all consultations** on page 1, and the **starting points for palliative consultations** at the beginning of this chapter.

Identification

Follow the **general guide for all consultations**.

Reason for Referral

The referral may seek to clarify the reasons for seeking hastened death and/or appropriate management.

History of Present Illness

Clarify the course in hospital (for inpatients): This includes clarifying the patient's initial presentation.

Clarify details of the leading palliative care diagnosis: Determine the date of diagnosis, dates of recurrence (if oncologic), disease progression, medications, treatments received (chemotherapy, radiation, surgery), and secondary complications.

Clarify details of the patient's wish for hastened death: Determine the timeline, triggers, motivations, evolution, and prior history.

Conduct a psychosocial review of systems: Ask about:
  › Psychiatric conditions: depression, anxiety, suicidal ideation, guilt, anticipatory grief
  › Social distress: loss of privacy, loss of control, burden to others, loss of autonomy, loss of dignity
  › Illness-related concerns: level of independence, death anxiety

Conduct a general review of systems: Follow the starting points on palliative consultations.

Identify actions demonstrating a desire to die: Examples include a voluntarily decreased oral intake and refusal of life-sustaining treatments (e.g., enteral feeding, debrillators).

Past Medical History
Follow the **general guide for all consultations** and the **starting points for palliative consultations.**

Past Surgical History
Follow the **general guide for all consultations** and the **starting points for palliative consultations.**

Medications
Ask about all current medications.

Allergies
Follow the **general guide for all consultations.**

Family History
Follow the **general guide for all consultations** and the **starting points for palliative consultations.**

Social History
In addition to standard questions, specifically review the patient's social support system:
- Do the patient's caregivers have conflicts of interest? For example, is there concern that caregivers have financial interest in a specific plan or outcome?
- What roles do the current caregivers have? Are there concerns about caregiver burnout?
- What community supports are in place for the patient?

Code Status
Follow the **general guide for all consultations** and the **starting points for palliative consultations.**

Physical Examination
Vital signs
Relevant signs: Perform a focused exam tailored to the patient's medical history and symptoms.
Psychiatric assessment:
› Look for an underlying primary or concurrent mood disorder.
› Consider standardized tools (e.g., Patient Health Questionnaire-9, Generalized Anxiety Disorder-7 scale).

Capacity assessment: Consider a formal capacity assessment.

Investigations

Pursue relevant blood work and imaging.

Impression and Plan

Describe the patient's disease status: Include staging, prognosis, and PPS.

Discuss the patient's wish for hastened death:
> The goal is to understand and communicate underlying factors.
> Give your clinical impression of what is driving the wish for hastened death. Is it a true wish to die, a plea for help, or an expression of suffering?
> If the patient is interested in medical assistance in dying (MAID):
>> For inpatients, the attending palliative care physician can provide guidance on initiating a discussion with the patient and relevant allied health team members.
>> The patient must be competent: they may require capacity assessment.
>> The patient requires assessment from 2 independent physicians.

Describe the patient's goals of care: Include:
> The preferred type of treatment: Options usually include: 1) palliative care (i.e., best supportive care); 2) palliative sedation therapy (when/if it's appropriate); and 3) MAID.
> The desire for symptom relief, life-prolonging measures, and/or MAID: *For example:* "The patient expresses that their main goal is to reduce symptoms of pain as much as possible in order to spend the time she has remaining with her family" or "The patient feels that their disease has caused intolerable suffering and wishes to die."
> Code status

Discuss the main physical and psychosocial impacts of the patient's disease as appropriate: Consider:
> additional treatments to address the physical and psychosocial impacts of their illness
> additional workup to identify the underlying causes of distress-inducing symptoms
> ways to help the patient find meaning in life
> symptom management (e.g., pain control, antiemetics, antidepressants, oncology consultation)
> psychosocial support (e.g., psychiatry or chaplain referral)

References

1. Puchalski C, Romer A. Taking a spiritual history allows clinicians to understand patients more fully. J Palliat Med. 2000;3(1):129-37. doi: 10.1089/jpm.2000.3.129
2. Anderson F, Downing G, Hill J, et al. Palliative performance scale (PPS): a new tool. J Palliat Care. 1996;12(1):5-11. PMID: 8857241

3. Oken M, Creech R, Tormey D, et al. Toxicity and response criteria of the Eastern Cooperative Oncology Group. Am J Clin Oncol. 1982;5(6):649-56. PMID: 7165009

4. Watanabe S, Nekolaichuk C, Beaumont C. The Edmonton Symptom Assessment System, a proposed tool for distress screening in cancer patients: development and refinement. Psychooncology. 2011;21(9):977-85. doi: 10.1002/pon.1996

5. Pereira J. The Pallium palliative pocketbook. 2nd ed. Ottawa: Pallium Canada; 2016. Chapter 8, Gastrointestinal problems; sections 8-1 to 8-22.

6. Hardy J, Glare P, Yates P, et al. Palliation of nausea and vomiting. In: Churney N, Fallon M, Kaasa S, et al, editors. Oxford textbook of palliative medicine. 5th ed. Oxford (UK): Oxford University Press; 2015. p. 661-73.

7. Webster L, Webster R. Predicting aberrant behaviors in opioid-treated patients: preliminary validation of the Opioid Risk Tool. Pain Med. 2005;6(6):432-42. doi: 10.1111/j.1526-4637.2005.00072.x

8. World Health Organization. Cancer pain relief [Internet]. Geneva: WHO; 1986 [cited 2022 Feb 27]. Available from: http://apps.who.int/iris/handle/10665/43944

9. Centers for Disease Control and Prevention (US). MME for commonly prescribed drugs [Internet]. [Atlanta]: Centers for Disease Control and Prevention; [updated 2021 Feb 17; cited 2022 Feb 23]. Available from: https://www.cdc.gov/opioids/providers/prescribing/guideline.html#anchor_1561563251

15

Respirology

Dr. Omri A. Arbiv
Dr. Shaun R. Ong
Dr. Mosaab Alam

REVIEWER
Dr. Janice M. Leung

Starting Points: Respirology Consultations

These notes are in addition to the **general guide for all consultations** on page 1.

Identification

Follow the **general guide for all consultations**.

Reason for Referral

The referral may seek to confirm a diagnosis of respiratory illness and/or clarify appropriate management.

History of Present Illness

Clarify the patient's current respiratory capacity:

> › This is usually quantified (e.g., with walking distance, ability to climb stairs).
> › Make sure that the limitation in respiratory capacity is not due to chest pain (which may indicate cardiac disease), or other nonrespiratory causes (e.g., osteoarthritis).
> › Ask about previous respiratory capacity and how this has changed over time.
> › Consider consulting the Modified Medical Research Council (mMRC) dyspnea scale[1] or the New York Heart Association (NYHA) classification.[2]
> › Ask about associated symptoms such as wheezing, orthopnea, and edema.

Assess coughing symptoms:
> Ask about frequency and triggers (e.g., scents, weather, exercise, pets, occupation), and whether the cough is productive.
> If it is productive, identify the quantity and colour of sputum; ask about hemoptysis.
> Ask how the cough compares to any usual cough or previous exacerbations.

Past Medical History

Ask about:

- **Respiratory conditions:** Determine results of previous pulmonary function testing if available (FEV_1, FVC, FEV_1/FVC, TLC, and diffusing capacity for carbon monoxide; 6-minute walk test).
- **Current or previous respirology follow-up**
- **Other conditions:** Key conditions include thromboembolic disease, rheumatologic disease (especially seropositive conditions), cardiac disease (dyspnea may be secondary to HF), and immunosuppressive conditions (these predispose patients to infections).

Medications

Ask about:

- **Oxygen:** Determine flow rate (in litres) at rest and with activity; and hours per day of use.
- **Inhalers:** Assess the patient's technique and frequency of use.
- **Antibiotics**
- **Immunosuppressive medications:** If the patient is immunosuppressed, is *Pneumocystis jiroveci* prophylaxis used?
- **Medications that can cause interstitial lung disease:**
  > Common agents include amiodarone, bleomycin, busulfan, methotrexate, and nitrofurantoin.
  > Consult www.pneumotox.com.

Allergies

Follow the **general guide for all consultations**.

Family History

Ask about relevant respiratory disease (e.g., lung cancer, asthma).

Social History

Ask about:

- **Smoking:**
  > Clarify cigarettes smoked per day and total pack-years for patients who smoked; if a patient stopped smoking, determine when.

> Ask about other substances (e-cigarettes, marijuana, recreational drugs).
- **Use of biofuels in the home:** For example, does the patient have a wood-burning oven indoors?
- **Organic material that may cause lung disease (i.e., hypersensitivity pneumonitis [HP]):**
  > Ask about regular interactions with animals (e.g., pets).
  > Assess for exposure to other organic material (e.g., hot tubs, molds).
- **Inorganic material that may cause lung disease (i.e., pneumoconioses):** Ask about exposures through sandblasting, hard rock mining, quarry work, and stonecutting (this is relevant to silicosis); coal mining (coal worker pneumoconiosis); asbestos mining, shipyard work, construction, and work with insulation and brake linings (asbestos); work with fluorescent light bulbs, with nuclear weapons, with electronics, and in the aerospace industry (berylliosis).
- **Infection risks:**
  > Ask about risk factors for TB (contact with known TB cases, incarceration, time on Indigenous reserves, time in low or middle-income countries).
  > Ask about recent travel, sick contacts.

Physical Examination

Vital signs: Specifically check oxygen saturation and mode, temperature, and respiratory rate.

General impression: Assess respiratory effort and sentence length, and check for purse-lipped breathing and clubbing.

Cardiovascular:
> Auscultate the heart.
> Assess the patient's volume status: check for peripheral edema and ascites, and assess JVP.

Respiratory:
> Auscultate and percuss the lungs.
> Inspect and palpate the chest for abnormal breathing patterns.

Investigations

LABORATORY INVESTIGATIONS

CBC with differential: Don't forget the differential for WBCs (eosinophils can provide an important clue).

ABG: If this is not available, order venous blood gas.

Electrolytes, creatinine, liver enzymes: These may be important for treatment options.

BNP, CRP: Pursue these based on clinical context.

Rheumatologic workup: This may be important, especially for seropositive disease (review the patient's prior investigations to see if a workup has already been done).

IMAGING

Imaging is of utmost importance in respirology. Make sure you look at all imaging and reports yourself. Call the radiologist directly if your specific questions are not addressed in the report or if further information is required.

Chest x-ray:
› Pursue this for every patient, preferably a posterior-anterior view and a lateral view.
› Compare current imaging to previous imaging.

CT of the chest:
› It is important to review previous radiology: How has the disease progressed over time? Was it seen previously?
› Previous CTs of the abdomen or head sometimes provide views of the chest if no previous chest CTs are available.

Echocardiogram:
› This may be helpful in determining risk for pulmonary edema.
› Review prior studies; consider ordering a new study if there is a specific indication.

OTHER INVESTIGATIONS

Pulmonary function tests (PFTs): Compare current and previous results to establish a pattern over time.

Cultures and pathology: Check for recent investigations and order new investigations as indicated.

ECG: Assess for signs of right heart strain (e.g., right axis deviation, RBBB or incomplete RBBB, inferior and anterior T wave inversions).

Impression and Plan

- Consider common and uncommon causes of the patient's symptoms.
- Most respiratory symptoms can be explained by 1 of the following:
  › pulmonary edema
  › infection (usually pneumonia)
  › obstructive diseases (asthma or COPD)
  › pulmonary emboli
- Make sure to address the common diseases that cause respiratory symptoms.
- Imaging often guides decision-making and planning.

Hemoptysis

These notes are in addition to the **general guide for all consultations** on page 1, and the **starting points for respirology consultations** at the beginning of this chapter.

Identification

Follow the general guide for all consultations.

Reason for Referral

- The referral may seek to clarify the cause of hemoptysis and/or appropriate management.

- The referral may quantify the hemoptysis if it is massive (definitions vary between >100–600 mL over 24 hours; usually enough hemoptysis to cause desaturations is concerning).

History of Present Illness

Determine the progression of the hemoptysis over time.

Quantify the hemoptysis: Is it teaspoons? Is it cups?

Ask about the colour of the sputum:
> Dark red indicates older blood; bright red indicates an ongoing bleed and is more worrisome.
> Pus mixed with blood suggests an infectious etiology.

Ask about exercise capacity.

Assess for rheumatologic symptoms: Ask about:
> joint stiffness (RA)
> skin thickening, Raynaud phenomenon, dysphagia, digital ulceration (scleroderma)
> proximal muscle weakness, photosensitive rash (dermatomyositis, polymyositis)
> sicca symptoms (i.e., dry mouth or dry eyes [Sjögren syndrome])

Assess for symptoms of vasculitis: Examples include active sediment, peripheral edema, and purpuric rash.

Ask about key risk factors: These include infection, PE, malignancy, and coagulopathy.

Try to rule out a GI bleed:
> GI bleeds are much more common and can masquerade as hemoptysis.
> Ask about nausea, vomiting, diarrhea, and hematochezia.
> Ensure that bleeding is associated with coughing.

Past Medical History
- Ask about previous hemoptysis history.
- Pay special attention to:
  - › respiratory conditions, particularly structural lung disease (e.g., bronchiectasis)
  - › conditions that predispose to HF
  - › systemic infections or predisposition to infections (TB can be a common culprit in high-risk populations)

Medications
Focus on new medications and anticoagulants.

Allergies
Follow the **general guide for all consultations**.

Family History
Ask about:
- lung cancer and lung disease
- rheumatologic disease
- hereditary hemorrhagic telangiectasia
- cystic fibrosis

Social History
Focus on lung cancer risk and smoking history.

Physical Examination
Vital signs: Take particular note of oxygen saturation and respiratory rate.

Nose: Examine the nostrils for polyps.

Cardiovascular: Assess for murmurs (especially mitral stenosis), symptoms of cor pulmonale, and HF.

Respiratory: Follow the starting points for respirology consultations.

Extremities: Look for clubbing, signs of DVT, and palpable purpura.

Joints: Perform a joint exam as clinically indicated.

Dermatological: Assess for telangiectasia and rash.

Investigations
LABORATORY INVESTIGATIONS
CBC, INR, PTT

Electrolytes, creatinine, urinalysis, urine microscopy: In pulmonary-renal syndrome, expect to see RBCs and protein in the urine.

Sputum culture, blood culture: Pursue these if appropriate.

Other:
> **On concern for diffuse alveolar hemorrhage:** ANA, rheumatoid factor, anti-cyclic citrullinated peptide (anti-CCP), C3, C4, CK, antineutrophil cytoplasmic antibody, HBV, HCV, HIV, antiphospholipid antibodies, anti-glomerular basement membrane
> **On concern for TB:** 3 sputum acid-fast bacilli and mycobacterial cultures

IMAGING

Chest X-Ray
Assess for masses, lobar atelectasis (could indicate a mass), cavitation, and consolidation.

CT of the Chest
Order specific x-rays based on clinical suspicion (almost all patients will need a chest x-ray).
CT PE protocol: Pursue this on high suspicion of PE.
CT angiogram:
> Pursue this if you don't order a CT PE protocol.
> It can help identify the source of bleeding and may guide interventions.
CT without contrast:
> This can help identify large lesions, bronchiectasis, and consolidations.
> Consider the impact on kidney function, depending on the magnitude of hemoptysis.

OTHER INVESTIGATIONS
Echocardiogram: Check in particular for mitral stenosis as a cause for hemoptysis.

Impression and Plan
Triage quickly:
> Massive hemoptysis is a medical emergency.
> Begin immediate monitoring of the patient and establish goals of care.
> Involve critical care early.
  » **Asphyxiation from hemoptysis:** It will be very difficult to secure the airway: involve a clinician skilled with airway management.
  » **Intubation plan:** Use the largest bore endotracheal tube; consider single lung ventilation to protect the unaffected lung or a bronchial blocker.
Position the patient with the bleeding side facing down: This directs blood away from the nonbleeding side.

Identify the cause of hemoptysis:
> The cause may be clear from previous investigations (e.g., if a large cancer or bronchiectasis is identified).
> The most-common causes are bronchitis, bronchiectasis, and lung cancer.

Consider bronchoscopy:
> This can be useful in select instances.
> If oxygenation is tenuous, wait until the patient is intubated.
> Uses for bronchoscopy include:
>> confirming diffuse alveolar hemorrhage (serial lavages will show increasingly bloody returns)
>> identifying the site of bleeding
>> advance workup for infection or malignancy
>> certain therapeutic interventions as a bridge to a hemostatic procedure (e.g., involve interventional pulmonology, interventional radiology, or thoracic surgery early)

Consider angiography: This is often used to embolize bleeding, especially in emergencies.

Treat the underlying cause: For example, treat infection and reverse coagulopathy.

Consider tranexamic acid: This is not well studied, but is unlikely to do harm.

Interstitial Lung Disease

These notes are in addition to the **general guide for all consultations** on page 1, and the **starting points for respirology consultations** at the beginning of this chapter.

Identification

Key information in the identification statement includes the patient's chief complaint and the primary radiographic pattern.

Reason for Referral

The referral typically seeks assessment and management of changes in interstitial lung disease (ILD) identified on imaging, which may or may not manifest with clinical abnormalities in gas exchange.

‖‖

BEFORE YOU SEE THE PATIENT

Review the patient's radiology: the radiographic pattern often guides the differential diagnosis and assessment.

- Chest x-ray lacks sensitivity as a screening tool, but is usually a first-line test.
  - › Look for volume loss or gross architectural distortion.
  - › Look for coarse reticular lines.
- What is the radiographic pattern of the ILD on CT?
  - › **Definite usual interstitial pneumonia (UIP):** honeycombing
  - › **Probable UIP:** subpleural or basal-predominant changes
  - › **Indeterminate for UIP:** changes that are not typical of UIP, or not yet differentiated enough
  - › **Changes consistent with an alternate diagnosis**
- In radiographic changes consistent with an alternate diagnosis or indeterminate for UIP, consider whether the changes fit other patterns of ILD, including:
  - › nonspecific interstitial pneumonia
  - › organizing pneumonia
  - › respiratory bronchiolitis-ILD or desquamative interstitial pneumonia
  - › lymphoid interstitial pneumonia
- Consider whether any features suggest a diagnosis (whether fibrotic lung disease or not).
  - › HF and atypical infection-related changes are common.
  - › Peribronchovascular nodules and hilar adenopathy may be consistent with sarcoidosis.
  - › Centrilobular nodules and gas trapping suggest HP.
- Are the radiographic features more in keeping with acute or chronic changes?
- Is there a previous imaging study to compare with?

History of Present Illness

Assess presenting symptoms: These are typically:
- › dyspnea
- › cough
- › decreased exercise tolerance

Establish the time course of the disease.

Ask about symptoms consistent with HF.

Ask about symptoms or risk factors for infection: Check for:
> purulent sputum, fever, acute cough
> sick contacts, recent travel, immunocompromised states

Ask about symptoms that suggest an underlying connective tissue disease (CTD):
> joint stiffness (RA)
> skin thickening, Raynaud phenomenon, dysphagia, digital ulceration (scleroderma)
> proximal muscle weakness, photosensitive rash (dermatomyositis, polymyositis)
> sicca symptoms (i.e., dry mouth or dry eyes [Sjögren syndrome])

Ask about symptoms that suggest GERD.

Past Medical History

Ask about:
- CTD, and whether it is well or poorly controlled
- malignancy (especially adenocarcinoma) and how it was treated (e.g., pneumotoxic agents, radiation)
- GERD

Medications

- If the patient has been previously treated with chemotherapy, determine the details of the regimen (e.g., bleomycin, cyclophosphamide) and its duration.
- Ask about exposure to other pneumotoxic medications (e.g., methotrexate, nitrofurantoin).

Allergies

Follow the **general guide for all consultations.**

Family History

Ask about ILD, particularly familial idiopathic pulmonary fibrosis (IPF).

Social History

Key information includes agents that cause HP or pneumoconioses.

Physical Examination

Vital signs: Note that patients usually have an elevated respiratory rate; those on home oxygen usually have advanced disease.

General impression: Patients usually exhibit increased work of breathing.

Cardiovascular: Screen for HF.

Respiratory:
> Listen for coarse "velcro" crackles, generally associated with honeycombing.

> Assess for preserved to decreased inspiratory-to-expiratory ratio.

Neurological: Look for proximal muscle weakness.

Hands: Check for:
> clubbing
> digital ulceration, Raynaud phenomenon, sclerodactyly, calcinosis cutis
> inflamed joints
> nicotine stains

Dermatological: Check for:
> skin changes in dermatomyositis (shawl sign, holster sign, Gottron papules, "mechanic's hands," heliotrope rash)
> general skin changes associated with CTD

Investigations

LABORATORY INVESTIGATIONS

CBC: Assess for evidence of infection.

Standard screening labs for metabolic disease

BNP: Pursue this to exclude CHF (note that RV failure can confound this assessment).

CK: Assess for myositis (note that CK can be normal in amyopathic disease).

CTD screen: Order:
> ANA by ELISA (if negative, consider ANA by immunofluorescence in the context of a high pretest probability of CTD)
> rheumatoid factor, anti-CCP antibodies
> C3 and C4
> myositis panel

PULMONARY FUNCTION TESTING

- In ILD, PFTs primarily show a pattern consistent with restrictive lung disease.
- ILD is associated with a decreased diffusing capacity for carbon monoxide.
- Look for gas trapping, which may indicate HP.

Impression and Plan

Consult specialists:
> ILD requires assessment by a respirologist.
> It often also requires a multidisciplinary approach (respirology, pathology, and radiology) to determine if surgical lung biopsies are necessary for diagnosis and further management.

Aim to answer 5 questions:
1) Is there an underlying ILD?

» This is usually indicated by changes evident on CT that have no other probable explanation (i.e., reticular lines without evidence of HF).

2) If so, what is the most likely etiology based on clinical, biochemical, and radiographic information?

» If no etiology is found, the disease could be idiopathic, but consider whether a surgical lung biopsy is required and whether the patient would tolerate this procedure.

3) Is there a component of disease that is active and/or may be reversible with steroids?

» HP is an example of steroid-reversible disease.

» Active disease is usually indicated by a decline in function assessed clinically and associated with "ground glass" changes on CT.

» For findings of active disease, consider steroids after ruling out infection.

» Monitor patients on steroids via radiographic data, clinical data, and spirometric data (if available) to assess whether the disease responds to steroids.

4) Is there a component of the disease that may need immunosuppression?

» This is usually indicated in the context of CTD.

» Mycophenolate mofetil or azathioprine are typically used due to the lower risk of lung toxicity.

5) Is there chronic disease management that the patient has not yet had?

» **Pharmacologic therapy:** IPF and progressive fibrotic lung disease are known to benefit from antifibrotic agents (i.e., nintedanib or pirfenidone); consider starting this therapy in the outpatient setting as guided by a respirologist.

» **Nonpharmacologic therapy:** This can include vaccinations, exercise, pulmonary rehabilitation, home oxygen, and advanced care planning.

Obstructive Airway Disease

These notes are in addition to the **general guide for all consultations** on page 1, and the **starting points for respirology consultations** at the beginning of this chapter.

Identification

Key information in the identification statement includes the patient's chief complaint and the degree of obstructive disease (i.e., mild, moderate, severe).

Reason for Referral

The referral typically seeks to confirm a diagnosis of asthma or COPD and/or clarify appropriate management.

History of Present Illness

ASTHMA

Ask about typical symptoms: These include shortness of breath,
cough, wheezing with variability, and decreased peak flows.

Ask about common triggers:
> infections (typically URTI)
> allergens (e.g., pets, mold, pollen, dust, perfumes)
> irritants (e.g., dry or cold air, smoking, biomass fuels, fumes)
> NSAIDs, beta-blockers
> medication nonadherence

Assess for factors associated with worse outcomes:
> comorbidities: chronic rhinosinusitis, GERD, obesity
> no prescribed inhaled corticosteroid (ICS), poor adherence to
  medications
> lack of asthma action plan
> more than 1 canister of short-acting beta agonist (SABA) per month
> smoking, allergen exposure, air pollution
> socioeconomic challenges
> FEV_1 less than 60% of predicted value
> history of intubation or ICU admission
> nocturnal symptoms

COPD

Ask about symptoms typical of an exacerbation: These include
worsening shortness of breath, wheezing, cough, and sputum
production.

Identify triggers for an exacerbation:
> infection (most exacerbations have a viral or bacterial etiology)
> pneumothorax, atelectasis, pulmonary edema, or malignancy
  (consider these etiologies in worsening symptoms)
> medication nonadherence
> GERD

Past Medical History

ASTHMA

Ask about:
• the patient's asthma diagnosis (when it was diagnosed and whether the
  diagnosis was confirmed with PFT)
• their most recent PFT
• the level of asthma control
• known triggers; environmental and occupational exposures
• limitations of daily activity

- the number of exacerbations and their severity (admission to hospital; history of ICU admission or intubation)

Table 15.1. Level of Asthma Control

In the past 4 weeks, assess for any of the following:
1. Daytime symptoms > 2 times/week?
2. Any night waking due to asthma?
3. Reliever needed more than twice/week?
4. Any activity limitation due to asthma?
One point for each question with a "yes."

No points = well controlled; 1-2 points = partially controlled; 3-4 points = poorly controlled

GINA ©2021 Global Initiative for Asthma, reprinted with permission. Available from www.ginasthma.org

COPD
Ask about:
- the etiology of the patient's COPD (e.g., tobacco, α_1-antitrypsin deficiency)
- the patient's COPD grade, based on the mMRC dyspnea scale or the Global Initiative for Chronic Obstructive Disease (GOLD) criteria
- comorbidities (CHF, lung cancer, bronchiectasis)
- baseline functional status and use of home oxygen
- complications (cor pulmonale, pulmonary hypertension)
- exacerbation frequency and severity

Medications
Follow the **general guide for all consultations** and the **starting points for respirology consultations**.

Allergies
Ask about allergens causing atopy.

Family History
Ask about eczema, allergic rhinitis, and food and drug allergies.

Social History
Focus on smoking history, including e-cigarettes, marijuana, illicit substances, and biomass exposure.

Physical Examination
Vital signs: pulsus paradoxus

General impression: tripod position, use of accessory muscles, ability to speak in full sentences, diaphoresis, cyanosis, increased anteroposterior (AP) chest diameter

Cardiovascular:
› Assess for elevated JVP.
› Palpate for subcutaneous emphysema (pneumothorax), displaced apical cardiac impulse, decreased tactile vocal fremitus, and pitting edema.
› Auscultate for wheeze, rhonchi, prolonged expiratory phase, loud pulmonic valve closure (P2), and crackles.
   » A loud P2 may indicate pulmonary hypertension.

Signs of airflow obstruction: maximal forced expiratory time (highest sensitivity if more than 9 seconds), subxiphoid impulse, increased AP diameter, loss of cardiac dullness

Signs of CHF and DVT

Investigations

ALL PATIENTS

CBC
Electrolytes
Creatinine, urea
Sputum culture
Nasopharyngeal swab
Chest x-ray
ABG: Pursue this if indicated.

ASTHMA

Blood work to measure eosinophils and IgE levels: Eosinophilia and elevated IgE levels suggest asthma, but have their own differentials that should be considered.

Peak flow spirometry:
› Results of 50% to 70% indicate moderate airflow limitation.
› Results of less than 50% indicate severe airflow limitation.

COPD

Review previous investigations, if available, including sputum cultures (this will guide empiric antibiotic therapy) and transthoracic echocardiogram (assess for pulmonary hypertension, CHF).

Electrolytes or blood gas: Typically, elevated bicarbonate indicates carbon dioxide retention.

CT PE protocol: Pursue this if indicated.

Impression and Plan

GENERAL APPROACH

• Summarize the presenting complaint with comparison to baseline asthma or COPD symptoms.

- Provide a working diagnosis of the likely exacerbating precipitant, and a differential diagnosis (e.g., CHF, PE).
- Always ask yourself if the patient requires bilevel positive airway pressure (BiPAP) or a higher level of care.
- Always think of the differential diagnosis for wheezing: not all wheezing is asthma (the differential diagnosis includes vocal cord dysfunction, airway tumours, CHF, and bronchiectasis).

ASTHMA

Consider whether the patient needs admission to hospital:
> Most asthma exacerbations are managed in the ED.
> Consider admission for patients who have been previously admitted to ICU or intubated.

Identify modifiable risk factors: Examples include treatment of GERD, avoidance of allergens.

Provide the patient with an asthma action plan.

Consider ICS therapy: New guidelines suggest use of ICS as first-line therapy.[3]

Consider single maintenance and reliever therapy (SMART)[3]: This applies to patients with significant as-needed SABA use.

Provide appropriate treatment:
> Mild-to-moderate asthma exacerbation:
  » Provide SABA 4–10 puffs or 2.5–5 mg nebulized every 20 minutes for 1 hour: peak expiratory flow should improve to 60% to 80% of predicted value (reassess in 1 hour: if no improvement, treat as severe asthma).
  » Prescribe prednisone 40–50 mg daily for 5 days (consider extending in patients with frequent exacerbations or steroid dependency).
> Severe asthma exacerbation:
  » To the management of mild-to-moderate asthma, add ipratropium: 2 puffs of 80 mcg, or 250 mcg nebulized, every 20 minutes.
  » Consider adding IV magnesium 2 g over 20 minutes.
  » Add antibiotics if pneumonia is suspected.

COPD

Provide appropriate treatment:
> First-line treatment includes:
  » salbutamol 2.5–5 mg every 1 to 2 hours initially, then 2.5–5 mg every 4 hours as needed
  » ipratropium 0.25–0.5 mg every hour initially, then every 4 hours
  » prednisone 40–50 mg orally every day for 5 days
> Provide antibiotics on evidence of an infectious trigger.
> Target oxygen saturation is 88% to 92% for patients with evidence of hypercapnia.
> Consider BiPAP in severe exacerbation.

Pleural Effusion

These notes are in addition to the **general guide for all consultations** on page 1, and the **starting points for respirology consultations** at the beginning of this chapter.

Identification

Follow the general guide for all consultations.

Reason for Referral

The referral may seek to clarify the etiology of pleural effusion and/or clarify appropriate management.

History of Present Illness

Ask about typical symptoms of pleural effusion:
> › shortness of breath
> › decreased exercise tolerance
> › pleuritic chest pain

Ask about conditions associated with transudative effusion:
> › CHF (ask about dyspnea on exertion, orthopnea, paroxysmal nocturnal dyspnea, pedal edema)
> › cirrhosis (alcohol use, viral hepatitis, ascites)
> › nephrotic syndrome
> › hypothyroidism

Ask about conditions associated with exudative effusion:
> › malignancy (weight loss, decreased appetite, risk factors for malignancy)
> › parapneumonic effusion or empyema (recent pneumonia, sick contacts, fever, cough)
> › trauma (hemothorax, rib fractures)
> › TB (fever, chills, night sweats, weight loss, hemoptysis)
> › RA and SLE (joint pain, joint stiffness, skin manifestations)
> › drugs (methotrexate, amiodarone, phenytoin, nitrofurantoin, beta-blockers)
> › benign asbestos effusion (asbestos exposure)
> › pancreatitis

Past Medical History

Ask about:
- previous effusions (clarify type: complicated versus uncomplicated, transudative versus exudative), previous thoracentesis
- pleurodesis (this is usually done for refractory effusions)
- malnutrition and/or malabsorption (this is relevant to hypoalbuminemia)

- peritoneal dialysis
- recent MI or CABG
- conditions associated with transudative effusions (see History of Present Illness)
- conditions associated with exudative effusions (see History of Present Illness)

Medications

Ask about:
- recent antibiotic use (if used to treat pneumonia)
- anticoagulants (these may delay thoracentesis if indicated)

Allergies

Note that allergies are less relevant in pleural effusions.

Family History

Ask about:
- malignancy
- autoimmune disease

Social History

Key information includes alcohol use, smoking history, and occupation.

Physical Examination

Vital signs: Patients may have an increased respiratory rate or hypoxemia; hypoxemia may worsen if the patient lies on the affected side.

General impression: Assess for accessory muscle use and decreased chest rise on the side of the effusion.

Signs of pleural effusion:
› Assess for weight loss and/or muscle wasting (this suggests malignancy or TB); clubbing (malignant effusion, empyema); ascites (hepatic hydrothorax); and elevated JVP (CHF).
› Examine the skin for autoimmune-related effusion.
› Perform a joint exam for autoimmune-related effusion.
› Palpate for tracheal deviation away from the side of the effusion and for decreased tactile vocal fremitus.
› Percuss for dullness over the effusion.
› Auscultate for decreased breath sounds over the effusion.

Investigations

LABORATORY INVESTIGATIONS

CBC with differential

ABG

Electrolytes, creatinine, liver enzymes
BNP, CRP
HIV
ANA, anti-double stranded DNA, rheumatoid factor, anti-CCP:
Consider these on suspicion of autoimmune disease.
Sputum and blood cultures: Consider these on suspicion of an
infectious etiology.

IMAGING

Chest x-ray:
> A posterior-anterior view detects > 200 mL of fluid.
> A lateral view detects > 50 mL of fluid.
CT: Assess for features that suggest an infectious consolidation or
malignant features (e.g., pleural nodularity, pleural thickening,
mediastinal pleural thickening).[4]
US of the lungs: This may identify loculation, which indicates a
complicated effusion.

PLEURAL FLUID ANALYSIS

• This is indicated in pleural effusion of unclear etiology: sampling is
not required in cases of obvious etiology (e.g., CHF that responds to
diuresis).
• Contraindications to pleural fluid sampling include: small effusions;
overlying skin or soft tissue infection; INR greater than 1.5; a platelet
count < 50 x 10^9/L; and therapeutic anticoagulation.
• Send pleural fluid for: cell count, differential, Gram stain, acid-fast
bacilli, culture (including fungal culture), pH (collect the sample in
an ABG syringe and analyze it within 1 hour), protein, LDH, glucose,
amylase, triglyceride, cholesterol, cytology, and adenosine deaminase
(in suspected TB).

Interpretation
• Apply Light's criteria; an effusion is exudative if any of the following is
true:
> The ratio of pleural to serum protein is greater than 0.5.
> The ratio of pleural to serum LDH is greater than 0.6.
> Pleural fluid LDH is more than two-thirds of the ULN of serum
LDH.
• The following results also suggest exudative effusion[5]:
> cholesterol > 1.4 mmol/L
> LDH > 200 U/L
> ratio of pleural to serum cholesterol greater than 0.3
> serum-pleural albumin gradient < 12 mmol/L
• Parapneumonic pleural effusions should be classified as 1 of:

> simple effusions (these tend to be free flowing, but still meet Light's criteria; they are likely culture negative with normal glucose and pH)
> complicated effusions (these tend to be loculated, have a low glucose level, and pH < 7.2)
> empyema, which is frank pus in the pleural space
- The differential diagnosis of lymphocyte-predominant effusions (i.e., with a lymphocyte fraction of 85% to 95%) includes:
  > malignancy
  > TB (adenosine deaminase > 40 U/L)
  > lymphoma
  > rheumatoid pleurisy
  > chylothorax
- The differential diagnosis of eosinophilic-predominant effusions (i.e., with an eosinophil fraction greater than 10%) includes:
  > TB, fungal infections (coccidioidomycosis, *Cryptococcus*, histoplasmosis), parasite infection
  > malignancy
  > eosinophilic pneumonia, eosinophilic granulomatosis with polyangiitis
  > pneumothorax, hemothorax
  > drug-induced effusion

Impression and Plan
Describe the etiology:
> This is key: it guides further management.
> Discuss relevant history, investigations, and pleural fluid analysis.

Describe management based on etiology:
> **Transudative effusions:** Treat with diuretics, as indicated.
> **Exudative effusions:** These have many possible etiologies: treat the underlying etiology.
> **Malignant effusions:** These may require repeat thoracenteses or a long-term indwelling catheter; they should not be treated with a short-term chest tube.
> **Parapneumonic effusions:** These may require chest-tube drainage and antibiotics; complicated parapneumonic effusions require antibiotics for at least 4 to 6 weeks, and may require lytic therapy with tissue plasminogen activator and deoxyribonuclease.

Describe next steps if an etiology is not found:
> In patients with a high pretest probability of malignancy, a second drainage is useful, but further repeated drainages have marginal benefits.
> If a second drainage does not clarify a diagnosis, consider a pleural biopsy or pleuroscopy.

References

1. Mahler D, Wells C. Evaluation of clinical methods for rating dyspnea. Chest. 1988;93(3):580-86. doi: 10.1378/chest.93.3.580
2. Goldman L, Hashimoto B, Cook E, et al. Comparative reproducibility and validity of systems for assessing cardiovascular functional class: advantages of a new specific activity scale. Circulation. 1981;64(6):1227-34. doi: 10.1161/01.cir.64.6.1227
3. Global Initiative for Asthma. Global strategy for asthma management and prevention, 2021. Available from: www.ginasthma.org
4. Leung A, Müller N, Miller R. CT in differential diagnosis of diffuse pleural disease. Am J Roentgenol. 1990; 154:487-92. doi: 10.2214/AJR.154.3.2106209
5. Wilcox M, Chong C, Stanbrook M, et al. Does this patient have an exudative pleural effusion? The Rational Clinical Examination systematic review. JAMA. 2014;311(23):2422-31. doi:10.1001/jama.2014.5552

16

Rheumatology

Dr. Derin Karacabeyli
Dr. Jocelyn Chai
Dr. Lauren Eadie
Dr. Siavash Ghadiri
Dr. Navjeet Gill
Dr. Xenia Gukova
Dr. Ahmad Abdullah

REVIEWERS
Dr. Kam Shojania
Dr. Shahin Jamal

Starting Points: Rheumatology Consultations

These notes are in addition to the **general guide for all consultations** on page 1.

Identification

Follow the **general guide for all consultations**.

Reason for Referral

The referral may seek to confirm a rheumatic condition and/or clarify appropriate management.

History of Present Illness

Conduct a rheumatology review of systems: Ask about the onset of the patient's condition and associated symptoms, with emphasis on the following 4 categories:

1) **Constitutional or systemic symptoms:** Check for fever, chills, weight loss (determine how much over how long), drenching night sweats, fatigue, malaise, myalgias, and lymphadenopathy.

2) **Seropositive review of systems:** Check for symptoms of:
   › **RA:** swollen, painful joints (determine how many and whether DIP joints are spared), morning stiffness (determine how long it lasts)

> **SLE:** patchy hair loss; malar or discoid rash; oral ulcers; Raynaud phenomenon; arthralgia; chest pain (relevant to serositis); photosensitivity; miscarriages or VTE; seizures; psychosis
> **Sjögren syndrome:** sicca symptoms (dry eyes and/or mouth), vaginal dryness, paresthesia, weakness
> **Scleroderma:** skin tightening, pruritus, GERD, dysphagia, abdominal pain, shortness of breath (relevant to interstitial lung disease)
> **Myositis:** rashes around the eyes, on the fingers, or on the upper back and/or chest; proximal muscle weakness

3) **Seronegative review of systems (for psoriatic arthritis [PsA], ankylosing spondylitis, inflammatory bowel disease [IBD], reactive arthritis):** Ask about psoriasis (elbows, scalp, knees, umbilicus, buttocks); enthesitis (elbow, Achilles tendon, plantar fascia, sacroiliac joint [SI joint]); dactylitis ("sausage digits"); inflammatory back pain (morning stiffness that lasts longer than 30 minutes; night pain; pain that is better with activity, not better with rest); uveitis (eye pain, photophobia, increased lacrimation); conjunctivitis; IBD symptoms (abdominal pain; tenesmus or urgency; diarrhea with blood or mucous); urethritis or cervicitis; and recent infection (particularly GI or GU).

4) **Miscellaneous review of systems:** Check for symptoms of:
> **Gout or calcium pyrophosphate dihydrate (CPPD) deposition:** i.e., monoarthritis
> **Sarcoidosis:** ankle periarthritis, cough, shortness of breath, uveitis, erythema nodosum (and others)
> **Behçet syndrome:** mouth and genital ulcers
> **Antineutrophil cytoplasmic antibody (ANCA) vasculitis:** sinusitis, hematuria, hemoptysis, asthma, palpable purpura (and others)
> **Giant cell arteritis (GCA) and polymyalgia rheumatica (PMR):** jaw claudication; headache; vision changes; shoulder and/or hip stiffness

Past Medical History

Ask about:
• **Previous rheumatologic history:** This includes (but is not limited to):
> **Arthritis:** RA, osteoarthritis (OA), gout, and others (determine the type)
> **Connective tissue disease:** SLE, Sjögren syndrome, scleroderma, myositis, mixed connective tissue disease (MCTD)
> **Diseases associated with seronegative arthritis:** psoriasis, IBD
> **Vasculitis:** GCA, ANCA vasculitis, cryoglobulinemia
> **Other:** sarcoidosis, adult-onset Still disease
• **Other autoimmune conditions:** These include thyroid conditions (Graves disease, Hashimoto thyroiditis), autoimmune hepatitis,

primary biliary cholangitis, primary sclerosing cholangitis, and vitiligo.

- **Previous chronic infections:** Some can cause positive tests for rheumatoid factor (RF), ANA, and ANCA, and they are also relevant in the context of plans for immunosuppression.
  - › **HIV:** Determine the date diagnosed, the most recent CD4 count or viral load, and treatment history.
  - › **HBV and HCV:** Determine the date diagnosed, viral load, and treatment history.
  - › **TB:** Determine the date of screening tests, the date diagnosed, and treatment history.
- **Malignancy:** Obtain a history, including treatment.
- **Osteoporosis:** Obtain a history, including fracture history.

Past Surgical History
Pursue this when relevant (e.g., joint replacements).

Medications
Ask about:
- immunosuppressive agents (e.g., corticosteroids, biologics), including dose
  - › Determine DMARDs tried (and if stopped, and why they were stopped).
  - › Determine prednisone history (dose, taper schedule, side effects, complications).
- pain medications (e.g., acetaminophen, NSAIDs)
- OTC medications (e.g., vitamins, herbal supplements, glucosamine)
- drugs associated with drug-induced lupus (e.g., hydralazine, procainamide, thiazides, CCBs, TNFα inhibitors, statins, ACEIs)

Allergies
Follow the **general guide for all consultations.**

Family History
Ask about PsA, ankylosing spondylitis, IBD, RA, SLE, gout, lymphoma, and MS (if planning anti-TNFα therapy).

Social History
Ask about:
- alcohol use, recreational drug use, smoking
- occupation
- travel history
- ADLs and IADLs
- drug coverage

- TB risk factors (ethnicity; living conditions; immigrant and refugee status)

Physical Examination

Vital signs: fever

Head, ears, eyes, nose, throat: dry eyes or mouth; nasal ulcers or crusting; saddle nose deformity (relevant to GPA); oral ulcers (SLE)

Cardiovascular and respiratory: muffled heart sounds (pericardial effusion), friction rub (pericarditis), dullness to percussion at bases (pleural effusion)

Neurological: patchy sensorimotor findings (mononeuritis multiplex)

Musculoskeletal: swollen or tender joints; symmetry; DIP joint involvement; hand and/or foot deformities; spinal or SI joint tenderness

> **RA:** symmetric inflammatory arthritis (bilateral wrists; metacarpophalangeal [MCP] joints and PIP joints without DIP joints) with or without hand and foot deformities (swan neck, boutonnière deformity, volar subluxation, ulnar deviation, Z-deformity, pes planus, hallux valgus)
> **SLE:** symmetric, nonerosive, inflammatory polyarthritis; reducible ulnar deviation of the MCP joints (Jaccoud arthropathy)

Dermatological:

> **Dermatomyositis:** Gottron papules, shawl sign, V-sign, holster sign, heliotrope rash, "mechanic's hands," dilated capillary loops
> **PsA:** dactylitis, nail changes, psoriatic plaques
> **RA:** subcutaneous nodules
> **Scleroderma:** skin thickening, calcinosis, telangiectasia on fingers, toes, and/or face
> **SLE:** malar rash that spares nasolabial folds, discoid rash, photosensitivity rash, nonscarring alopecia
> **Vasculitis:** palpable purpura; livedo reticularis and/or mottling; petechiae; digital infarcts

Investigations

LABORATORY INVESTIGATIONS

CBC with differential: Assess for anemia, leukocytosis, leukopenia, eosinophilia, thrombocytosis, and thrombocytopenia.

> Consider a hemolysis workup if both anemia and thrombocytopenia are present.

Electrolytes, extended electrolytes, creatinine, urea: Assess for renal dysfunction.

Liver enzymes, liver function tests, CRP (or ESR), CK

Urinalysis and microscopy: Assess for hematuria and proteinuria.

Infection: Relevant tests include HIV; syphilis; HBV and HCV screens; EBV; CMV IgM; TB skin test or interferon-gamma release assay (IGRA); blood cultures (2 sets); and *Strongyloides* serology, and stool ova and parasites (3 sets), on suspicion of parasitic infection.

Malignancy: Order serum and urine protein electrophoresis (SPEP, UPEP) and serum free light chains.

AUTOIMMUNE WORKUP WITH SEROLOGY CORRELATES

SLE:
› ANA (this is positive on multiplex immunoassay or ≥ 1:80 on immunofluorescence assay)[1,2]
› double-stranded DNA (dsDNA) (this correlates with disease activity and lupus nephritis)[3]
› extractable nuclear antigens (ENA) (SLE is positive for anti-Smith antibodies, RNP, SSA, and SSB)
› C3 and C4 (these are typically low during flares)[4] with or without antiphospholipid antibody syndrome antibodies (associated with anti-cardiolipin, anti-ß2 glycoprotein, lupus anticoagulant)

Drug-induced lupus: antihistone antibodies (from ENA)[4]

RA: RF IgM (this is about 70% to 75% specific)[5] and anti-cyclic citrullinated peptide (this is about 95% specific and a sign of worse prognosis)[6]; CRP (this is elevated with increased RA activity)

ANCA-associated vasculitis: proteinase 3 (cANCA) with granulomatosis with polyangiitis (GPA); myeloperoxidase (pANCA) with microscopic polyangiitis (MPA) and eosinophilic granulomatosis with polyangiitis (EGPA)[7]

MCTD: RNP (from ENA)

Sjögren syndrome: SSA and SSB (from ENA)

Diffuse and limited scleroderma: Scl-70 and anticentromere, respectively (from ENA)

Myositis: Jo (from ENA, associated with antisynthetase syndrome)

IMAGING

Chest x-ray or CT of the chest: Consider this to assess for fibrosis, lung nodules, infiltrations, cavitary lesions, pneumonitis, pleural effusions, and interstitial lung disease.

X-ray or MRI of joints: Consider this to assess for joint space narrowing, erosions, osteopenia, and soft tissue swelling.

Echocardiogram: Consider this to assess for myocarditis and pericarditis.

OTHER INVESTIGATIONS

Skin, renal, or arterial biopsy: Assess for vasculitis.

Arthrocentesis: Send fluid for cell count and differential, Gram stain and culture, and crystals (with or without cytology).

Impression and Plan

Provide a diagnosis. Consider the patient's age, gender, past medical history, family history, symptoms, signs, and serology. Is the patient's presentation consistent with a seropositive, seronegative, or miscellaneous rheumatic disease?

- ANA positivity can be associated with an "organ specific" autoimmune disease (e.g., thyroid disease, autoimmune hepatitis, vitiligo, primary biliary cholangitis) or a systemic autoimmune rheumatic disease (e.g., SLE, Sjögren syndrome, scleroderma, myositis).
- Positivity for ANA, RF, and ANCA has many possible causes: rule out malignancy (paraneoplastic or lymphoproliferative), chronic infection (endocarditis, HBV, HCV, HIV, EBV, syphilis), and drug-related causes.
- Positivity for ANA or RF can indicate a normal variant: consider this if the patient's history and physical exam are unremarkable.

Acute Monoarthritis

These notes are in addition to the **general guide for all consultations** on page 1, and the **starting points for rheumatology consultations** at the beginning of this chapter.

Identification

Key information in the identification statement includes relevant comorbidities (e.g., prosthetic joints, type 2 diabetes, dyslipidemia, obesity, and CKD for gout).

Reason for Referral

The referral may seek to confirm acute monoarthritis and/or clarify appropriate management.

History of Present Illness

Characterize the presenting illness:

  › Determine when the symptoms began, the joint involved (ensure true monoarthritis), and whether the symptomatic joint is native versus prosthetic.
  › Ask about swelling, pain, range of motion, and fever.

Assess for relevant risk factors:
> **Gonococcal septic arthritis:** sexual activity
> **Nongonococcal septic arthritis (mainly *Staphylococcus aureus*, *Streptococcus*, and gram-negative bacteria):** IV drug use, bacteremia, trauma, active skin and soft tissue infection, diabetes, underlying inflammatory arthritis, immune compromise (e.g., chronic steroids, chemotherapy, cancer)
> **Gout:** history of gout, dyslipidemia, hypertension, diabetes, CKD, obesity; use of diuretics, low-dose acetylsalicylic acid (ASA), or alcohol; high fat or fructose intake; recent surgery or illness

Assess for triggers (e.g., trauma, activity): These include fracture, OA, and injuries of bursa, ligaments, menisci, and tendons.

Conduct a rheumatology review of systems: A key aspect of the review is seropositive and seronegative screening (see the **starting points for rheumatology consultations** at the beginning of this chapter).

Past Medical History

Ask about:
- **Gout:** Determine if the gout is tophaceous and whether the patient is taking urate-lowering therapy (determine the last outpatient urate level); clarify recent flares and treatments (colchicine versus NSAID versus glucocorticoid, and whether oral or injected).
- **Joint prosthetics:** Determine surgery dates and complications.
- **Coagulopathy and thrombocytopenia**
- **Bacteremia:** Identify the organisms and complications (e.g., endocarditis, osteomyelitis, abscess, septic arthritis).
- **Diabetes mellitus:** Check the patient's last HbA_{1c}, and ask about micro- and macrovascular complications.
- **CKD:** Identify the cause, and determine the patient's eGFR, and urine albumin-to-creatinine ratio.
- **OA:** Ask about recent injections.

Medications

Ask about:
- immunosuppressives (e.g., glucocorticoids, synthetic DMARDs, biologic DMARDs, chemo)
- urate-lowering agents (allopurinol, febuxostat)
- diuretics (these may trigger gout, especially thiazides)
- ASA (low dose ASA may trigger gout, but high dose is uricosuric)
- recent antibiotic use (this increases the risk of resistant organisms)
- recent NSAID, colchicine, or steroid use (this is relevant to gout)

Allergies
Follow the **general guide for all consultations**.

Family History
Follow the **general guide for all consultations** and the **starting points for rheumatology consultations**.

Social History
Ask about:
- sexual activity, and history of STI or STI screening (this is relevant to gonococcal infection)
- IV drug use (*Streptococcus* or *Staphylococcus aureus*)
- travel history and TB risk factors (other infections)
- alcohol use (especially beer), fatty or high purine foods (e.g., shellfish, organ meats, red meat), and high-fructose intake (gout)

Physical Examination
Vital signs and level of consciousness: Assess for signs of sepsis: consider scoring the patient with qSOFA.

Head, ears, eyes, nose, throat: Assess for lymphadenopathy, eye redness (uveitis, conjunctivitis, and/or episcleritis), and oral ulcers.

Cardiovascular, respiratory: Assess for murmur and signs of heart failure (elevated JVP, crackles, peripheral edema).

GU: Look for urethral discharge, and penile or vulvar lesions.

Musculoskeletal:
  › Assess for asymmetry of symptoms.
  › Perform a joint exam: assess active and passive range of motion, feel for warmth, and test for effusion (e.g., swipe test, patellar tap).
  › Assess neurovascular status (distal pulses, sensation, and strength).

Dermatological: Look for track marks, cellulitis, psoriasis, nail changes, and tophi (common sites include fingers, toes, wrists, Achilles tendon, olecranon, knees, outer ear).

Investigations
LABORATORY INVESTIGATIONS
CBC with differential: In findings of low platelets, consider hemarthrosis.

Electrolytes, extended electrolytes: Low Mg, low PO_4, and elevated parathyroid hormone are secondary causes of pseudogout.

Creatinine (eGFR): These may be relevant for antibiotic dosing and selecting acute gout treatment.

INR, PTT: In abnormal findings, consider hemarthrosis.

Serum uric acid: This is of limited utility in acute gout because proinflammatory states promote renal urate excretion (thus, urate levels may be low, normal, or high); however, assessing serum uric acid is part of the "acute gout diagnosis rule" and, in the correct clinical context, very high urate levels may facilitate diagnosis without joint aspiration.

CRP: This is a nonspecific inflammatory marker.

MICROBIOLOGY AND SEROLOGIES

Blood culture and sensitivity

Urinalysis, and urine culture and sensitivity

Urine nucleic acid amplification test (NAAT) for gonorrhea and chlamydia

Treponina pallidum EIA

HIV, HBV, HCV

IMAGING

Joint x-ray: This may demonstrate osteomyelitis, erosions, or tophi.

Dual energy CT: Assess for crystal deposition in joints.

ARTHROCENTESIS (DIAGNOSTIC AND THERAPEUTIC)

- Before performing arthrocentesis, check the patient's INR/PTT: anticoagulation is typically safe in the context of arthrocentesis, but consider holding warfarin in patients with INR greater than 5.5.
- Perform arthrocentesis before antibiotic therapy if the patient is stable.
- Send samples for culture (order bacterial with Gram stain; consider acid-fast bacilli and fungi), cells (with differential), and crystals.
  › Gram stain yield is low (around 30%).
  › Culture yield can also be low (less than 50% in gonococcal infections).
  › Crystals do not rule out infection: patients can have concurrent septic and crystal arthritis.
  › Intracellular crystals suggest acute flare.
  › WBCs > 100 000/μL have a LR of +28 for diagnosing septic joints (WBCs > 50 000/μL have a LR of +7.7).[8]
  › Monosodium urate crystals (needle-shaped, negative birefringence) are consistent with gout.
  › CPPD deposition (rhomboid-shaped, positive birefringence) is consistent with pseudogout.

Impression and Plan

GENERAL APPROACH

- Outline the provisional diagnosis and trigger in the context of patient-specific risk factors.

- Provide a differential diagnosis:
  › Consider trauma, hemarthrosis, OA, malignancy, and extraarticular causes.
  › Note that olecranon and prepatellar bursitis (both of which can be septic) can closely resemble elbow and knee arthritis.
- *For example:* "Issue 1. Acute native knee monoarthritis with fever, concerning for septic arthritis. Differential diagnosis includes hemarthrosis, bursitis, and gout. Arthrocentesis for diagnosis and source control, blood cultures then empiric ceftriaxone and vancomycin. Acetaminophen and naproxen as needed."

MANAGEMENT OF SEPTIC ARTHRITIS

- **Identify the source of infection with arthrocentesis:** If the fluid is purulent or if the affected joint is prosthetic, consult an orthopedic surgeon.
- **Provide empiric antibiotics:** Prescribe IV ceftriaxone (or ceftazidime in patients with *Pseudomonas* risk factors such as IV drug use, previous *Pseudomonas* infection, or a prosthetic joint that is infected more than 1 year after surgery) and vancomycin (use nomogram).
- **Treat pain:** Provide acetaminophen and opioids with or without NSAIDs, as needed.

MANAGEMENT OF GOUT

Acute Pharmacologic Options

Prednisone: 0.5 mg/kg/day (30–40 mg orally every day) for 5 to 10 days (prednisone is safe in renal disease)

Methylprednisolone: 40–80 mg intraarticular injection

Colchicine: 1.2 mg oral load, then 0.6 mg 1 hour later, then 0.6 mg orally twice a day until resolution (e.g., 5 to 10 days)
  » Adjust the dose for renal impairment if eGFR < 30 mL/min; observe for GI side effects.
  » Avoid in ESRD (consider a single dose of 0.6 mg every 14 days in patients on hemodialysis).

NSAIDs: naproxen 500 mg orally twice per day or indomethacin 50 mg orally 3 times per day until resolution (e.g., 5 to 10 days)
  » Avoid in patients with GI, renal, or cardiac disease.

Allopurinol

- Do not stop allopurinol during an acute attack or acute kidney injury (consider adjusting the dose for renal impairment).
- Strong indications to initiate allopurinol include: 2 or more flares per year; tophi on exam or imaging; or findings of damage on imaging.[9]

- Conditional indications to initiate allopurinol include: more than 1 lifetime flare; first flare plus CKD (eGFR < 60 mL/min); urate > 535 μmol/L; or urolithiasis.
  - › Start the patient on a low dose and titrate the dose in an outpatient setting to achieve serum urate targets (< 357 μmol/L).[9]
  - › Provide prophylaxis (e.g., colchicine 0.6 mg/day) for at least 3 months while titrating.[9]
- Test for the HLA-B*58:01 allele in patients of Southeast Asian or African American descent before starting allopurinol (these patients are at increased risk for allopurinol hypersensitivity syndrome).
- Consider nonpharmacologic treatments including a modified diet (low purine, low fructose) and, if possible, cessation of offending medications.

Giant Cell Arteritis and Polymyalgia Rheumatica

These notes are in addition to the **general guide for all consultations** on page 1, and the **starting points for rheumatology consultations** at the beginning of this chapter.

Identification

Key information in the identification statement includes history of PMR.

Reason for Referral

Examples of reason for referral include headache, vision changes, high CRP, and suspected GCA.

History of Present Illness

Clarify why the patient has sought care: In an inpatient setting, why was the patient admitted to hospital?

Assess for GCA symptoms: Ask about:
- › **New temporal headaches or scalp tenderness:** Patients with a previous history of headaches or migraines may report a "different" type of headache (e.g., more intense, constant, only partially responsive to analgesics without prednisone).
- › **Abrupt onset of visual disturbances:** Specifically ask about transient monocular visual loss (amaurosis fugax) and diplopia (diplopia has high positive LR for GCA).[10]

> Jaw claudication: Patients might describe this as soreness, achiness, and heaviness along the mandible with prolonged chewing (e.g., chewing steak); distinguish these symptoms from TMJ pain.
> Scalp tenderness: Clarify if the patient has pain when they brush their hair.
> Unexplained fever, anemia, or other constitutional symptoms and signs: GCA is a common cause of fever of unknown origin in adults older than 65.[11]
> Chest pain or limb claudication: This may indicate GCA with large-vessel involvement (e.g., AAA, thoracic aortic aneurysm, other aneurysms).
> Cough: Often patients with GCA get a mild dry cough of unknown etiology.
> Stroke-like symptoms: Stroke is a complication of GCA.

Ask about a current or previous diagnosis of PMR: Does the patient have proximal hip and shoulder girdle pain and stiffness?

Conduct a rheumatology review of systems: Pay particular attention to screening for vasculitis.

Past Medical History
Ask about:
- PMR (proximal myalgia, constitutional symptoms, and elevated ESR or CRP)
- previous vasculitis (clarify as small-, medium-, or large-vessel vasculitis)
- neurological and cardiac history (especially aortic aneurysms or aortic arch syndrome)

Medications
Follow the **general guide for all consultations** and the **starting points for rheumatology consultations.**

Allergies
Follow the **general guide for all consultations.**

Family History
Ask about GCA, PMR, RA, and other types of vasculitis.

Social History
Key information includes current or past smoking because this is associated with GCA complications (e.g., aneurysms).

Physical Examination
Vital signs: In particular, check for tachycardia, fever, and difference in BP between arms (systolic BP difference > 20 mmHg or diastolic BP difference > 10 mmHg).

Signs of superficial temporal artery involvement: Assess for erythema, nodularity, "beading," pain on palpation, and reduced pulsation.

Eyes: Assess visual acuity, pupillary reflexes, and visual fields, and perform funduscopy.

Ear, nose throat: Include assessment for carotid bruits, oral ulcers, and alopecia.

Cardiovascular: Bruits and asymmetric pulses suggest large-vessel involvement.
› Assess 4 pulses for asymmetry.
› Check for abnormal heart sounds, murmurs, and displaced apical beats.
› Listen for the following bruits: carotid, subclavian, midabdominal (relevant to AAA), renal, iliac, and femoral.

Respiratory: Assess for increased work of breathing, wheeze, and crackles.

Abdominal: Check for tenderness.

Neurological: Conduct a cranial nerve exam, looking for focal or patchy deficits (GCA may involve the CNS, causing seizures, strokes, and altered mental status).

Musculoskeletal:
› Examine the joints of the neck.
› Check the shoulder and hip girdle for PMR: get the patient to stand from a chair with their arms folded across their chest (patients with PMR are often unable to do this).

Dermatological: Check for rashes, erythema, nodules, petechiae, and discharge.

Investigations

URGENT TEMPORAL ARTERY ASSESSMENT
Temporal artery biopsy: This is the gold standard for diagnosing GCA.
» Colour Doppler US (CDUS) is also an option (this is an emerging modality).
» If the initial biopsy is negative, but clinical suspicion remains high, order a contralateral biopsy.
» If CDUS is the initial investigation and it is negative, proceed with temporal artery biopsy.

LABORATORY INVESTIGATIONS
CBC with differential: Patients may have anemia of inflammation and/or reactive thrombocytosis.

CRP, CK: Use this to rule out myositis in patients with muscle weakness.

› Consider adding troponin (in patients witb chest pain), ANA, ANCA, and cryoglobulins.

Electrolytes, extended electrolytes, urea, creatinine, urinalysis

Liver enzymes, albumin, bilirubin, INR, PTT

IMAGING

ECG, chest x-ray

CTA or MRA of the temporal artery: Consider pursuing this; MRA of the head often also captures temporal arteries and is validated for GCA.

CTA of the chest, abdomen, and pelvis:
› Pursue this in the context of high suspicion for GCA where temporal artery investigations are negative, and/or on suspicion of extracranial or large-vessel GCA.
› Assess aorta and first-order branches.

MICROBIOLOGY

Blood cultures: Pursue this on suspicion of infection as a cause of fever (e.g., endocarditis).

Impression and Plan

GENERAL APPROACH

Assess if the patient meets the criteria for GCA diagnosis: The presence of 3 or more of the following criteria has 94% sensitivity and 91% specificity:
› age 50 or older
› new-onset localized headache or pain
› temporal artery tenderness or decreased pulsation
› elevated ESR or CRP > 50 mg/L
› abnormal artery biopsy (e.g., mononuclear cell infiltration or granulomatous inflammation, usually with multinucleated giant cells and histiocytes; breakdown of internal elastic lamina; intimal thickening)

Treat suspected or confirmed GCA: Start high-dose prednisone 1 mg/kg for 2 to 4 weeks; begin taper once symptoms resolve.

Assess indications for IV pulse steroids: These include vision loss, visual symptoms, stroke, and suspected or confirmed large-vessel involvement (e.g., thoracic aneurysm).
› A typical example of pulse steroids is methylprednisolone 1000 mg IV daily for 3 days.

Consider alternative diagnoses on negative results from biopsy, CDUS, and imaging of aorta: Examples of alternative diagnoses include small- or medium-vessel vasculitides, primary angiitis of CNS, idiopathic aortitis, and infection.

TREATMENT

Consider ASA: This may benefit patients at high risk of TIA or with stroke-like symptoms.

Coprescribe medications with long-term prednisone: Prescribe vitamin D; calcium; bisphosphonate; and trimethoprim and sulfamethoxazole (TMP-sulfa) for *Pneumocystis jiroveci* pneumonia prophylaxis with or without a PPI.

Consider adding a DMARD early: Often patients will not be able to come off prednisone without a DMARD; options include methotrexate, azathioprine, leflunomide, and tocilizumab.[12]

EXAMPLE NOTE

"Suspected GCA. New temporal headache in 70-year-old male with elevated CRP. Administer pulse methylprednisolone because of visual symptoms. Order urgent temporal artery biopsy to confirm. Given chest pain, monitor BP in bilateral arms and order CTA chest/abdomen/pelvis to rule out aortic involvement. If GCA is confirmed, continue with high-dose prednisone, counsel on side effects and risks of long-term use, and coprescribe vitamin D, calcium, alendronate, and TMP-sulfa."

Polyarthritis

These notes are in addition to the **general guide for all consultations** on page 1, and the **starting points for rheumatology consultations** at the beginning of this chapter.

Identification

Follow the **general guide for all consultations**.

Reason for Referral

The referral may seek to confirm polyarthritis and/or clarify appropriate management.

History of Present Illness

Clarify why the patient has sought care: In an inpatient setting, why was the patient admitted to hospital?

Clarify the duration of joint issues: Has the patient had symptoms for more than 6 weeks or less than 6 weeks?

Determine the type of joints affected: Small, large, or axial?

Ask about inflammatory features: These include morning stiffness that lasts longer than 30 to 60 minutes; pain that is worse with rest,

better with activity; night pain; swelling; and pain that is responsive
to NSAIDs.

Ask about range of motion, symmetry, and pattern:
> Are the symptoms intermittent, additive, or migratory?
> Clarify arthralgia (pain) versus arthritis (inflammation).

Screen for associated symptoms: Conduct a rheumatology review of
systems.

Screen for gout and septic arthritis risk factors: See Acute
Monoarthritis in this chapter.

Past Medical History

Key information includes:
- specific past joint issues (prosthetics, surgeries, injections)
- recent STI or GI infection (these may indicate reactive arthritis)
- bacteremia (determine organisms and complications such as infective
  endocarditis, osteomyelitis, abscess, septic arthritis)
- dental health (gingivitis increases the risk of inflammatory arthritis)
- gout or pseudogout
  > Determine if the gout is tophaceous and whether the patient is taking
    urate-lowering therapy (ask about the last outpatient urate level);
    clarify recent flares and treatments (colchicine versus NSAID versus
    glucocorticoid, and whether oral or injected).

Medications

- Ask about all medications.
- Specifically ask about drugs causing polyarthritis: clindamycin,
  antithyroid drugs,[13] and certain immune modulators (durvalumab,
  nivolumab, ipilimumab, tremelimumab).[14]

Allergies

Follow the **general guide for all consultations.**

Family History

Follow the **general guide for all consultations** and the **starting points for
rheumatology consultations.**

Social History

Ask about:
- alcohol use, IV drug use, smoking
- occupation
- sexual history and travel history (this is relevant to reactive arthritis,
  TB, Lyme disease, and viral arthralgia)

- ethnicity
  - › In patients of Middle Eastern, East Asian, or Mediterranean descent who are younger than 40, consider Behçet syndrome.
  - › People of First Nations descent are at higher risk of RA, inflammatory arthritis, and overlap syndromes.

Physical Examination

Follow the **general guide for all consultations** and the **starting points for rheumatology consultations.**

Investigations

LABORATORY INVESTIGATIONS

CBC with differential

Electrolytes, extended electrolytes, urea, creatinine

Liver enzymes, liver function tests

CK: This assesses for myositis.

Inflammatory markers: These include CRP, ferritin, uric acid, and LDH; they are nonspecific tests, but may facilitate diagnosis if results are very high (e.g., ferritin in Still disease, uric acid in gout).

Viral testing: Test for syphilis; HIV; HBV, HCV (screen); *Parvovirus B19*; EBV; and CMV IgM (this is not routine but can be ordered on suspicion of infectious arthritis).

SPEP, UPEP, serum free light chains: Pursue these to rule out cancer.

HLA-B27: Pursue this on suspicion of seronegative arthritis.

MICROBIOLOGY

Blood culture and sensitivity

Urinalysis, and urine culture and sensitivity

Urine NAAT: This assesses for gonorrhea and chlamydia.

Stool culture and sensitivity, and ova and parasites: Consider this.

TB skin test or IGRA: Pursue this in planned immunosuppression.

Autoantibodies: Order these based on clinical suspicion (see the **starting points for rheumatology consultations** for test details)

Other microbiology:
  - › **RA:** RF, anti-cyclic citrullinated peptide (anti-CCP), JOINTstat
    - » JOINTstat measures serum protein 14-3-3-eta; it is a newer test for RA, similar to anti-CCP, and available in some Canadian centres.
  - › **Connective tissue disease:** ANA (plus ENA, if ANA is positive), dsDNA, C3, C4
  - › **Vasculitis:** ANCA, cryoglobulins, quantitative immunoglobulins

IMAGING

General Principles

- When possible, compare new imaging to past imaging to assess the progress of disease.
- It is not necessary to obtain imaging for every symptomatic joint.
- X-rays usually lack specificity in acute or early conditions.
- MRI has greater sensitivity than x-ray in detecting early RA (choose 1 hand only).
- CT scan is a good alternative to x-ray to assess erosions and damage; consider a dual energy CT for gout.
- Do not order bone scans for synovitis or sacroiliitis.

Specific Imaging

Hand, wrist, or foot x-rays: Order these to assess for lytic lesions and erosions.

Spinal x-ray or MRI: Pursue this in seronegative disease.
› Abnormalities in SI joints are an early finding of ankylosing spondylitis.
› Spine MRI is more sensitive in detecting early ankylosing spondylitis.

Joint US: This can detect subtle synovitis.

Radionuclide scans: Order these for malignancy, infection, and Paget disease.

OTHER INVESTIGATIONS

Arthrocentesis: Send fluid for cell count and differential, Gram stain and culture, and crystals (with or without cytology).

Biopsy:
› This is rarely needed.
› Provide tissue for fungal infection, Whipple disease, TB, or sarcoidosis; provide skin for vasculitis, psoriasis, SLE, or other connective tissue disease.

Impression and Plan

INFLAMMATORY VERSUS NONINFLAMMATORY PAIN

Differentiate inflammatory polyarticular pain (synovitis, joint gelling, prolonged morning stiffness) and noninflammatory polyarticular pain.

Inflammatory polyarticular pain: Use chronicity, age, history, physical exam, laboratory investigations, and imaging to differentiate between:
› Acute inflammatory polyarthralgia (symptoms for less than 6 weeks):
» infectious (viral, gonococcal, meningococcal)
» reactive (often after GI or GU infection)
» crystal-induced

» early systemic rheumatic disease
› Chronic inflammatory polyarthralgia (symptoms for more than 6 weeks):
  » crystal (gout or pseudogout)
  » seropositive systemic rheumatic disease (RA, SLE, scleroderma, myositis, Sjögren syndrome, MCTD, vasculitis)
  » seronegative systemic rheumatic disease (IBD, PsA, ankylosing spondylitis, reactive arthritis)
  » other (sarcoidosis, malignancy, chronic infection [e.g., TB, Whipple disease, subacute endocarditis, Lyme disease], Still disease)

Noninflammatory polyarticular pain: The differential diagnosis includes OA, fibromyalgia, Paget disease, and hemochromatosis.

TREATMENT
The differential is wide with a variety of treatments:
- Some rheumatic diseases are treated with low-dose systemic steroids and antimalarials.
  › Consider relative contraindications to steroids: peptic ulcers, uncontrolled hypertension, diabetes mellitus, CHF, systemic infection, and osteoporosis.
  › Consider important side effects with antimalarials (though mostly relevant in long-term use): arrhythmia, QTc prolongation, neuromuscular toxicity, and retinopathy.
    » Adjust the dose for renal impairment in acute kidney injury and CKD.

EXAMPLE NOTE
"Issue #1: Chronic symmetrical polyarticular arthritis involving MCPs and PIPs (sparing DIPs) with elevated CRP, consistent with RA. Differential diagnosis: connective tissue disease, OA. No recent travel, infection, or new sexual partners. No systemic features of vasculitis, psoriasis, or IBD. Pending RF, anti-CCP, ANA, and blood cultures x 2. Bilateral hand x-ray ordered. Symptomatic control with acetaminophen and NSAIDs. PT and occupational therapy referrals. Definitive treatment with DMARDs deferred until diagnosis is clear. TB skin test, HBV, HCV, and HIV serologies ordered in preparation for possible long-term immunosuppression."

Purpura or Possible Vasculitis
These notes are in addition to the **general guide for all consultations** on page 1, and the **starting points for rheumatology consultations** at the beginning of this chapter.

Identification

Follow the **general guide for all consultations.**

Reason for Referral

Examples of reason for referral include purpura and ruling out systemic vasculitis.

History of Present Illness

Clarify lesion characteristics: Ask about onset, distribution, presence on dependent areas (i.e., legs), pain or pruritus, associated nodules, ulcers, and urticaria (hives).

Screen for systemic manifestations of medium- and small-vessel vasculitis: Symptoms include:

> **Constitutional:** fever; weight loss; night sweats; severe myalgias or malaise

> **Neurological:** patchy limb paraesthesia or weakness (relevant to mononeuritis multiplex: polyarthritis nodosa [PAN], ANCA, cryoglobulinemia); blurry or double vision (cryoglobulinemia)

> **Head, ears, eyes, nose, throat:** rhinosinusitis (EGPA, GPA); epistaxis, nasal crusting, hearing loss, otorrhea (GPA); oral ulcers (Behçet syndrome; usual onset before age 40); eye redness or pain (scleritis, conjunctivitis, uveitis: PAN, GPA)

> **Respiratory:** dyspnea, hemoptysis, hoarse voice, stridor (ANCA)

> **Cardiovascular:** chest pain (myocarditis: EGPA; ischemia: PAN), heart failure symptoms

> **GI:** postprandial abdominal pain and bloody stool (mesenteric ischemia: PAN, IgA)

> **Renal, GU:** hematuria; tea- or cola-coloured urine; frothy urine or proteinuria (PAN, ANCA, cryoglobulinemia, IgA); scrotal or labial ulcers (Behçet syndrome)

> **Musculoskeletal:** arthralgias; joint swelling; myalgias; arm or leg claudication (PAN)

Screen for secondary causes of vasculitis: Apply the mnemonic MAID:

> **Malignancy:** Symptoms include bone pain (multiple myeloma), lymphadenopathy (lymphoma), and fatigue and/or recurrent infections or bleeding (pancytopenia).

> **Autoimmune:** Screen for RA, SLE, Sjögren syndrome, and myositis. Symptoms include patchy hair loss; eye pain and/or redness; oral ulcers; dry eyes and/or mouth; morning joint pain or stiffness lasting more than 30 to 60 minutes; photosensitive rash; Raynaud phenomenon; and proximal muscle weakness.

> **Infection:** Ask about HBV, HCV, and HIV risk factors (IV drug use, multiple sexual partners, unprotected sex, and tattoos and piercings) and exposure to children (*Parvovirus B19*).

> **Drugs:** Ask about hydralazine, propylthiouracil, methimazole, allopurinol, cocaine (cut with levamisole), phenytoin, and others.

Screen for causes of bleeding: Ask about trauma, and antiplatelet or anticoagulant use.

Ask about heating pad use: Erythema ab igne can mimic livedo reticularis.

Past Medical History

Ask about:

- asthma (adult onset raises suspicion for EGPA)
- RA, SLE, Sjögren syndrome, inflammatory myositis
- multiple myeloma, hairy cell leukemia (associated with PAN), or lymphoma
  > Clarify treatment.
- HBV, HCV, and HIV (all associated with cryoglobulinemia).
  > Clarify CD4 count and/or viral load, and treatment.
- venous thromboembolism
  > Clarify dates and anticoagulation therapy.
- hypercholesterolemia, recent vascular procedure (consider cholesterol emboli syndrome)

Medications

Key information includes:

- recent start of hydralazine, propylthiouracil, methimazole, allopurinol, or phenytoin
- antiplatelet or anticoagulant use

Allergies

Ask about atopy (this suggests EGPA).

Family History

Ask about RA, SLE, Behçet syndrome, ANCA vasculitides, hematologic malignancy, and asthma.

Social History

Ask about:

- smoking; alcohol use; cocaine use (specifically ask about snorting cocaine: if it is cut with levamisole, it can cause ANCA); and IV drug use
- travel history (this is relevant to infections such as rickettsial infections and *Strongyloides*)
- TB risk factors (these are important prior to starting biologics)
- heritage (e.g., people of Middle Eastern, East Asian, or Mediterranean descent have a higher risk of Behçet syndrome)

Physical Examination

Vital signs: fever, features of sepsis (consider screening with qSOFA)

General impression: alertness and orientation (consider CNS vasculitis in compromised level of consciousness)

Head, ears, eyes, nose, throat: scleral ulcers; conjunctivitis or eye redness; saddle nose deformity (relevant to GPA); nasal septal deformity (shine a light in 1 nostril and look in the other for a perforation); nasal polyps (EGPA); wet purpura on oral mucosa (this suggests imminent bleeding); mucosal ulcers, bullae, or purpura (oral and genital mucosal involvement may help rule out a drug eruption)

Cardiovascular, respiratory: crackles, wheeze, murmur (endocarditis, atrial myxoma); signs of HF (high JVP, crackles, peripheral edema)

GI: abdominal softness and tenderness

Neurological:
> Perform a sensorimotor screen in the limbs (patchy distribution suggests mononeuritis multiplex).
> Assess reflexes.
> Assess for reduced visual acuity (hyperviscosity) and stroke features (facial droop, dysarthria, asymmetric weakness).

Musculoskeletal: proximal muscle weakness; joint swelling, redness, tenderness, or reduced range of motion

Dermatological:
> Determine the distribution and character of purpura (palpable purpura suggests vasculitis).
> Look for petechiae, necrosis, ulceration, digital infarcts, mottling (livedo reticularis), and elbow papules (e.g., in palisaded neutrophilic granulomatous dermatitis).

Hematological: cervical, supraclavicular, axillary, and/or inguinal lymphadenopathy; hepatosplenomegaly

Investigations

LABORATORY INVESTIGATIONS

CBC with differential: Pancytopenia may indicate malignancy or viral suppression.

Hemolysis workup: Consider this if hemoglobin and/or platelets are low to rule out microangiopathic hemolytic anemia (MAHA).
> The workup includes: blood smear for schistocytes; reticulocytes; bilirubin, LDH, haptoglobin, fibrinogen, INR, PTT; and a direct antiglobulin test (DAT).
>> A positive DAT suggests autoimmune hemolytic anemia, which can arise from vasculitis.

› Include a heparin-induced thrombocytopenia (HIT) assay if the probability for HIT is intermediate or high based on the 4Ts score.[15]

Electrolytes, urea, creatinine, urinalysis with microscopy: Screen for glomerular disease.

Urine drug screen: Pursue this because patients may not disclose cocaine use.

Liver enzymes, liver function tests, CRP

Infection workup: Order HBV, HCV, and HIV serologies with or without serologies for CMV, EBV and *Parvovirus B19* IgM.

Rheumatologic workup: Order RF, anti-CCP, C3, C4, ANA, dsDNA, ENA, ANCA, CK, cryoglobulins, and quantitative immunoglobulins if the history and physical exam suggest an underlying systemic rheumatic disease.

› If ANCA is positive, screen for anti-glomerular basement membrane (anti-GBM).

› Consider tests for lupus anticoagulant, ß2 glycoprotein, and anticardiolipin (antiphospholipid syndrome can mimic vasculitis).

Malignancy workup: Order SPEP, UPEP, and serum free light chains if the history and physical exam suggest an underlying malignancy.

MICROBIOLOGY

Blood cultures: Consider these in most cases.

TB skin test or IGRA: Pursue these in anticipated biologic use.

Strongyloides **serology:** Pursue this in patients who have resided in or visited endemic locations.

IMAGING

Chest x-ray, ECG

CTA of the neck, chest, abdomen, and/or pelvis: Pursue this in the context of suggestive symptoms (assess for interstitial lung disease, malignancy, and vasculitis).

CT of the head: Consider this in patients with sinus or CNS symptoms.

PATHOLOGY

Skin biopsy: Consider also taking a biopsy specimen of an affected organ, if identified (e.g., kidney).

Impression and Plan

GENERAL APPROACH

Describe the likelihood of systemic small- or medium-vessel vasculitis: Base this on history and physical examination.

In cases of low likelihood, consider alternate causes: These include: thrombotic thrombocytopenic purpura; DIC; immune thrombocytopenic purpura; antiphospholipid syndrome; warfarin, heparin, or other drug-related cause; trauma; acute meningococcemia; and disseminated gonococcal or rickettsial infection.

In cases of medium to high likelihood, consider secondary causes: These include malignant, infectious, autoimmune, or drug-related causes. If relevant, treat the underlying cause (e.g., treat infection, remove offending drugs, tailor immune suppression, consult specialists in hematology or oncology).

TREATMENT

Primary Systemic Vasculitis

- Treatment varies by type.
- Classic small-vessel vasculitis limited to the skin, with no other organ involvement and no complications, may not require medications: observation, elevation, and time may be sufficient.

ANCA-Associated Vasculitis

- Severe ANCA-associated vasculitis is life- or organ-threatening.
- In consultation with specialists in respirology and nephrology, treat severe cases with pulse methylprednisolone 1 g/day IV daily for 3 days (followed by 1 mg/kg prednisone orally once a day with taper), plus either:
  › IV cyclophosphamide (e.g., 15 mg/kg every 2 weeks for a total of 3 doses, then every 3 weeks for a total of 3 to 6 doses)
  —or—
  › rituximab (1 g on day 0 and 14; avoid in EGPA)
- Plasma exchange is generally not recommended in light of the PEXIVAS trial.[16]
- Screen for anti-GBM in ANCA-positive patients: 5% of patients with ANCA-associated vasculitis also have anti-GBM antibodies, which are directly pathogenic and warrant plasma exchange[17]; also, GBM-GPA overlap exists.
- Counsel patients on potential adverse effects of chronic prednisone use (avascular necrosis, osteopenia, osteoporosis, infection risk, weight gain, diabetes, cataracts, glaucoma, GERD, and GI bleeding).
  › Coprescribe calcium, vitamin D, and bisphosphonate for bone health; TMP-sulfa (1 double-strength tablet 3 times per week or 1 regular-strength tablet daily) for *Pneumocystis jiroveci* pneumonia prophylaxis; and consider prescribing a PPI for gastric prophylaxis.

EXAMPLE NOTE

"Issue #1. Palpable purpura with hemoptysis and AKI, suspicious for small-vessel vasculitis. Pending ANA, dsDNA, C3, C4, ANCA, and anti-GBM. Start pulse methylprednisolone and add cyclophosphamide or rituximab if ANCA+ (plasma exchange if anti-GBM+). Screen for HBV, HCV, HIV and TB. Monitor BP and capillary blood glucose while on high-dose steroids."

References

1. Masi A, Hunder G, Lie J, et al. The American College of Rheumatology 1990 criteria for the classification of Churg-Strauss syndrome (allergic granulomatosis and angiitis). Arthritis Rheum. 1990;33(8):1094-1100. doi: 10.1002/art.1780330806

2. Satoh M, Tanaka S, Chan E. The uses and misuses of multiplex autoantibody assays in systemic autoimmune rheumatic diseases. Front Immunol. 2015;6:181. doi: 10.3389/fimmu.2015.00181

3. American College of Rheumatology. Antinuclear antibodies (ANA) [Internet]. Atlanta (GA): American College of Rheumatology; [updated 2019 March; cited 2020 April 27]. Available from: https://www.rheumatology.org/I-Am-A/Patient-Caregiver/Diseases-Conditions/Antinuclear-Antibodies-ANA

4. Hahn A. Systemic lupus erythematosus. In: Longo D, Fauci A, Kasper D, et al, editors. Harrison's principles of internal medicine. 18th ed. New York: McGraw-Hill Education; 2012. p. 2724-35.

5. Soroush M, Mojtaba Mahmoudi M, Akhlaghi M. Determination of specificity and sensitivity of rheumatoid factor and anti CCP tests in patients with RA in private clinic in Tehran, Iran. Biomed Pharmacol J. 2016;9(2):775-80. doi: 10.13005/bpj/1002

6. Shah A, St. Clair E. Rheumatoid arthritis. In: Longo D, Fauci A, Kasper D, et al, editors. Harrison's principles of internal medicine. 18th Ed. New York: McGraw-Hill Education; 2012. p. 2738-51.

7. Langford C, Fauci A. The vasculitis syndromes. In: Longo D, Fauci A, Kasper D, et al, editors. Harrison's principles of internal medicine. 18th ed. New York: McGraw-Hill Education; 2012. p. 2785-2801.

8. Margaretten M, Kohlwes J, Moore D, et al. Does this adult patient have septic arthritis? JAMA. 2007;297(13):1478-88. doi: 10.1001/jama.297.13.1478

9. FitzGerald J, Dalbeth N, Mikuls T, et al. 2020 American College of Rheumatology guideline for management of gout. Arthritis Care Res (Hoboken). 2020;72(6):744-60. doi: 10.1002/acr.24180

10. Smetana G, Shmerling R. Does this patient have temporal arteritis? JAMA. 2002;287(1):92-101. doi: 10.1001/jama.287.1.92

11. Knockaert D, Vanneste L, Bobbaers H. Fever of unknown origin in elderly patients. J Am Geriatr Soc. 1993;41(11):1187-92. doi: 10.1111/j.1532-5415.1993.tb07301.x

12. Stone J, Tuckwell K, Dimonaco S, et al. Trial of tocilizumab in giant-cell arteritis. N Engl J Med. 2017 Jul 27;377(4):317-28. doi: 10.1056/NEJMoa1613849

13. Nihei H, Tada H, Naruse Y, et al. Polyarthritis caused by methimazole in two Japanese patients with Graves' disease. J Clin Res Pediatr Endocrinol. 2013;5(4):270-2. doi: 10.4274/Jcrpe.1055

14. Smith M, Bass A. Arthritis after cancer immunotherapy: symptom duration and treatment response. Arthritis Care Res (Hoboken). 2019;71(3):362-66. doi: 10.1002/acr.23467

15. Crowther M. Clinical presentation and diagnosis of heparin-induced thrombocytopenia. Leung L, ed. UpToDate [Internet]. Waltham (MA); UpToDate Inc; 2022 Jan [cited 2022 Jan 24]. Available from: https://www.uptodate.com/contents/clinical-presentation-and-diagnosis-of-heparin-induced-thrombocytopenia

16. Walsh M, Merkel P, Peh C, et al. Plasma exchange and glucocorticoids in severe ANCA-associated vasculitis. N Engl J Med. 2020;382(7):622-31. doi: 10.1056/NEJMoa1803537

17. Jennette J, Nachman P. ANCA glomerulonephritis and vasculitis. Clin J AM Soc Nephrol. 2017;12(10):1680-91. doi: 10.2215/CJN.02500317

Abbreviations

AAA	abdominal aortic aneurysm
ABC	airway, breathing, and circulation
ABG	arterial blood gas
ABI	ankle-brachial index
ACE	angiotensin-converting enzyme
ACEI	angiotensin-converting enzyme inhibitor
ACh	acetylcholine
AChR	acetylcholine receptor
ACI	anemia of chronic inflammation
ACS	acute coronary syndrome
ACTH	adrenocorticotropic hormone
AD	Alzheimer disease
ADH	antidiuretic hormone
ADHF	acute decompensated heart failure
ADLs	activities of daily living
AEIOU	mnemonic for Acidosis, Electrolyte imbalance, Intoxication, overload (fluid), Uremia
AF	atrial fibrillation
AFP	α_1-fetoprotein
AG	anion gap
AGEP	acute generalized exanthematous pustulosis
AI	adrenal insufficiency
AI-CTD	autoimmune connective tissue disease
AIDP	acute inflammatory demyelinating polyneuropathy
AKI	acute kidney injury
aLOC	altered level of consciousness
ALP	alkaline phosphatase
ALT	alanine aminotransferase
ANA	antinuclear antibodies
ANCA	antineutrophil cytoplasmic antibody
anti-CCP	cyclic citrullinated polypeptide antibody
anti-TPO	anti-thyroid peroxidase
AP	anteroposterior

APLAS	antiphospholipid antibody syndrome
APS	antiphospholipid syndrome
ARB	angiotensin receptor blocker
ARDS	acute respiratory distress syndrome
ART	antiretroviral therapy
ASA	acetylsalicylic acid
AST	aspartate aminotransferase
AV	atrioventricular
AVM	arteriovenous malformation
β-HCG	beta subunit of human chorionic gonadotropin
BiPAP	bilevel positive airway pressure
BM	bone marrow
BMD	bone mineral density
BMI	body mass index
BMT	bone marrow transplantation
BNP	B-type natriuretic peptide
BP	blood pressure
BPH	benign prostatic hyperplasia
BPSD	behavioural and psychological symptoms of dementia
BSA	body surface area
BUN	blood urea nitrogen
C	complement; cervical nerve root
Ca	calcium
CABG	coronary artery bypass graft
CAD	coronary artery disease
CADASIL	cerebral autosomal dominant arteriopathy with subcortical infarcts and leukoencephalopathy
CAM	Confusion Assessment Method
CAPD	continuous ambulatory peritoneal dialysis
CBC	complete blood count
CBG	capillary blood glucose
CCB	calcium channel blocker
CCP	cyclic citrullinated peptide
CCPD	continuous cycling peritoneal dialysis
CCS	Canadian Cardiovascular Society
CCTA	coronary computed tomographic angiography
CD	clusters of differentiation (e.g., CD4)
CDUS	colour Doppler ultrasound
CEA	carcinoembryonic antigen
CF	cystic fibrosis

CGA	comprehensive geriatric assessment
CHD	congenital heart disease
CHF	congestive heart failure
CK	creatine kinase
CKD	chronic kidney disease
Cl	chloride
CMV	cytomegalovirus
CN	cranial nerve
CNS	central nervous system
COPD	chronic obstructive pulmonary disease
CPAP	continuous positive airway pressure
CPPD	calcium pyrophosphate dihydrate
CPR	cardiopulmonary resuscitation
CRAB symptoms	hypercalcemia; new renal failure; symptoms of anemia; bone or back pain
Cr	creatinine
CRP	C-reactive protein
CRRT	continuous renal replacement therapy
CSF	cerebrospinal fluid
CSVV	cutaneous small-vessel vasculitis
CT	computed tomography
CTA	computed tomography angiography
CTD	connective tissue disease
CTLA-4	cytotoxic T-lymphocyte antigen-4
CVD	cardiovascular disease
CVST	cerebral venous sinus thrombosis
D2 receptor	dopamine-2 receptor
DAPT	dual antiplatelet therapy
DAT	direct antiglobulin test
DIC	disseminated intravascular coagulation
DIF	direct immunofluorescence
DIMS-RE	mnemonic for Drugs, Infection, Metabolic abnormalities, Structural disease, Retention, Encephalopathy
DIP joint	distal interphalangeal joint
DKA	diabetic ketoacidosis
DOAC	direct oral anticoagulant
DRE	digital rectal exam
DRESS	drug rash with eosinophilia and systemic symptoms
dsDNA	double-stranded DNA
DVT	deep vein thrombosis

EABV	effective arterial blood volume
EBV	Epstein-Barr virus
ECG	electrocardiogram
ECOG	Eastern Cooperative Oncology Group
EGPA	eosinophilic granulomatosis with polyangiitis
ED	emergency department
EEG	electroencephalogram
EF	ejection fraction
EGD	esophagogastroduodenoscopy
eGFR	estimated glomerular filtration rate
EIA	enzyme immunoassay
ELISA	enzyme-linked immunosorbent assay
EM	erythema multiforme
EMG	electromyogram
ENA	extractable nuclear antigen
ENT	ear, nose, throat
EOE	eosinophilic esophagitis
EPS	extrapyramidal symptoms
ERCP	endoscopic retrograde cholangiopancreatography
ESKD	end-stage kidney disease
ESR	erythrocyte sedimentation rate
ESRD	end-stage renal disease
ETT	endotracheal tube
FEV	forced expiratory volume
FEV_1	forced expiratory volume in the first second of expiration
FFP	fresh frozen plasma
FIO_2	fraction of inspired oxygen
FIT	fecal immunochemical test
FSH	follicle-stimulating hormone
FTD	frontotemporal dementia
FVC	forced vital capacity
G-CSF	granulocyte colony-stimulating factor
G6PD	glucose-6-phosphate dehydrogenase
GBM	glomerular basement membrane
GCA	giant cell arteritis
GCS	Glasgow Coma Scale
GERD	gastroesophageal reflux disease
GFR	glomerular filtration rate
GGT	γ-glutamyltransferase
GH	growth hormone

GI	gastrointestinal
GLP-1	glucagon-like peptide 1
GN	glomerular nephritis
GO	Graves ophthalmopathy
GPA	granulomatosis with polyangiitis
GRACE score	Global Registry of Acute Coronary Events score
GTPAL	number of gestations, term pregnancies, preterm pregnancies, abortions, live births
GU	genitourinary
GVHD	graft-versus-host disease
H&E stain	hematoxylin and eosin stain
H1	histamine$_1$
HAV	hepatitis A virus
HbA$_{1c}$	glycated hemoglobin
HBV	hepatitis B virus
HCC	hepatocellular carcinoma
HCO$_3$	bicarbonate
HCV	hepatitis C virus
HDV	hepatitis D virus
HEV	hepatitis E virus
HF	heart failure
HFpEF	heart failure with preserved ejection fraction
HFrEF	heart failure with reduced ejection fraction
HHS	hyperosmolar hyperglycemic state
HHV	human herpesvirus
HIT	heparin-induced thrombocytopenia
HIV	human immunodeficiency virus
HLA	human leukocyte antigen
HP	hypersensitivity pneumonitis
HPV	human papillomavirus
HSV	herpes simplex virus
HTLV	human T-lymphotropic virus
HU	hydroxyurea
IADLs	instrumental activities of daily living
IBD	inflammatory bowel disease
ICD	implantable cardioverter-defibrillator
ICS	inhaled corticosteroid
ICU	intensive care unit
IDA	iron deficiency anemia
IgA	immunoglobulin A
IgE	immunoglobulin E

IGF-1	insulinlike growth factor 1
IgG	immunoglobulin G
IgM	immunoglobulin M
IGRA	interferon-gamma release assay
ILD	interstitial lung disease
IM	intramuscular
INR	international normalized ratio
IPF	idiopathic pulmonary fibrosis
IR	interventional radiology
IRIS	immune reconstitution inflammatory syndrome
ITP	immune thrombocytopenic purpura
IV	intravenous
IVC	inferior vena cava
IVF	in vitro fertilization
IVIG	intravenous immunoglobulin
JVP	jugular venous pressure
K	potassium
KUB	kidneys, ureter, bladder
L	lumbar nerve root (followed by a number: e.g., L1, L2)
LA	left atrium
LBBB	left bundle-branch block
LBD	Lewy body dementia
LDH	lactate dehydrogenase
LDL	low-density lipoprotein
LEMS	Lambert-Eaton myasthenic syndrome
LH	luteinizing hormone
LMWH	low-molecular-weight heparin
LOC	level of consciousness
LP	lumbar puncture
LR	likelihood ratio
LV	left ventricle
LVAD	left ventricular assist device
LVH	left ventricular hypertrophy
MAC	mycobacterium avium complex
mACh	muscarinic acetylcholine
MAHA	microangiopathic hemolytic anemia
MAID	medical assistance in dying
MAP	mean arterial pressure
MCI	mild cognitive impairment
MCP joint	metacarpophalangeal joint

MCTD	mixed connective tissue disease
MCV	mean corpuscular volume
MD	muscular dystrophy
MDS	myelodysplastic syndrome
MELD-Na	Model for End Stage Liver Disease with sodium
MEN	multiple endocrine neoplasia
MET	metabolic equivalent
Mg	magnesium
MGUS	monoclonal gammopathy of undetermined significance
MI	myocardial infarction
MIBI	myocardial perfusion imaging
MINS	myocardial injury after noncardiac surgery
MM	multiple myeloma
MME	morphine milligram equivalents
MMR	measles-mumps-rubella vaccine
mMRC	Modified Medical Research Council
MMSE	Mini-Mental State Examination
MoCA	Montreal Cognitive Assessment
MPA	microscopic polyangiits
MR	magnetic resonance
MRA	magnetic resonance angiography
MRCP	magnetic resonance cholangiopancreatography
MRI	magnetic resonance imaging
MRSA	methicillin-resistant *Staphylococcus aureus*
MS	multiple sclerosis
MTX	methotrexate
Na	sodium
NAAT	nucleic acid amplification test
NAFLD	nonalcoholic fatty liver disease
NIPPV	noninvasive positive pressure ventilation
NPH insulin	neutral protamine hagedorn insulin
NSAID	nonsteroidal antiinflammatory drug
NSTEMI	non–ST-segment elevation myocardial infarction
NT-proBNP	N-terminal pro–brain natriuretic peptide
NTIS	nonthyroidal illness syndrome
NYHA	New York Heart Association
OA	osteoarthritis
OAH	oral antihyperglycemic
OC	oral contraceptive
OCD	obsessive-compulsive disorder
ODS	osmotic demyelination syndrome

OG	osmolal gap
OPQRST AAA	mnemonic for **O**nset, **P**rovocation, **Q**uality, **R**adiation, **S**everity, **T**emporal changes, **A**lleviating measures, **A**ssociated symptoms, **A**ggravating factors
OTC	over the counter
$PaCO_2$	partial pressure of carbon dioxide
PAN	polyarthritis nodosa
PaO_2	partial pressure of oxygen
PBS	peripheral blood smear
PCI	percutaneous coronary intervention
PCP	*Pneumocystis jiroveci* pneumonia
PCR	polymerase chain reaction
PD	peritoneal dialysis
PD-1	programmed cell death protein 1
PD-L1	programmed death ligand 1
PDD	Parkinson disease dementia
PE	pulmonary embolism
PEEP	positive end-expiratory pressure
PEG	percutaneous endoscopic gastrostomy
PET	positron emission tomography
PFT	pulmonary function test
PICC	peripherally inserted central catheter
PIP joint	proximal interphalangeal joint
PLEVA	pityriasis lichenoides et varioliformis acuta
PMN	polymorphonuclear leukocyte
PMR	polymyalgia rheumatica
PNH	paroxysmal nocturnal hemoglobinuria
PO_4	phosphate
POCUS	point-of-care ultrasound
PPI	proton pump inhibitor
Pplat	plateau pressure
PPM	permanent pacemaker
PPS	Palliative Performance Scale
PRES	posterior reversible encephalopathy syndrome
PSA	prostate-specific antigen
PsA	psoriatic arthritis
PT	physical therapy
PTSD	posttraumatic stress disorder
PTT	partial thromboplastin time
PUD	peptic ulcer disease
PUVA	psoralen-UV-A

qSOFA	quick Sequential Organ Failure Assessment
RA	rheumatoid arthritis
RAI	radioactive iodine
RBBB	right bundle-branch block
RBC	red blood cell
RCRI	revised cardiac risk index
RCVS	reversible cerebral vasoconstriction syndrome
RF	rheumatoid factor
RNA	ribonucleic acid
RUDAS	Rowland Universal Dementia Assessment Scale
RV	right ventricle
RVR	rapid ventricular response
S	sacral nerve root (followed by a number: e.g., S1, S2)
SABA	short-acting beta agonist
SAH	subarachnoid hemorrhage
SC	subcutaneous
SCAR	severe cutaneous adverse reaction
SCID	severe combined immunodeficiency
SDH	subdural hematoma
SE	status epilepticus
SGLT2	sodium-glucose cotransporter-2
SI joint	sacroiliac joint
SIADH	syndrome of inappropriate antidiuretic hormone secretion
SIGECAPS	mnemonic for **S**leep, **I**nterest, **G**uilt, **E**nergy, **C**oncentration, **A**ppetite, **P**sychomotor symptoms, **S**uicidal ideation
SIRS	systemic inflammatory response syndrome
SJS	Stevens-Johnson syndrome
SLE	systemic lupus erythematosus
SOBOE	shortness of breath on exertion
S_{Osm}	serum osmolality
SPEP	serum protein electrophoresis
SSRI	selective serotonin reuptake inhibitor
SSTI	skin and soft tissue infection
STEMI	ST-segment elevation myocardial infarction
STI	sexually transmitted infection
STOP BANG	mnemonic for **S**noring, **T**ired, **O**bserved, **P**ressure, **B**ody mass index, **A**ge, **N**eck size, **G**ender
T	thoracic nerve root (followed by a number: e.g., T1, T2)
T_3	triiodothyronine

T_4	thyroxine
TAC	trigeminal autonomic cephalalgia
TB	tuberculosis
TBI	traumatic brain injury
TCA	tricyclic antidepressant
TEN	toxic epidermal necrolysis
TIA	transient ischemic attack
TIBC	total iron-binding capacity
TIMI risk score	thrombosis in myocardial infarction risk score
TLC	total lung capacity
TLS	tumour lysis syndrome
TMJ	temporomandibular joint
TMP-sulfa	trimethoprim and sulfamethoxazole
TNF	tumour necrosis factor
tPA	tissue plasminogen activator
TPN	total parenteral nutrition
TPO	thyroid peroxidase
Tsat	transferrin saturation
TSH	thyroid-stimulating hormone (thyrotropin)
TSS	toxic shock syndrome
TTP	thrombotic thrombocytopenic purpura
UA	urinalysis
UIP	usual interstitial pneumonia
ULN	upper limit of normal
U_{Osm}	urine osmolality
UPEP	urine protein electrophoresis
URTI	upper respiratory tract infection
US	ultrasound
UTI	urinary tract infection
UV	ultraviolet
V/Q scan	ventilation-perfusion scan
VAP	ventilator-associated pneumonia
VD	vascular dementia
VDRL	Venereal Disease Research Laboratory test
VT	tidal volume
VT	ventricular tachycardia
VTE	venous thromboembolism
VZV	varicella-zoster virus
WBC	white blood cell

Contributors

EDITORS
Brandon Tang, MD, MSc
Meiying Zhuang, MD
James Tessaro, MD, MHPE, FRCPC

1 GENERAL INTERNAL MEDICINE
Mitchell Vu, MD
Elina Liu, BASc, MD
Justin Lambert, MD
Ben Schwartzentruber, BA, MD
Yu Chiao Peter Chen, MD

2 ALLERGY AND IMMUNOLOGY
Arun Dhir, MD
Pauline Luczynski, MSc, MD
Jian Weng, BSc(Pharm), MD
Juan Camilo Ruiz, MD, FRCPC
Raymond Mak, MD, FRCPC

3 CARDIOLOGY
Eric Wong, BSc(Pharm), MD
Jaihoon Amon, MD
Shekoofeh Saboktakin Rizi, MD, MSc
Ren Jie Robert Yao, MD
Abdulaziz Alshaibi, MBBS
Soohyun Alice Chang, MD, FRCPC Cardiology
Christopher B. Fordyce, MD, MHS, MSc, FRCPC

4 CRITICAL CARE MEDICINE
Jing Ye (Carol) Bao, MD
Keir Martyn, MD
Amanallah Montazeripouragha, MD, MSc
Matthew Renwick, MD, MSc
Amanda Bettle, MD, BSc
Cheryl L. Holmes, MD, FRCPC, MHPE
Constantin Shuster, MD
Daniel Ovakim, MD, MSc, FRCPC

5 DERMATOLOGY
Linghong Linda Zhou, MD
Sheila Au, MD, FRCPC

6 ENDOCRINOLOGY AND METABOLISM
Ahsen Chaudhry, MD, BSc
Jusung Hwang, MD, BSc
Alexa Clark, BSc, MD, FRCPC
Sadiq Juma Al Lawati, MD, FRCPC, ABIM Certified in Internal Medicine
Jordanna Kapeluto, MD, FRCPC, Dipl. ABOM

7 GASTROENTEROLOGY
Amrit Jhajj, MD, BSc
Ciarán Galts, MD, BSc
Eric Sonke, MDCM, MSc
Harjot Bedi, MD, MHSc, MSc, BSc
Sepehr Nassiri, MD, BSc

Marcel Tomaszewski, MD, FRCPC
Rohit Pai, MD, FRCPC
Dustin Loomes, MD, FRCPC

8 GERIATRIC MEDICINE
Clara Tsui, MD, FRCPC
Lindsay Schnarr, MD
Claire Wu, MD
Mark Fok, MD, MAS, BSc(PHARM)

9 HEMATOLOGY
Angelina Marinkovic, MD
WanLi Zhou, MD
Julia Varghese, MD
Katherine Ng, MD, FRCPC

10 INFECTIOUS DISEASES
Rahel Zewude, MD
Marie JeongMin Kim, MD
Stephan Saad, MD, FRCPC
Natasha Press, MD
William J. Connors, MD, MPH, FRCPC, ABIM

11 MEDICAL ONCOLOGY
Lidiya Luzhna, MD, PhD
Arkhjamil Angeles, BSc, MD
Meredith Li, MD
Howard J. Lim, MD, PhD, FRCPC

12 NEPHROLOGY
Jordan Friedmann, MD, BSc
Julia Zazoulina, BSc(PHARM), MD, FRCPC
Teresa Tai, MD
Alastair K. Williams, MD
Sabina Freiman, MD

Wayne Hung, MD, FRCPC
Nadia Zalunardo, MD, SM, FRCP(C)

13 NEUROLOGY
Sina Marzoughi, MD
Olivia Marais, MD, BASc
Meshari Alsaeed, MD
Jason Jeet Randhawa, MD, FRCPC
Tychicus Chen, MD, FRCPC

14 PALLIATIVE MEDICINE
Arunima Soma Dalai, MD
Adrianna Gunton, MD
Jowon L. Kim, MD
Natanya S. Russek, MD
Hayden Rubensohn, BSc, MD, FRCPC
Rose Hatala, MD, MSc, FRCPC

15 RESPIROLOGY
Omri A. Arbiv, MD
Shaun R. Ong, MD, FRCPC
Mosaab Alam, MD
Janice M. Leung, MD

16 RHEUMATOLOGY
Derin Karacabeyli, MD
Jocelyn Chai, MD
Lauren Eadie, MD, BSc
Siavash Ghadiri, MD
Navjeet Gill, MD
Xenia Gukova, MD
Ahmad Abdullah, MD
Kam Shojania, MD, FRCPC
Shahin Jamal, MD, FRCPC, MSc

Index